Studies in Autonomic, Data-driven and Industrial Computing

The book series Studies in Autonomic, Data-driven and Industrial Computing (SADIC) aims at bringing together valuable and novel scientific contributions that address new theories and their real world applications related to autonomic, data-driven, and industrial computing. The area of research covered in the series includes theory and applications of parallel computing, cyber trust and security, grid computing, optical computing, distributed sensor networks, bioinformatics, fuzzy computing and uncertainty quantification, neurocomputing and deep learning, smart grids, data-driven power engineering, smart home informatics, machine learning, mobile computing, internet of things, privacy preserving computation, big data analytics, cloud computing, blockchain and edge computing, data-driven green computing, symbolic computing, swarm intelligence and evolutionary computing, intelligent systems for industry 4.0, as well as other pertinent methods for autonomic, data-driven, and industrial computing.

The series will publish monographs, edited volumes, textbooks and proceedings of important conferences, symposia and meetings in the field of autonomic, data-driven and industrial computing.

More information about this series at http://www.springer.com/series/16624

Debabrata Samanta · Amit Banerjee

Computationally Intensive Statistics for Intelligent IoT

Springer

Debabrata Samanta
Department of Computer Science
CHRIST (Deemed to be University)
Bangalore, Karnataka, India

Amit Banerjee
Department of Physics
Bidhan Chandra College
West Bengal, India

ISSN 2730-6437 ISSN 2730-6445 (electronic)
Studies in Autonomic, Data-driven and Industrial Computing
ISBN 978-981-16-5935-5 ISBN 978-981-16-5936-2 (eBook)
https://doi.org/10.1007/978-981-16-5936-2

This Springer imprint is published by the registered company Springer Nature Singapore Pte Ltd.
The registered company address is: 152 Beach Road, #21-01/04 Gateway East, Singapore 189721, Singapore

To my parents Mr. Dulal Chandra Samanta and Mrs. Ambujini Samanta, my elder sister Mrs. Tanusree Samanta, my brother-in-law Mr. Soumendra Jana, and daughter Ms. Aditri Samanta.

—Dr. Debabrata Samanta

This work is dedicated to my Father Late Mr. Asit Baran Banerjee, whose vibrant persona, guidance, encouragement, and profound enthusiasm for life have been the source of inspiration for me and the people around him.

—Dr. Amit Banerjee

Preface

The book, *Computationally Intensive Statistics for Intelligent IoT*, focuses on devising an efficient methodology to obtain quantitative solutions for problems that are devised quantitatively. This subject brings together the computational capability and statistical advanced thought process together to solve some of the problems efficiently. Some of the interesting areas of the subject are optimization techniques in the process of statistical inferencing, algorithms of expectation maximization, and Monte-Carlo simulation, to name a few. Advances in simulation and graphical analysis also add to the pace of the statistical analytics field.

Intelligent IoT plays a key role in financial applications, particularly risk management and derivative pricing, biological applications that include bioinformatics and computational biology, and computer network security applications that touch the lives of people. With high impacting areas such as these, it becomes important to dig deeper into the subject and explore the key areas and their progress in the recent past. Also, the applications of new advances in computational statistics are explored.

Introduction to intelligent IoT is dealt with in Chap. 1. Modern computer systems, data centers, and digital strategies generate terabytes of data every day via numerous means in order to handle the growing number of internet-connected devices. Despite the vast amounts of data available, gathering information and making decisions from it requires a tremendous deal of effort on many levels. As a result, advanced analytics has gone to the top of the priority list for research and development. The statistical analysis of data from the Internet of Things is the subject of this article, which looks at cutting-edge research (IoT). The primary purpose of this paper is to call attention to the potential ramifications of big data issues, as well as research efforts focused on Internet of Things statistical analysis and the technologies that go with it, in this context. As a result, this article recommends tools for evaluating big data at various phases and better comprehending the information we may get from it, opening up new opportunities for scientists to deliver discoveries based on open research subjects and themes. When faced with the problems of evaluating diverse data sequences and identifying sophisticated samples in real time, the use of complicated event processing (CEP) has emerged as a viable solution for several Internet of Things (IoT) operations. Despite the fact that CEP is a dependable and scalable method for analyzing massive streams of data on the fly, it is meant for responsive systems because it works with near-real-time data and does not rely on previously gathered or confirmed data. In this regard, we propose a dynamic infrastructure that utilizes historical data and forecasts future outcomes using machine learning and cognitive engineering approaches. We propose an adaptive forecast technique for active IoT records called adaptive moving window regression (AMWR) that, when tested against a real-world application situation, yields an efficiency of over 98%. Because of its lower complexity, which allows it to make real-time decisions, we may employ it in conjunction with CEP in our design. Using open-source tools specifically designed for big data integrations development, we developed and tested our proposed architecture on a real application from the smart transportation systems sector. When it comes to complicated event prediction, we suggest an architecture that is both reliable and applicable to a wide range of applications.

Chapter 2 deep dives with ML and information advancement platform in intelligent IoT. The lack of adaptive learning systems is a disincentive to the proliferation of smart IoT structures, given the prominence of IoT applications. Nothing is looked at as to how computers will exchange knowledge regardless of where the information comes from. As a result, this section proposes a model for how nodes would independently share information, develop new information, and adaptively comprehend from knowledge in order to be relevant through diverse applications. Individuals' acquisition and categorization of information inform the structure. To begin with, this study examines the various methodologies used in IoT smart big data analysis.

Chapter 3 intends various applications of machine intelligence and data science for intelligent IoT. The Internet of Things has spawned an abundance of applications, resulting in a massive amount of data that requires clever data translation. The development of acute IoT techniques is hampered by the proliferation of IoT frameworks (e.g. edge, fog, and cloud) as well as protocol limitations at the IoT application level in the transmission and reception of messages. Existing acute IoT frameworks are unable to learn from other IoT applications in an adaptable manner due to the challenges. In this chapter, we critically examine how machine learning research handles data supplied by IoT devices and emphasizes the challenges of developing intelligent IoT solutions. In addition, the authors propose a basis for IoT frameworks to learn from other IoT frameworks appropriately, as well as a timeline for how to apply the technique to specific literature surveys. Finally, we respond to the critical aspects that influence possible IoT intelligent frameworks.

In Chap. 4, various approaches of data analytics in intelligent medicare utilizing IoT are presented. The intelligent healthcare network is a game-changing means of combining the benefits of sensors, the Internet of Things, and big data analytics to provide high-quality supervised care while lowering medical costs. The medical industry will have significant challenges in saving and analyzing data in order to extract information in the future. The expanding volume of health records generated by IoT devices, e-health, m-health, and telemedicine necessitates the development of newer techniques for their management. In this work, most medical difficulties and big data analysis breakthroughs are briefly explored in this fast-growing field of study, with an emphasis on those addressed by remote tracking to intelligent healthcare. Individuals will benefit from the use of a sensor and IoT system to track the status of their healthcare. The purpose of this study is to make medical aid for the sick and unstable population easier by employing clever algorithms, software, and procedures to provide good curing suggestions via remote observation with faster analysis and expert intervention. The distribution of healthcare services has improved dramatically as a result of technological integration. This research proposes a new big data system for smart healthcare that allows for remote control of both healthy and unhealthy communities' physical daily habits. A specific scenario that tracks the physical operations of an athlete with sensors on the wrist, ankle, and chest checks the structure. The receiver sends messages to the human body on a regular basis. On the other side, signals processed and analyzed by big data analytic approaches and machine learning techniques are used at the receiver end to understand the operation. Based on the contender's body behaviors, the proposed method predicts whether the contestant is busy or idle. Our proposed framework has a 99.96% accuracy rate and can be adjusted by nurses for remotely tracking fitness difficulties in elderly victims in cases of Alzheimer's disease, recuperation, obesity control, and remote tracking, among other applications. Athletes' physical activity can also be used for remote monitoring of chronic illnesses that need physical, biochemical, and genetic expertise.

The world's population is quickly increasing, prompting a transition toward more environmentally friendly farming methods. Food security is a serious concern for most countries due to dwindling natural resources, limited arable land, and highly unpredictable weather patterns. As a result, data analytics (DA) and the Internet of Things are being leveraged to boost agricultural productivity and operational efficiency. As a key driver of smart agriculture, wireless sensor networks (WSNs) have given way to IoT and DA. Wireless sensor networks, radio frequency recognition, cloud networking, middleware platforms, and end-user applications are all part of the Internet of Things. The advantages and disadvantages of IoT have been covered in this article. The Internet of Things (IoT) environment is examined, as well as how IoT and DA may improve intelligent agriculture. The most recent innovations, as well as prospects, are frequently offered and are divided into four categories: technological developments, deployment scenarios, business, and marketability in Chap. 5.

Renewable energy consolidation and energy efficiency are essential elements of sustainable energy transformations and climate change mitigation. New technology, such as the Internet of Things (IoT), can be employed in a variety of ways in the power industry, including power supply, communication, and demand. The Internet of Things could be used to improve energy efficiency, boost the use of renewable energy, and reduce the environmental impact of power use. This paper focuses on a recent review on the use of IoT in power systems, with a focus on smart grids in particular. We also look at some of the IoT's enabling technologies, such as cloud computing and several data analysis platforms. We also look at some of the challenges of integrating IoT in the power sector, such as security and privacy, as well as a few solutions, such as blockchain technology. This manuscript provides an overview of the importance of IoT in power system optimization for legislators, financial specialists, and business owners. Transformation of intelligent IoT in the energy sector is reviewed in Chap. 6.

In Chap. 7, *Abnormality Diagnosis from Ambient Data: IoT Data Sequences in Real Time* is presented. The Internet of Things (IoT) paradigm is propelling modern sensor networks to track a wide range of phenomena, including environmental control, medical care, manufacturing processes, and intelligent city. These meshworks serve as pivot facilitators for a digital earth nervous system, providing a continual pulse of the nearly infinite events occurring in physical space. Nonetheless, the fast transformation of these sensor data sequences poses a dilemma for traditional data-handling procedures, prompting the development of alternative approaches. We propose a broad solution to this issue that might be applied to all areas of dispensed instantaneous inspection. This unbiased method uses a brokering strategy and web-based protocols to enable interoperability while interacting with diverse sorts of record origins. As a proof of concept, we employed the technique to detect anomalies in real time and linked it to the subject of atmospheric management. The developed framework is capable of detecting anomalies, issuing alerts, and displaying the current status to the user.

Chapter 8 takes the *Future of Intelligent IoT*. Sensor data gathered as a time series can be used to examine unusual events in the environment. The data collected by the sensors make this possible. The data collected by the sensors can be analyzed using statistical tools and methodologies in conjunction with the textual and numerical data collected by the sensors. The trigger points of the data series can be used to determine how well the other sensors were working at the time of the trigger point. Reverse engineering approaches are also impressive when it comes to identifying someone's presence in their environment. The presence of someone can be used to illustrate that something is wrong with the system because the presence of someone gives logically supported evidence, as evidenced by the Boolean values from the PIR movement sensor. When a PIR motion sensor detects movement, it can be used to confirm the presence of someone nearby. A probability distribution is used while seeking to locate a certain person. While numerical and textual data alone are insufficient for sensor analysis, multimedia data can be employed as a backup to numerical and textual data.

Bangalore, India Debabrata Samanta
West Bengal, India Amit Banerjee

Acknowledgments

It is with great pleasure that we express our sincere gratitude and appreciation for all those who significantly helped in the completion of this book with their contributions and support. We are sincerely thankful to Dr. Siddhartha Bhattacharyya, Principal, Rajnagar Mahavidyalaya, Birbhum 731 130, India, for his encouragement, support, guidance, advice, and suggestions toward the completion of this book. Our sincere thanks to Dr. Fr Benny Thomas, Professor, Computer Science and Engineering, School of Engineering and Technology, Kengeri Campus, CHRIST (Deemed to be University), and SK Hafizul Islam, Department of Computer Science and Engineering, Indian Institute of Information Technology Kalyani, India, for their continuous support, advice, and cordial guidance from the very beginning to the completion of this book.

We would also like to express our honest appreciation to our colleagues at CHRIST (Deemed to be University), Bengaluru, Karnataka, India and Physics Department, Bidhan Chandra College, Asansol, West Bengal 713303, India for their guidance and support.

We are very grateful to the entire publishing team at Springer Publishing, who extended their kind cooperation, timely response, expert comments, and guidance. Finally, we sincerely express our special and heartfelt respect and gratitude to our family members and parents for their endless support and blessings.

Contents

About the Authors

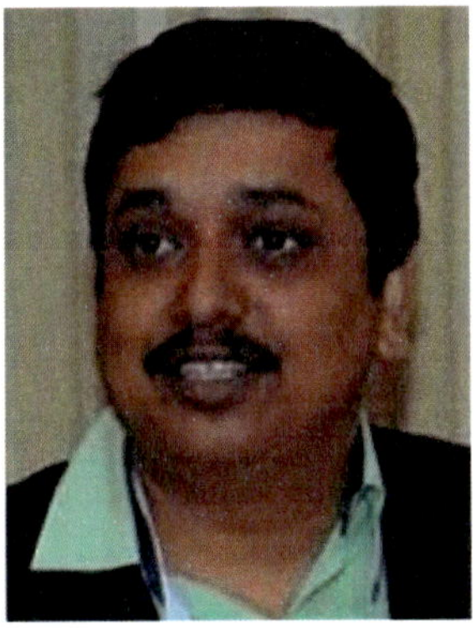

Dr. Debabrata Samanta is presently working as Assistant Professor, Department of Computer Science, CHRIST (Deemed to be University), Bangalore, India. He obtained his Bachelors in Physics (Honors), from Calcutta University; Kolkata, India. He obtained his MCA, from the Academy of Technology, under WBUT, West Bengal. He obtained his PhD in Computer Science and Engg. from National Institute of Technology, Durgapur, India, in the area of SAR Image Processing. He is keenly interested in Interdisciplinary Research & Development and has experience spanning fields of SAR Image Analysis, Video surveillance, Heuristic algorithm for Image Classification, Deep Learning Framework for Detection and Classification, Blockchain, Statistical Modelling, Wireless Adhoc Network, Natural Language Processing, V2I Communication. He has successfully completed six Consultancy Projects. He has received funding under International Travel Support Scheme in 2019 for attending conference in Thailand. He has received Travel Grant for speaker in Conference, Seminar etc for two years from July, 2019. He is the owner of 18 Patents (2 Design Indian Patent and 2 Australian patent Granted, 14 Indian Patent published) and 2 copyright. He has authored and coauthored over 155 research papers in international journal (SCI/SCIE/ESCI/Scopus) and conferences including IEEE, Springer and Elsevier Conference proceeding. He has received "Scholastic Award" at 2nd International conference on Computer Science and IT application, CSIT-2011, Delhi, India. He is a co-author of 10 books and the co-editor of 7 books, available for sale on Amazon and Flipkart. He has presented various papers at International conferences and received Best Paper awards. He has author and co-authored of 20 Book Chapters. He also serves as acquisition editor for Springer, Wiley, CRC, Scrivener Publishing LLC, Beverly, USA. and Elsevier. He is a Professional IEEE Member, an Associate Life Member of Computer Society Of India (CSI) and a Life Member of Indian Society for Technical Education (ISTE). He is a Convener, Keynote speaker, Session chair, Co-chair, Publicity chair, Publication chair, Advisory Board, Technical Program Committee members in many prestigious International and National conferences. He was invited speaker at several Institutions.

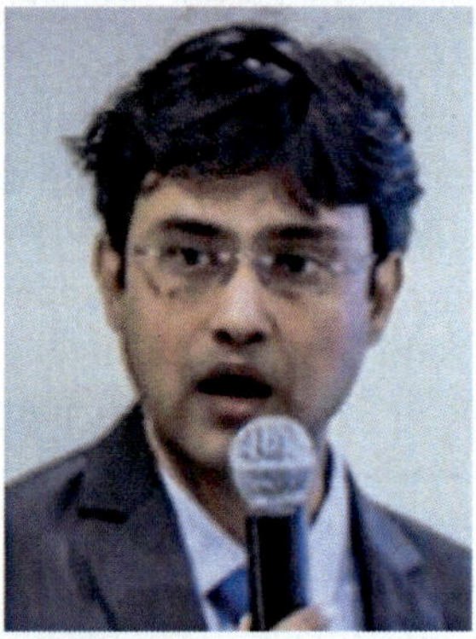

Dr. Amit Banerjee joined the Advanced Device Research Division, Research Institute of Electronics, Japan as a Scientific Researcher in 2016 and was also part of the Innovative Photonics Evolution Research Center at Hamamatsu, Japan. He later joined the Microelectronic Technologies & Devices, Department of Electrical and Computer Engineering of the prestigious National University of Singapore, as Scientist in 2017. Currently Amit is member of 40+ international advisory boards with global MNCs, deep-tech startups, technical program committees, in various countries, co-authored several scientific papers, presented in several international conferences as plenary and keynote speaker, received 8 international awards, authored & edited nine deep-tech books with prominent international publishers. Amit received Ph.D. degree in Semiconductor Technology from Energy Research Unit, Indian Association for the Cultivation of Science (D.S.T., Govt. of India) and has extensively worked on design and development of high vacuum plasma CVD reactors, which are used in industrial manufacturing of solar cells, coatings and TFTs. His recent work on antenna-coupled microbolometer arrays, are compatible with the state-of-the-art medium-scale semiconductor device fabrication processes, and technologically competitive with commercial viability as on-chip integrable detector arrays for terahertz imaging. He is currently associated with the Physics Department, Bidhan Chandra College, West Bengal, India.

Chapter 1
Introduction to Intelligent IoT

Abstract In order to accommodate the increasing number of internet-connected appliances, modern computer systems, the data center, and digital strategies generate terabytes of data every day via various means. Although enormous quantities of data are available, collecting information and making choices from them take a great deal of work on many different levels. As a consequence, advanced analytics has risen to the top of the research and development priority list. This article examines cutting-edge research on the statistical analysis of data from the Internet of Things (IoT). The main goal of this manuscript is to draw attention to the possible consequences of big data problems, as well as to research efforts centered on the Internet of Things statistical analysis and the technologies that go along with it, in this context. Thus, systems for analyzing big data at different stages and better comprehending the information we may get from it are recommended in this article, bringing up new possibilities for scientists to provide findings that are based on open research topics and themes. The use of complicated event processing (CEP) has evolved as a feasible alternative for several Internet of Things (IoT) activities when confronted with the difficulties of analyzing various data sequences and noticing complicated samples in real time. In spite of the fact that CEP is a dependable and scalable solution for studying large streams of data on the fly, it is designed for responsive systems since it works on close to real-time information and therefore does not make use of previously collected data or confirmed data. Regarding this, we suggest a dynamic infrastructure that makes use of historical data and predicts future outcomes via the use of machine learning in addition to cognitive engineering principles. With adaptive moving window regression (AMWR), we suggest an adaptive forecast technique for active IoT records that achieves an efficiency of over 98% when tested against a real-world application scenario. We may utilize it in combination with CEP in our design because of its reduced complexity, which allows it to make conclusions in real time. We developed and tested our proposed architecture on a real application from the smart transportation systems sector, utilizing open-source software that was specifically designed for big data integrations development. We propose an architecture that is reliable and can be used across a broad variety of fields when it comes to complex event prediction.

D. Samanta and A. Banerjee, *Computationally Intensive Statistics for Intelligent IoT*, Studies in Autonomic, Data-driven and Industrial Computing,
https://doi.org/10.1007/978-981-16-5936-2_1

1.1 Introduction

By expanding the advantages for both businesses and people, the growth of big data and the IoT is exerting an impact on a broad span of scientific sectors, together with business. With the increase in data generated by the IoT, the big data environment has seen a substantial increase in its size. Because these data are often accessible in semi-structured or unstructured formats, database management data inspection framework processing software has a tough time dealing with them [1]. It is possible to categorize big data into three categories: volume, variety, and velocity. Gartner was the organization that devised this categorization system to explain the many distinct aspects of big data problems. A variety of choices become accessible with the capacity to analyze and utilize huge quantities of Internet of Things data, such as that produced by intelligent cities, intelligent transportation, and intelligent energy meters, as well as remote monitoring devices for medical treatment. A lack of communication between databases and analytical methods including data mining and statistical analysis makes large-scale data analysis difficult. This becomes much more difficult to resolve when the goal is to acquire finding and presentation knowledge for particular applications rather than general information [2]. A number of publications on big data and related trends were discovered online, which served as the basis for this investigation. When we talk about significant data analysis, we're talking about the techniques that are used to analyze a huge quantity of Internet of Things data in order to find patterns that were previously undiscovered, connections that were previously unknown, along with newer facts. IoT big data analysis attempts to assist businesses along with various other organizations in preferably comprehending data and concluding more informed decisions by using big data [3, 4]. It is possible that data miners and scientists may turn to big data analysis for help when considering huge quantities of unstructured data which can be accessible using conventional methods. Big data analysis, which focuses to extricate accurate intelligence as quickly as possible, involves the utilization of data mining methods in helping to generate forecasts, the diagnosis of current trends, the discovery of hidden information, and the making of choices. IoT data differs from traditional big data gathered via systems in that it has a high set of devices and objects that are engaged in the data collection process, as well as unpredictability, noise, diversity, and fast expansion. By 2030, the number of sensors may have increased by a ratio of a trillion to a trillion billion, representing a tenfold increase. In order to combine big data analysis and the IoT, a significant investment of time and money is needed, and the IoT has the potential to facilitate an outstanding solution. In order to solve storage, processing, data analysis, and visualization issues, the Internet of Things (IoT) and big data integration could be a great help. This service may be helpful in a variety of situations, including intelligent green surroundings, intelligent transportation, intelligent networks, intelligent buildings, and logistics management, to name a few. We will concentrate our attention in this article on the refining of data produced by IoT utilizing existing technical explanations, which are primarily connected with big data, rather than on the data processing generated by IoT at the enterprise extent [5].

When conducting regular company operations, it is necessary to inspect a variety of health sites on a daily basis. Sensitive locations include places like homes, production plants, sensitive research labs, major roads, airlines, supply chain yards, campus buildings, hospitals, international borders, and the perimeters of factory buildings, among other things. International borders and the perimeters of factory buildings are instances of critical areas, as are international borders. Physical site monitoring is more than simply doing a basic task; it also entails putting in place the required remedial measures after performing a thorough investigation in order to prevent future material loss and environmental hazards from happening. A comprehensive sensor-based data gathering system is thus needed for decision-making in the subsequent phases. In spite of the fact that data is critical for companies to operate effectively, the vast quantity of data that must be kept in the cloud pushes up storage prices considerably. Optimization is required in the context of physical tests due to the fact that it includes not only text and image data but also pictures and streaming live video recordings, which makes it difficult to use conventional methods of data storage [6, 7].

However, there is one drawback to the controller-based system: sensor detection is real time rather than preset, which means that in the summertime, the refrigerating system will be activated whenever an individual comes into the room and not earlier, resulting in the area being cooled for 10–15 min after the human has entered. Machine learning techniques may be used to estimate the amount of time needed for a variety of regular tasks as well as for predicting the duration of unexpected circumstances [8]. It is possible to collect information on a person's behaviors, like entering and exiting a room, as well as turning on and off various pieces of equipment. Those estimates are kept in the controller as data records, and this information relates to prolonged-term activities that can last anything from one month to many months in length. As an illustration, various climatic circumstances may be found in various areas of the same nation.

In the Internet of Things-based initiatives, the choice of equipment and the preparation of such hardware are important responsibilities. In order to be ready for the Internet of Things applications, one must first select the sensors that will be used to solve the problem domain in question [9–11]. This is followed by steps such as using SD cards and LAN wires to allot the internet between laptops or personal computers in the advancement habitat, associating the sensors with the appropriate voltage measurement, and remote login to single board computers (SBC) or microcontrollers, among other things. Furthermore, the many methods in which industrial buses may interact with lengthy units such as Zigbee and Z-Wave, as well as data exchange mechanisms like Bluetooth low energy or Wi-Fi on the Raspberry Pi, will be discussed in detail. After comparing and contrasting the Raspberry Pi, Arduino, and BeagleBone Black, some researchers came up with the conclusion that, among the four platforms examined, the Raspberry Pi is the most cost-effective option.

Because of the need for accuracy, it is essential to evaluate the large number of data points received from the sensor. Precise figures cannot be disregarded as a result of this requirement. Specifically, the issue may arise when the sensors connect with the frameworks stationed in the single board computers, and/or when the sensor records are gathered in the SBC and sent to a web-server or the cloud. When enforced to the specimen records collected during the first evaluation, the handshaking and synchronization issues that were identified may be recognized and evaluated by using statistical tools and methods that were used to analyze the sample data obtained during that testing via basic programming or machine learning algorithms. The analysis and design of IoT-based physical tests results present a method for collecting data and giving a prediction for a particular location using the IoTs [12]. In the heart of the so-called Internet of Things is anything from items which links to sensors and collect data from things that connect with neighbors and utilize mobile, wireless, and internet technologies, as well as other technologies (IoT). This article covers a fundamental geographic space: a living room in a person's house, which is utilized for the collection and analysis of data collected by sensors and devices.

1.2 Background of Intelligent IoT

As a method of anticipating the number of individuals who might be in the lab before they came, some researchers proposed vertical framework coordination. For this purpose, the technology-labeled sensor data with additional information created a larger dataset and conducted machine learning computations on that dataset in order to provide results. Upon seeing how forecasts have been broken down due to the inherent and extended data, the system believes that the number of individuals can be predicted and collected by the sensor data, which is backed by the data. The chance of success for each of the three ML computations may also be increased if additional data is used in each of the three calculations. Using a method that was developed to restrict the estimates of the class of 0 or no individuals, it was possible to enhance the accuracy of the expected outcome when the class of 0 or no people was limited [13, 14].

Aspects such as application and expected outcomes must be taken into account when deciding on the most suitable machine learning technique to use to process sensor data. More research on larger datasets, however, is needed before any general implications can be made from the findings. Direct relapse produces worse results than decision trees and Bayesian algorithms, which are much more efficient methods of prediction. In terms of functionality, it was discovered that the decision tree model was the most transferrable and successful. As a result of the discoveries made, the growth of the framework may be aided by the creation of a sensor system that would allow for the collection of even more information. The possibility of supplementing the current framework with semantic improvements is also being explored in order to expand the data available for extended and highly exact assumptions [15].

Internet of Things innovation is quickly growing and expanding its branches all over the world, particularly in developing countries like India. Many sectors, both directly and indirectly, benefit from it as a significant source of revenue. When transistors are used to connect electronic devices such as a microprocessor, a DMA control system, CC cameras, cognitive storage systems, and other enhancements, they make a contribution to the centralization of framework understanding in the Internet of Things because they allow them to communicate with one another. Whenever end-user devices are employed, the information acquired is put to use in the form of activity or strength. Unlike conventional electrical appliances, these devices are not powered by electricity. Actuators, engines, motors, transformers, cylinders, and a range of other non-electrical devices are regulated to meet the needs and expectations of customers. Directed calculations, such as hereditary computations and swarm optimization calculations, may be utilized to improve the reliability of the framework interface. Hereditary analyses and swarm optimization computations are examples of such computations [16, 17].

It is used in a case study on meteorological data grouping that is discussed in more detail below. The expanded Internet of Things framework developed by various researchers, which includes the knowledge recovery, preparation, and learning layers, is used in the case study. As part of the system's learning phase, a grouping unsupervised learning method is used to the learning model that is generated with the aim of making the most of the associated huge data in order to optimize its performance. Log books are used to collect meteorological data at much more than 8000 climate stations situated across North America. With three wind speed clusters and one sensor failure, the process of learning has been advanced to the next stage. Data on ambient temperature, air temperature, relative wetness, deceit, and weight are all used in this research as part of a data analysis process to determine the outcome of the study's findings. Many standard k-implies grouping calculations have been combined to get the results that are shown here [18]. When the information bunching was being calculated, the system kept track of how well it was matching up with the topographical layout of the units that was a tremendous marvel of engineering in itself. According to the current situation, many of the most important geographical areas on the North American continent (as well as the continental United States) are classified into numerous climatic groupings that are easily distinguished from one another by their geographic location. Further use of the grouping method is in the investigation of the potential of sensor inadequacies and anomalies in the future. As a result of this use case, we were able to demonstrate how an Internet of Things big data system could be put to use for this purpose [19].

The researchers utilize both naive Bayesian classifier (NBC) and tree-augmented naive Bayesian classifier (TAN) computations while doing an additional truss analysis to determine whether or not it is acceptable to speed up sensors in an NBC analysis. An auxiliary truss investigation is performed in order to ensure that the calculations are accurate. In this study, the goal is to show that the methods mentioned in this article are effective when used in conjunction with NBC and TAN. Another finding of the research is that the binned quantity has an effect on the accuracy rate of grouping, which is another important finding. Because of this, the precision of grouping falls in a decreasing way as the binning amount is raised. Other kinds of suspicions may be more strongly matched with the requirements of the truss test dataset, while Gaussian suspicions may be less well-aligned [20, 21].

Huge information-based gadget control makes the storage and retrieving of information much more convenient. The transliteration process will be aided by the preparation component of the procedure. Because of the huge quantity of data saved, it may decide to terminate any other processes that are currently running. A consequence of this is that dedicated memory controllers, like direct access stockpiling, get overloaded with information [22, 23]. When information is transmitted via the internet, it may be handled in ways that are potentially harmful. It is used to transmit and retain information in order to make long-distance communication more convenient and efficient. To guarantee that either the web and storage systems operate at the same pace at all times, a pipeline is implemented. Aside from that, the pipeline sends information to be processed in serial at the storage device, resulting in an overall performance improvement even further.

Researchers used Internet of Things (IoT) devices, connection, analysis, and user interfaces to demonstrate the major elements of smart home systems that make use of IoT technology. To enable the system to construct more flexible and aware house frameworks for its users, the SLASH (self-learning and adaptive smart home) arrangement was developed as a theoretical framework for the system to utilize. By starting with no predetermined configuration, Slice differs from previous work in the smart home area in that it grows and develops like another created baby, collecting experiences from a number of different settings as it grows. In addition, it analyzes how the smart home should collaborate with the tenant based on the generally consistent actions of different clients, captures and stores Internet of Things tracking devices, and prosecutes why the smart home should collaborate with the tenant using machine learning and massive data analysis techniques [24, 25]. The use of this framework may enable the realization of a new vision of shining homes, one that offers more and more customized participation based on the routines of residents. The SLASH system gathers and analyzes data from a variety of sources for each individual home in order to improve the experience for the inhabitants of that institution. The article concluded by highlighting the difficulties associated with such a structure, as well as an intelligent home survey point with regards to opening zones that are experiencing concerns and recommendations that, among other things, are limiting the evolution of the Internet of Things in an individual's daily lives.

"Internet of Underwater Things" and "Internet of Everything" are the things that are used to describe things that are similar to the Internet of Things. Researchers compared and contrasted sensor network topologies for tracking underwater pipelines, and also explained the distinctions that exist between the different designs. Sensor networks, including wired sensor networks, acoustic wireless sensor networks, radio frequency wireless sensor networks, and hybrid wired, are all accounted for these two technologies. Researchers describe the observation and tracking of undersea sound along with pressure waves produced by demolishing and pile driving having the assistance of hydrophones along with other dynamic pressure sensors in accordance with environmental science and technology. For water surface communications, researchers proposed a three-tier architecture that combines the use of Zigbee and Wi-Fi technologies. They also discuss the importance of choosing the right MAC layer for the application. To better understand aquatic vehicle sensor networks for underwater monitoring, researchers provide an explanation of the architecture of the marine vehicle sensor network for ocean observation that utilizes static and dynamic frameworks for route monitoring along with evaluating ocean features. Researchers presented an ANN-based system for undersea sensor data prediction that they have developed. It is shown that the suggested architecture has a low computational cost and is appropriate for usage in the absence of data [26, 27].

Since the introduction of the IoT, the number of products that are affixed to the Internet has increased significantly. These gadgets vary from devices and data phones to increasingly softer characteristics like crowd detection or individuals serving as sensors as technology progresses farther. In sectors like supply chain, smart transportation systems, and intelligent cities, for example, the analysis of information produced by these many sensors has produced newer scopes for new implementations. In order to make informed decisions, the majority of Internet of Things implementations, like vehicular control systems or supply chain operations in large supermarkets, produce enormous amounts of information that have to be analyzed quickly and accurately. The Internet of Things generates real-time events from data collected by different sensors, which frequently combine to create complex patterns, each of which represents a distinct occurrence. To be able to make decisions in the situation of the current circumstances, it is necessary to comprehend these one-of-a-kind events with the smallest feasible time delay. An investigation domain known as complex event processing was established to address the requirement for transforming, analyzing, and deducing meaningful data from these complicated structures in factual time. It is possible to combine, evaluate, and compare event streams from many different sources of data in order to infer more important phenomena in near real time via event stream processing and correlation. According to examples accessible, the inherent distributed nature of CEP makes many Internet of Things applications feasible, such as analyzing instantaneous congestion data and facilitating automated management appliances for intelligent buildings. In terms of predictive capacity, CEP falls short of various machine learning algorithms along with quantitative data scrutiny techniques, despite the fact that it provides solutions for dealing with data sequences in substantial time [28, 29]. The vast majority of CEP programs are planned to facilitate reactive reactions by associating information packets according to pre-built criteria as incidents occur, rather than proactive replies. Because of the restricted amount of memory available, the majority of CEP systems do not make use of previously collected information. Many applications, on the other hand, have discovered that anticipating a future occurrence is much helpful than recognizing it thereafter it has happened. To avoid traffic congestion, rather than just detecting it, it will be more advantageous to foresee the problem rather than simply detect it so that transportation management may take preventive measures to avoid it from happening. Knowing when a natural catastrophe will occur or a pandemic disease will strike becomes more obvious when we examine the advantages of being able to anticipate occurrences in advance. Various literature works have discovered several methods based on machine learning along with analysis that have the potential to facilitate inventive and anticipating remedies in a variety of systems. For example, predicting passenger travel time for intelligent transportation systems and power consumption for homes are two of the numerous domains that have been discovered [30, 31]. However, one disadvantage of utilizing them is that they need historical data to be utilized in order to train the models, making them unsuitable for assessing and correlating different data sources in near real time. Machine learning methods make use of historical data to create predictions about the future. They use a range of disciplines, including statistics, linear algebra, and probability to instruct prototypes and improve them over time. They have the potential to be used as the basis for an optimization program for Internet of Things applications, but they lack the scalability and the ability to handle a large number of data sources in real time that CEP provides [32, 33].

Insights on the importance of motivation using CEP, it is possible to correlate data from a wide range of sources and to withdraw foremost information from the records. Query languages comparable to SQL are utilized in most CEP systems, allowing users to perform operations like filtering, aggregating, coupled with sliding window actions on various data sequences, and then merging them with the help of uncomplicated regulations to create new data streams. CEP varies from batch processing methods that reserve information and then execute queries on them, in that it reserves questions and then executes information through them, rather than the other way around. If anyone is working with Internet of Things applications, CEP's built-in ability is to manage a large amount of seemingly unconnected data and correlate it in order to deduce important phenomena that offer it an edge over machine learning methods. Since the transition from reactive to proactive Internet of Things applications in recent years, many research efforts have been focused on blended solutions that include machine learning and cognitive engineering [34]. There has been an increasing amount of interest among researchers in the academic community in integrating CEP with machine learning for the purpose of forecasting complex events; however, the vast majority of the research done in this area has been theoretical and has not included system architecture or real-world application examples. As far as the authors are aware, no prior work has addressed the numerous confrontations and open experimentation issues connected with the improved execution of ML prediction using CEP in a systematic way, and this is authentic to the best of the researchers' understanding. Machine learning algorithms are sophisticated and increasingly advanced approaches that are not only unsuitable for actual forecasting but also incapable of dealing with the speedy and productive data sequences produced by the Internet of Things. Because of the increasing speed of streaming regression techniques (e.g., Spark Streaming), which are focused on micro account information, the accuracy of these algorithms is decreased as a consequence of the increased speed. A solution that addressed these problems was proposed and early results were presented as part of our prior study. Our initial approach is expanded upon in this paper, as is our innovative assessment, and the whole framework is built utilizing open source modules that are well-suited for mass-scale Internet of Things data gathering and processing. According to this article, the following factors have an impact on the outcome: a general framework depending on open source constituents for blending machine learning with cognitive event prediction for anticipating complicated occurrences for dynamic Internet of Things approaches has been suggested and developed. We suggest an adaptive prognosis technique for determining the authenticity of dynamic IoT data streams. A moving window regression model, which we tested on a real ITS use case and found to be 96% correct, is included in this article. An innovative technique for identifying the ideal span of a training window in our research study was created by analyzing the spectrum components of time series data and applying it to our data. A parametric distribution is used to characterize the error generated by our prediction method. As a consequence of this modeling, we are able to derive equations for the inherent fault of the framework as the inaccuracy spreads across the CEP [35].

1.3 Big Data with Intelligent IoT

There are a number of possibilities for statistical analysis and data analytics now since the Internet of Things (IoT) is becoming more prevalent; this section gives an overview of different technologies. In computing, the phrase "Big Data" describes information that is enormous in quantity and scope. In the context of conventional software, "big data" refers to large quantities of data (processed, unorganized, and quasi) that can be collected, stored, and processed in a reasonable period of time by conventional software. Numerous petabytes of data were predicted to be collected in a given data collection in 2012, ranging from just a few hundred gigabytes to many pet bytes of data. When it comes to big data, the MIKE2.0 approach, which is devoted to studying problems connected with information management, characterizes it in spells of usable permutations and the difficultness of deleting every piece of data. In accordance with the McKinsey Global Institute, "big data" is defined as "the scale of data sets that can be handled more efficiently by database system tools than by conventional tools for the collection, storage, manipulation, and assessment of information". Conventional database management systems are inefficient when dealing with large amounts of data, also referred to as big data that must be saved, processed, and assessed in a short period of time. Big data is defined as data that must be stored, analyzed, and assessed fast [36]. The new inception of mechanization and frameworks aimed at extracting practicality from a large quantity of information in several structures, according to the book "The Digital Universe", are described as follows: "a new generation of architectures targeted at extracting value from a large amount of data in multiple formats, ensuring higher gathering, discovery, and analysis". According to the results of a previous study, big data may be classified into three categories: (a) sources of data, (b) data analysis, and (c) display of outcomes. Beyer proposes a framework for comprehending big data that is based on the three Vs (volume, variety, and velocity). It is important to understand that data volume signifies the bulk quantity of information produced every day, while data velocity refers to the pace at which the amount of data increases and the velocity with which it is collected for analysis. The term "variety" refers to the many various kinds of data that exist, including organized, unstructured, and semi-structured information, among other things [37].

Because of the Internet of Things (IoT), sensors and gadgets may interact in a seamless way inside an intelligent environment. The IoT also provides for the easy transmission of data across different platforms. Because of the recent adoption of many wireless technologies, the Internet of Things (IoT) is poised to become the next breakthrough technology, one that will fully exploit all of the opportunities presented by internet technologies. Industrial sectors have incorporated the Internet of Things in their development considering intelligent workplaces, intelligent retail, intelligent agriculture, intelligent transportation, e-health, and intelligent energy. It is possible to collect data from devices such as mobile phones, public transportation systems, public infrastructure, and appliances, culminating in the Internet of Things becoming a major trend currently [38].

1.3.1 Big Data Analytics in IoT

The internet has enabled the remote control of a wide range of electrical equipment, including wristwatches, convenience stores, safety alarms, door locks, washing machines, air conditioning units, and water heaters, among many others. Integration of communication devices into data collecting equipment allows for the transmission of data through various wireless technologies, like Wi-Fi, ZigBee, Bluetooth, GSM, along with other wireless technologies. Researchers transmitted and received data from remotely operated equipment, allowing connection with the actual globe via computer networks, and thus improving livelihood qualities across the globe [39].

Estimates predict that in the next few years, 60 billion electronic gadgets-like sensors, laptop computers, smart-phones, and gaming consoles will access the internet through a wide range of diverse access networks made possible by innovations like radio frequency identification (RFID) and WSNs. In general, the Internet of Things (IoT) may be classified into three categories: those that are internet-oriented, those that use sensors, and those that are knowledge-based. Because of the widespread use of various wireless technologies in recent years, the Internet of Things (IoT) is poised to become the next technological breakthrough that will have most of the advantages presented by web technology [40].

Analysis of large amounts of big data analytics, in its broadest sense, is the technique of analyzing large datasets containing different types of data in order to determine missing data patterns, hidden connections, industry trends, consumer trends, and other essential business information previously unknown to the analyst (BDA). It comprises data collection, data mining, and data analysis, all of which are intended to improve the overall performance of the company in which it is used. Big data analytics (BDA) is a solution to these problems because of its focus on improving the capacity to collect, store, analyze, and display millions of data sources which would otherwise be unreachable using traditional analytic methods or instruments. In order to assist researchers in any field to better understand their data and make more effective and informed choices as a result of this information and decision-making, the BDA has established a number of goals. It is feasible to analyze large amounts of data with BDA, which would otherwise be impossible to do using conventional data analysis methods [41].

A significant quantity of processed, semi-structured, and unstructured data must be converted into complete data along with metadata form that can be utilized for analytics before BDA can be implemented. It is essential to detect patterns, tendencies, and connections in the data using the techniques used by these analysis instruments across a broad range of time periods in order to be successful. This software presents results in the form of spreadsheets, diagrams, and graphs to aid in decision-making once the data has been processed and analyzed. Performance of existing BDA techniques that does not increase linearly with increased availability of computer resources is the primary subject of this discussion. Three-dimensional methodology is a method of thinking in three dimensions.

Because the light-dependent resistor (LDR) converts the intensity of light into a resistor (i.e. the lesser the resistance, the more light beam which reflects on the LDR, the LDR is very accurate when estimating light intensity (i.e. the lower the resistance, the more light falls on the LDR). The sensor will detect motion and sends an alert to the user's phone as soon as an item passes within the sensor's detection range [42, 43]. The temperature sensor detects the temperature of the air environment or the temperature of a specific item in the environment. We need an external analog to digital converter (ADC) in converting the analog sensor readings to digital data as the Raspberry Pi doesn't even have an inbuilt ADC and because majority of the sensor data are analog, and thus controller can thereby comprehend digital data. ADC MCP3204 is used for the conversion of analog signals to digital signals in a digital system. Because it is the primary controller, when the Raspberry Pi is utilized, it gathers data from all multiple controllers and saves it on the computer [44].

PCs, laptops, and portable devices were all considered while designing the user interface. The interface was designed to work on a number of platforms. Sensors linked together by jumper cables are a method of tracking a person's physical position. A range of sensors, comprising heat, air temperature, physical presence, and gas monitoring sensors, have also been attached to the Raspberry Pi in order to increase the precision of the physical position tracking system [45]. In particular, the system is designed to collect data through sensors in real time. ADC is used to link all of the sensors to the Raspberry Pi, with the exception of the PIR sensor, which is linked back to the Raspberry Pi through USB. Getting the sensor readings for heat, LDR, and air is accomplished via the use of ADC channels 0, 1, and 2, respectively.

Four things we have discovered as a result of my data-gathering efforts.

The gathering of multi-factor sensor data is a critical job in an Internet of Things system because it regulates critical components that coordinate programming operations and is thus critical. The data analysis, which is carried out privately utilizing ML approaches, necessitates the use of processor pipelines for time-sensitivity conclusion-making, and delay-dependent processing is needed in information acquisition.

A local server repository, which again is accessible over the internet, is used to store sensor data gathered on a daily basis and to store it. Because of the quad-core CPU of the Raspberry Pi, data is gathered in accordance with the delay specified in the code, eliminating the need for an extra synchronization delay. You can process data considerably more quickly when utilizing multithreading programming, which allows you to receive truer sensor data or add more features to your application.

The aim of this article is to look at the relationship between heat and LDR in more depth. The amount of light emitted by the Sun has an impact on the temperature and LDR values; the greater the amount of light emitted, the higher the temperature will become. Light-detecting resistors have a higher sensitivity than photodiodes and phototransistors, which have a lesser sensitivity. In contrast to temperature fluctuations, which may induce the resistance to fluctuate considerably, the devices may be considered temperature-sensitive even when the visible light is maintained constant. To put it in its most basic form, the following is the temperature calculation equation:

$$\text{Temperature} = (\text{sensor}_{\text{val}} \times 5 \times 10)/1023 \tag{1.1}$$

Here, $\text{sensor}_{\text{val}}$ denotes the output for LM36 (type of sensor).

The equation for light intensity calculation is

$$\text{V1} = 5 \times (\text{RL}) / (\text{RL} + \text{R1}) \tag{1.2}$$

$$\text{L} = [(2500/\text{V1}) - 500] / \text{R1} \tag{1.3}$$

where L = light intensity; V1 = O/P voltage of the light-dependent resistor; R1 = resistance attached to the voltage divider.

In terms of functionality, the overwhelming majority of the tools offered are geared toward batch processing, flow storage, and interactive analysis, to name a few applications. A majority of batching solutions, like Mahout and Dryad, are built on the Apache Hadoop architecture, which is free and open source. Flow data frameworks are often utilized in real-time analysis, which is one of the most popular applications. Splunk is an instance of a bulk-scale streaming framework that is completely free to use. Big data platforms Dremel and Apache Drill are two examples of big data frameworks which enable the collective analysis of massive quantities of data to be carried out. The use of these technologies in the creation of big data projects may turn out to be very advantageous. Hadoop projects based on the Apache software Hadoop and MapReduce are two examples of this kind of technology.

For storing huge amounts of data, many open-source frameworks are commonly utilized, including the Apache Hive, MapReduce, Hadoop kernel, and the Hadoop distributed file system (HDFS), among others. It is possible to manage big datasets effectively using Map Reduction, which is a split-and-conquer programming technique. Companies like Facebook, Google, and Yahoo make use of them in order to analyze and manage huge quantities of data effectively. When it comes to storage and parallel systems for big clustered datasets, the Hadoop library relies on fundamental programming principles once again, ensuring redundancy while simultaneously making use of a huge number of computing instances. On each cluster node is a distributed file system (HDFS), which is based on the multiple MapReduce algorithm. HDFS is a distributed file system that is used to store and manage data in a distributed manner. The combination of these frameworks makes it feasible for data to be duplicated and spread over N nodes, allowing for high-volume access to data. If we are conducting a distributed data records action, Hadoop is supervising for managing every portion of the data records at the node which is in possession of that part of it. In order to increase total capacity, it is necessary to include additional nodes. Processing is manipulated by MapReduce, while storing and transferring of data are handled by the Hadoop distributed file system (HDFS). Master nodes and worker nodes are two kinds of nodes that make up Hadoop's high-level architecture, in general. At this point, the primary node breaks down the incoming data into minute sub-problems, then disseminates it to the secondary nodes to work on. A single output from the master node is produced during the reduction phase, which is comprised of the results of the entire sub-problems combined [46].

Apache Spark is a programming language developed by Apache Software Foundation (ASP). Apache Spark is a strong open-source processing engine completely free to use, with a focus on speed, simplicity, and advanced analytics. AMP Lab at the University of California, Berkeley created this architecture as a reaction to constraints in the MapReduce storage framework, which is based on Hadoop's two-stage disc storage technology. While retaining MapReduce's linear scalability and fault tolerance, the team sought to increase computing capacity in four specific domains: in-memory analysis, data federation, iterative analysis, along with near-real-time analysis. As a consequence of its resilient distributed dataset (RDD) abstraction, in-memory analytics provides in-memory access to intervening findings in a multi-level processing pipeline, resulting in performance that is up to 100 times quicker than that of the traditional MapReduce approach. For data federation, there is a plethora of tools and APIs available, including a wide collection of tools and APIs that enable developers to rapidly build analytic processes for any kind of data source, such as HDFS, object storage, NoSQL, or relational databases [47].

Because iterative graph analysis is integrated with ETL and interactive analysis in Spark's GraphX libraries, automated learning and graph analysis are made possible. The use of Spark Streaming allows for the execution of near-real-time survey for Hadoop ecosystem consolidation, as well as the creation of a unified platform for processing Kafka data sequences in micro-packages [48]. An application execution begins with the Driver Program of the Spark Cluster, which is the first program that is executed. Whenever there is a requirement for data processing, Cluster Manage is in charge of resource and worker node allocation. Each application will be given a group of executors who will be in charge of carrying out their responsibilities. A major benefit of this technology is the ability to install Spark applications on top of an existing Hadoop cluster.

As an underworld dweller, the legendary creature Dryad may be found in many cultures.

The data flow graph is a common programming paradigm for creating parallel and distributed systems that must cope with vast context bases of information when applied to a graph of data. A computer cluster is a collection of computer nodes that enables you to run a distributed application while making use of the resources available on the cluster. A Dryad user has access to thousands of computers, each of which has a huge number of processors or cores, all at his or her fingertips [49]. A significant benefit of this approach is that it does not need users to have any prior knowledge of concurrent programming in order to be successful. With the help of Dryad, a programmer may manage the functioning of an algorithmic directed graph that has computational vertices and communication channels, among other functions. The result of this is that Dryad is capable of providing a wide range of features, including task graph creation, machine scheduling for available processes, cluster transition fault management, performance metrics collection, and visualization.

A distributed system that enables interactive big data study, Apache Drill is currently available in version 5.4. As compared to earlier versions, it is more flexible in terms of the number of query languages, data formats, and data origins that it can support. Moreover, it is intended to take advantage of information that has been nested inside other information. A key element of the company's expansion plan is the acquisition of at least 10,000 new computers with the capability of processing petabyte-scale data and trillion-scale records in less than one millisecond per server. Data is saved in HDFS and batch analysis is performed on the data using Drill, which makes use of MapReduce [50].

It is, in essence, a fault-tolerant distributed real-time computer system that is capable of handling very huge amounts of transmission data without crashing. In terms of performance, the Hadoop Cluster and the Storm Cluster are comparable. Storm tasks are carried out utilizing a number of topologies, while MapReduce jobs are used on the Hadoop platform to carry out the same applications as the Storm tasks. There are two kinds of nodes in a Storm Cluster: the master node and the worker node, both of which are different from one another. Implementing Nimbus and supervising workers fall to the responsibility of the master and worker nodes, respectively. These two jobs have duties that are comparable to one another, in accordance with the Jobtracker and Tasktracker of the MapReduce structure. Nimbus is in charge of spreading code across the Storm Cluster, scheduling along with allocating jobs to worker nodes, along with overseeing general system management. Nimbus delegated duties to the supervisor, who was in charge of seeing that they were fulfilled. Additionally, various Nimbus instructions are utilized to start and stop the operation as necessary. Work activities are divided into groups, each of which implements a piece of the topology, and the majority of the computing system is split and dispensed between these groups as well.

In the search engine world, Splunk may be described as follows:

Heterogeneous, intelligent platform for the exploitation of machines that is driven by big data in real time makes the use of cloud-based and Big Data technologies. A web-based interface is also available, which allows users to search for and monitor data produced by the computer, as well as analyze the data that has been collected. Results are presented in a clear and understandable manner using graphs, reports, and alerts, among other tools. A number of features distinguish Splunk from other flow analysis tools. Machine-generated structured along with semi-structured data indexing, real-time exploration, analytical outcomes reporting, and dashboards are just a few of the capabilities available with this product. In addition to being able to create a range of applications, it can also identify system and information infrastructure issues and offer intelligent business assistance.

As a result of this open-source data analysis software, real-time analysis, database column reporting, and rapid data visualization are all supported on popular storage systems, such as Mongo DB, Redis, and Cassandra. Large amounts of data may be examined without the requirement for extraction, modification, or loading. This is one of the most significant characteristics of big data (ETL). It is capable of producing interactive HTML reports from huge datasets without a requirement for ETL or data transformation. It is available for free. Anybody inside or outside the organization for which the individual works may get these reports.

1.4 Conclusion

In particular, big bata is focused on the creation of scalable algorithms for autonomous learning systems, which is a primary focus of this open-source initiative. It is possible to carry out tasks like sorting, batch-based collaborative filtering, clustering, pattern extraction, dimensional reduction, evolutionary algorithms, and regression, via the use of the MapReduce framework, which is built on top of the Hadoop platform. Its main goal is to provide people with a tool that will help them in coping with difficult situations in the future. As a consequence of its accessibility, companies like Twitter, Amazon, Google, IBM, Yahoo, and Facebook have all utilized it to build scalable ML approaches.

References

1. Pramanik S, Samanta D, Bandyopadhyay S, Ghosh R, A new combinational technique in image steganography. Int J Inf Secur Privacy (IJISP) 15(3). ISSN: 1930-1650|EISSN: 1930-1669
2. Rao KR, Samanta D, Somashekara MT, Gurunath R, Paul A (2019) Automatic segmentation based graphical interface for recognition of tomography image analysis of damage cell. In: 2019 third international conference on inventive systems and control (ICISC), Coimbatore, India, 2019, pp 52–55. https://doi.org/10.1109/ICISC44355.2019.9036343
3. Gurunath R, Agarwal M, Nandi A, Samanta D (2018) An overview: security issue in IoT network. In: 2018 2nd international conference on I-SMAC (IoT in social, mobile, analytics and cloud) (I-SMAC), 2018 2nd international conference on I-SMAC (IoT in social, mobile, analytics and cloud) (I-SMAC), Palladam, India, 2018, pp 104–107. https://doi.org/10.1109/I-SMAC.2018.8653728
4. Ghosh G, Samanta D, Paul M (2016) Approach of message communication based on twisty "Zig-Zag". In: 2016 international conference on emerging technological trends (ICETT), Kollam, 2016, pp 1–5. https://doi.org/10.1109/ICETT.2016.7873676
5. Dhanush V, Mahendra AR, Kumudavalli MV, Samanta D (2017) Application of deep learning technique for automatic data exchange with air-gapped systems and its security concerns. In: 2017 international conference on computing methodologies and communication (ICCMC), Erode, India, 2017, pp 324–328. https://doi.org/10.1109/ICCMC.2017.8282701

6. Hossain MA, Samanta D, Sanyal G (2012) Extraction of panic expression depending on lip detection. In: 2012 international conference on computing sciences, Phagwara, India, 2012, pp 137–141. https://doi.org/10.1109/ICCS.2012.35
7. Hossain MA, Samanta D, Sanyal G (2012) A novel approach for panic-face extraction based on mutation. In: 2012 IEEE international conference on advanced communication control and computing technologies (ICACCCT), Ramanathapuram, India, 2012, pp 473–477. https://doi.org/10.1109/ICACCCT.2012.6320825
8. Saha AK et al, IOT-based drone for improvement of crop quality in agricultural field. In: IEEE 8th annual computing and communication workshop and conference (CCWC), pp 612–615. https://doi.org/10.1109/CCWC.2018.8301662
9. Sai PY, Harika P (2017) Illustration of IoT with big data analytics. Global J Comput Sci Technol 17(3)
10. Salloum SA, Khan R, Shaalan K (2020) A survey of semantic analysis approaches. In: Hassanien AE, Azar A, Gaber T, Oliva D, Tolba F (eds) Proceedings of the international conference on artificial intelligence and computer vision (AICV2020). AICV 2020. Advances in intelligent systems and computing, vol 1153. Springer, Cham. https://doi.org/10.1007/978-3-030-44289-7_6
11. Sanchez-Huertas W, Víctor Gómez V, Hernández C (2018) Machine learning techniques and smart grid applications: a review. Int J Appl Eng Res 13(21):14876–14885
12. Saleem TJ, Chisthi MA (2019) Deep learning for Internet of Things data analytics. Procedia Comput Sci 163:381–390. https://doi.org/10.1016/j.procs.2019.12.120
13. Santamaria AF, Raimondo P, Tropea M, Rango FD, Aiello C (2019) An IoT surveillance system based on a decentralized architecture. Sensors 19:1469. https://doi.org/10.3390/s19061469
14. Shirke A, Chandane MM (2018) IoT data based predictive modeling for energy usage of appliances in smart home. Int J Eng Technol 7:931–934
15. Biswal AK, Singh D, Pattanayak BK, Samanta D, Yang M-H (2021) IoT-based smart alert system for drowsy driver detection. Wireless Commun Mobile Comput 2021:13. Article ID 6627217. https://doi.org/10.1155/2021/6627217
16. Pramanik S, Samanta D, Dutta S, Ghosh R, Ghonge M, Pandey D (2020) Steganography using improved LSB approach and asymmetric cryptography. In: 2020 IEEE international conference on advent trends in multidisciplinary research and innovation (ICATMRI), Buldhana, India, 2020, pp 1–5. https://doi.org/10.1109/ICATMRI51801.2020.9398408
17. Maheswari M, Geetha S, Kumar SS, Karuppiah M, Samanta D, Park Y, PEVRM: probabilistic evolution based version recommendation model for mobile applications. IEEE Access. https://doi.org/10.1109/ACCESS.2021.3053583
18. Kumar R, Kumar R, Samanta D, Paul M, Kumar V (2017) A combining approach using DFT and FIR filter to enhance impulse response. In: 2017 international conference on computing methodologies and communication (ICCMC), Erode, India, 2017, pp 134–137. https://doi.org/10.1109/ICCMC.2017.8282660
19. Gomathy V, Padhy N, Samanta D et al (2020) Malicious node detection using heterogeneous cluster based secure routing protocol (HCBS) in wireless adhoc sensor networks. J Ambient Intell Human Comput 11:4995–5001. https://doi.org/10.1007/s12652-020-01797-3
20. Ghosh G, Samanta D, Paul M, Janghel NK (2017) Hiding based message communication techniques depends on divide and conquer approach. In: 2017 international conference on computing methodologies and communication (ICCMC), Erode, 2017, pp 123–128. https://doi.org/10.1109/ICCMC.2017.8282658
21. Sivakumar P, Nagaraju R, Samanta D et al (2020) A novel free space communication system using nonlinear InGaAsP microsystem resonators for enabling power-control toward smart cities. Wireless Netw 26:2317–2328. https://doi.org/10.1007/s11276-019-02075-7
22. Samanta D, Sanyal G (2012) A novel approach of SAR image classification using color space clustering and watersheds. In: 2012 fourth international conference on computational intelligence and communication networks, Mathura, India, 2012, pp 237–240. https://doi.org/10.1109/CICN.2012.27

23. Khamparia A, Singh PK, Rani P, Samanta D, Khanna A, Bhushan B (2020) An internet of health things-driven deep learning framework for detection and classification of skin cancer using transfer learning. Trans Emerging Tel Tech e3963. https://doi.org/10.1002/ett.3963
24. Hossain MA, Samanta D, Sanyal G (2012) Statistical approach for extraction of panic expression. In: 2012 fourth international conference on computational intelligence and communication networks, Mathura, India, 2012, pp 420–424. https://doi.org/10.1109/CICN.2012.189
25. Althar RR, Samanta D (2021) The realist approach for evaluation of computational intelligence in software engineering. Innov Syst Softw Eng. https://doi.org/10.1007/s11334-020-00383-2
26. Singh RK, Begum T, Borah L, Samanta D, Text encryption: character jumbling. In: 2017 international conference on inventive systems and control (ICISC), Coimbatore, India, 2017, pp 1–3. https://doi.org/10.1109/ICISC.2017.8068691
27. Guha A, Samanta D (2021) Hybrid approach to document anomaly detection: an application to facilitate RPA in title insurance. Int J Autom Comput 18:55–72. https://doi.org/10.1007/s11633-020-1247-y
28. Agarwal M, Sarkhel D, Samanta D (2018) Architecture of 'loop' without 'for' & 'while'. In: 2018 2nd international conference on inventive systems and control (ICISC), Coimbatore, India, 2018, pp 491–494. https://doi.org/10.1109/ICISC.2018.8399121
29. Samanta D, Sivaram M, Rashed A, Boopathi CS, Amiri IS, Yupapin P (2020) Distributed Feedback Laser (DFB) for signal power amplitude level improvement in long spectral band. J Optical Commun. https://doi.org/10.1515/joc-2019-0252
30. Chakrabarti S, Samanta D (2015) Notice of removal: a novel approach to digital image steganography of key-based encrypted text. In: 2015 international conference on electrical, electronics, signals, communication and optimization (EESCO), Visakhapatnam, India, 2015, pp 1–6. https://doi.org/10.1109/EESCO.2015.7254009
31. Stergiou C, Psannis KE, Kim BG, Gupta B (2018) Secure integration of IoT and cloud computing. Futur Gener Comput Syst 78:964–975. https://doi.org/10.1016/j.future.2016.11.031
32. Sundaravadivel P, Kesavan K, Kesavan L, Mohanty SP, Kougianos E (2018) Smart-log: a deep-learning based automated nutrition monitoring system in the iot. IEEE Trans Consum Electron 64(3):390–398. https://doi.org/10.1109/TCE.2018.2867802
33. Sun S, Luo C, Chen J (2017) A review of natural language processing techniques for opinion mining systems. Inf Fusion 36:10–25. https://doi.org/10.1016/j.inffus.2016.10.004
34. Sun Y, Song H, Jara AJ, Bie R (2016) Internet of Things and big data analytics for smart and connected communities. IEEE Access 4:766–773. https://doi.org/10.1109/ACCESS.2016.2529723
35. Sun P (2020) Security and privacy protection in cloud computing: discussions and challenges. J Netw Comput Appl 160. https://doi.org/10.1016/j.jnca.2020.102642
36. Sunhare P, Chowdhary RR, Chattapadhyay MK (2020) Internet of Things and data mining: an application oriented survey. J King Saud Univ-Comput Inf Sci. https://doi.org/10.1016/j.jksuci.2020.07.002
37. Szilagyi I, Wira P (2016) Ontologies and semantic web for the Internet of Things—a survey. In: IECON 2016—42nd annual conference of the IEEE industrial electronics society, Florence, 2016, pp 6949–6954. https://doi.org/10.1109/IECON.2016.7793744
38. Raptis TP, Passarella A (2017) A distributed data management scheme for industrial IoT environments. In: IEEE 13th international conference on wireless and mobile computing, networking and communications (WiMob), pp 196–203. https://doi.org/10.1109/WiMOB.2017.8115846
39. Uy NQ, Nam VH (2019) A comparison of AMQP and MQTT protocols for Internet of Things. In: 6th NAFOSTED conference on information and computer science (NICS), Hanoi, Vietnam, pp 292–297. https://doi.org/10.1109/NICS48868.2019.9023812
40. Wang X, Ellul J, Azzopardi G (2020) Elderly fall detection systems: a literature survey. Front Robot AI. https://doi.org/10.3389/frobt.2020.00071

41. Wukkadada B, Wankhede K, Nambiar R, Nair A (2018) Comparison with HTTP and MQTT in Internet of Things (IoT). In: International conference on inventive research in computing applications (ICIRCA), Coimbatore, pp 249–253. https://doi.org/10.1109/ICIRCA.2018.8597401
42. Xiao S, Liu T, Wang X, Liu X, Zhou C (2020) Tailoring the absorption bandwidth of graphene at critical coupling. Phys Rev B. https://doi.org/10.1103/PhysRevB.102.085410
43. Xingyuan W, Suo G (2020) Image encryption algorithm for synchronously updating Boolean networks based on matrix semi-tensor product theory. Inf Sci 507:16–36. https://doi.org/10.1016/j.ins.2019.08.041
44. Xu X, Zhong M, Wan J et al (2016) Health monitoring and management for manufacturing workers in adverse working conditions. J Med Syst 40:222 (2016). https://doi.org/10.1007/s10916-016-0584-4
45. Yacchirema DC, Sarabia-Jácome D, Palau CE, Esteve M (2018) A smart system for sleep monitoring by integrating iot with big data analytics. IEEE Access 6:35988–36001
46. Yahaya AS, Javaid N, Fahad A, Rehman A, Ullah I, Shahid A, Shafiq M (2020) Blockchain based sustainable local energy trading considering home energy management and demurrage mechanism. Sustainability 12:3385. https://doi.org/10.3390/su12083385
47. Yang C (2020) The inequity of conscientious objection: refusal of emergency contraception. Nurs Eth 27(6). https://doi.org/10.1177/0969733020918926
48. Yuan X, Wang Y, Liu J, Xu X, Yuan X (2018) Experimental and numerical study of airflow distribution optimization in high-density data center with flexible baffles 140:128–139. https://doi.org/10.1016/j.buildenv.2018.05.043
49. Zhang C, Liu Z (2019) Application of big data technology in agricultural Internet of Things. Int J Distrib Sensor Netw 15(10). https://doi.org/10.1177/1550147719881610
50. Zhang P, Yin ZY, Jin FY, Chan THT (2020) A novel hybrid surrogate intelligent model for creep index prediction based on particle swarm optimization and random forest. Eng Geol 265. https://doi.org/10.1016/j.enggeo.2019.105328

Chapter 2
ML and Information Advancement Platform in Intelligent IoT

Abstract Given the prevalence of IoT applications, the scarcity of adaptive learning systems is a deterrent to the multiplication of smart IoT structures. Nothing is examined as to how computers will exchange knowledge independently where the information arrives from various applications. This section, therefore, suggests a paradigm for how nodes will share information independently, produce innovative information, and understand from expertise adaptively, in such a way that they will be relevant through various applications. The structure is drawn from the way how information is acquired and categorized by individuals. To start with, this research discusses the different techniques relevant to IoT smart big data analysis.

2.1 Introduction

It portrays the different domains which, using machine learning methods, have supported big data analysis for solving IoT problems. The research could be divided into four major areas: intelligent city, agriculture, maintenance of buildings, and health. The studies given in this section are listed in the following discussions. The intelligent city concept is dependent on delivering everyday life experiences that are productive and enjoyable. Some examples include having an optimal traffic path, foreseeing the trend of garbage heap loading for assemblage, proposing a location-dependent product, and predicting smart meter energy consumption. Help vector machines have been used in energy prediction to evaluate historical energy use and building condition data such as warmth and moisture, deriving in a projected power utilization of 2.5 kWh discrepancies between real and forecast energy use over a 25-day segment.

In the field of agriculture, the authors suggested finding signs of lameness in dairy buffaloes and cows. Unhealthy cows control milk development, having their signs basically seen for a period of time by inactive activities such as lying down. Thus, to gather data of their operations like lying time, interchanges every hour, with phase count, IoT sensors were mounted on cows. Three varieties of practices including active, regular, along with inactivity in cows were discovered through

D. Samanta and A. Banerjee, *Computationally Intensive Statistics for Intelligent IoT*, Studies in Autonomic, Data-driven and Industrial Computing,
https://doi.org/10.1007/978-981-16-5936-2_2

machine learning techniques. Random forest [1] has an accuracy of 89%, exposed 1 day earlier it was possible to observe any visual signs; and KNN showed an accuracy of 78%, determined 2 days earlier to the visual signs noted their symptoms.

In the manufacturing area, the repair of machinery is necessary to eliminate output disruptions when motors are broken. Therefore, in order to gather vibration information like motor frequency and amplitude, a study mounted three-axis accelerometers on factory tools. With ANN [2], the research recognized defects from typical motor circumstances having 99% accuracy.

Construction management should be regarded as an area linking the intelligent city and the industrial realm, as both domains can be linked to their solutions. A research estimated a building's occupancy level by analyzing temperature, CO_2, volume of air, and air conditioning data. To identify the data, random forest was used and gave 94% accuracy in estimating the degree of accommodation of rooms inside the building. Further research gathered apartment sensor information like warmth, moisture, dust, fires, and carbon dioxide to furnish with construction having a speedy tracking structure for toxic fumes, including the risk of fire monitoring. Four threat layers, from no threat to high threat, were arranged in the study; the technique of regression trees [3] obtained 99.86% precision for estimating threat layers.

Since IoT devices are connected to humans, the wellbeing domain could be the most prevalent software. Applications forecast the level of sugar for the control of diabetes, estimate the level of thermal comfort at work, and predict whenever a human collapses at residence. DL was used to track postural control activities like irregular loitering patterns, behaviors while sleeping, and trips to the bathroom. The research offers a real-time approach from wearable tracker data capturing pulse rate, breathing rate, and so on to identify anomalous health hazards and produced 93% perfection [4, 5].

2.2 Training Through Contact with Humans and Machines

How a person should communicate web pages will show you how computers can communicate with different computers. A website's most important property is that its presentation can be interpreted by humans. To achieve the necessary objectives of a mission, users can semantically access websites. Websites consist of vocabulary assisted by individual users in the language underlying them. Further, webpage formats are structured in a relevant framework so that visitors may originally traverse to locate the data that is looked for.

There exist two features for exchanging information that may be extracted from contact with humans and computers. Thus, we suggest the theorems that follow.

Lemma 2.1 Identification of an individual (like a person, services, relationship, and property) should utilize vocabulary recognized by persons.

Lemma 2.2 Knowledge can be structured syntactically in such a possible manner that following its arrangement enables humans to infer meaning.

Instead of abbreviations, passwords, or binary mapping, naming an object would use words in human language that can only be understood by computers, even if the latter is theoretically extra effective in the sense of physical space or bandwidth of a network. The use of ontology is the paradigm itself in organizing knowledge semantically [6–8].

2.3 Epistemologies

Awareness philosophy, or epistemology, offers the breakdown of how knowledge is obtained by a person. Fundamental awareness is "a priori" and "a posteriori" in this area. By meanings, such as grouping, a priori is acquired; apples are fruits. A posteriori, as apples being red, is obtained through experience and findings [9].

For the description of concepts and human comprehension, deviations from the aforementioned meaning are often used [10, 11]. A priori and a posteriori are parallel to the primary and secondary quality of human comprehension by researchers [12]. The primary attribute involves the features for an entity irrespective of the overseer, e.g., the mass, dimension, and color of an orange. Secondary quality oranges, according to an observer, to certain entity properties, e.g., oranges are orange in color. An extra word, i.e., conceived, indicates a plan obtained through creativity, such as mermaids and unicorns, was used by researchers [13]. Primary information is integrated into ontology, like the concept of "When the mud is damp, then crops grow well". The IoT sensors, like "The mud is dehydrated", acquire secondary information. Discovered information is produced after presumptions of abduction, comprehending the ideas that show the measurements for the flourishing of crops under sunbeam and composts. When the quality it represents can be extended, supplementary information could become main information [14, 15].

2.4 A Computer Awareness System

The concept is adapted from the philosophy of verifications that offers a decomposition of the techniques of research. It is an idea where experimentally tested observations obtain information. As culture has evolved along this scientific pathway, it is possible to borrow the structure for knowledge acquisition through observations in accordance with the construction of self-learning systems. A computer awareness structure suggested for the manuscript exists in Fig. 2.1. A system explains the way intelligent objects (SOs) may share information from other SOs autonomously. The Ontology, Parameters, and Hypotheses databases consist of three repositories. SOs mark the resources indicating the main or the second level of information when submitting data from the databases. SOs share information with other SOs through advertising and looking for resources [16, 17]. Figure 2.1 express intelligent entities

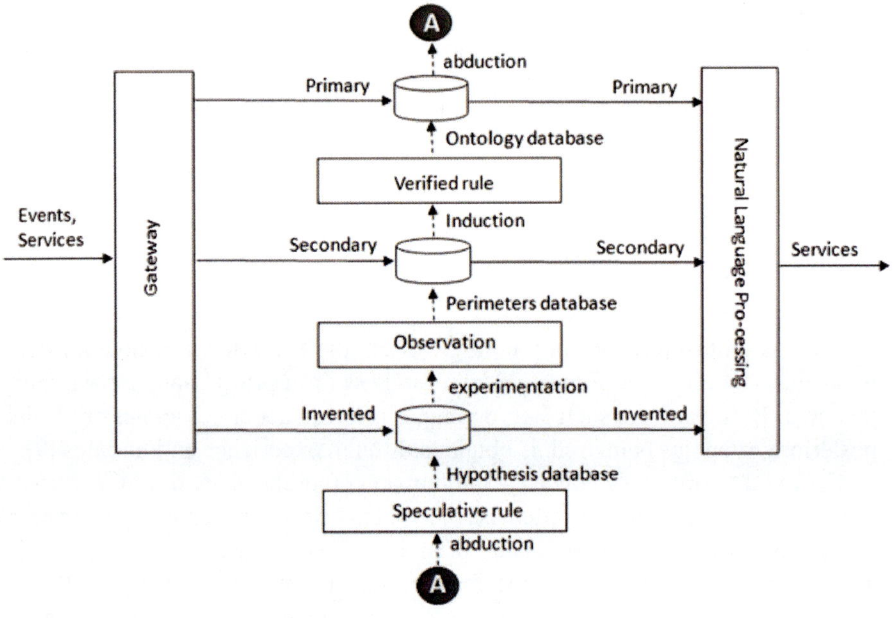

Fig. 2.1 Intelligent entities allot their assistances, enhancing them to master the breakdown of regulations to a bunch of jobs and circumstances

allot their assistances, enhancing them to master the breakdown of regulations to a bunch of jobs and circumstances.

After the hypothesis in the repository has been checked by certain preliminary studies, secondary knowledge may become primary knowledge. For the preliminary study, various ML algorithms like clustering and Bayesian algorithm may be utilized [18–20]. The repository of theories includes laws of inferences not confirmed. It requires guidelines from many other SOs explicitly, like smart information, or from some concept of ontology, or from the ontology repository. After such discoveries that the calculations have connected to a pattern, invented knowledge will become secondary knowledge. To observe the distribution of data, statistics may be used.

The Hypothesis database is also provided by the Ontology database. After the generation of laws based on speculation by various approaches, basic learning from the Ontology repository may cause imagined information. Provided the hypothesis "apples are red" for example, the hypothesis aims to when "red" is seen, assume that the object is an "apple". In this case, abduction is caused when the class fails to infer an observable attribute (i.e. red) (i.e. apple).

The structure applies two theorems previously discussed in establishing speculative laws [21]. Next, to comprehend human language, it uses natural language processing (NLP) techniques. The NLP can locate a word's synonyms, homonyms, and groups. The NLP learns in "apples are red", indicating "red" denotes a color, while "apple" indicates noun in grammar. Therefore, this thing tries in locating different nouns, thereby establishing a law like "[noun] are red". Usage of natural language processing implements Lemma 2.1. Second, like other SOs, the system shares ontologies. Ontologies are structured in such a manner that people can grasp the laws of inference. While SOs are devices, the ontological structure must convey significance. The Ontology of the Semantic Web, seen playing this function, as in the physical world, the properties it represents embody the model. Therefore, it enforces Theorem 2.

2.5 Case Studies

An overview of how the structure can be applied is given in this section. It accepts the ontology and metrics from research papers and modifies them using the proposed structure so that SOs can autonomously construct expertise.

2.5.1 Initialization

Due to the intention of dispatching warnings for help in the intelligent home dominion, a recent research indicated detecting an incident when a human fell [22]. From irregular behaviors such as when the individual slips, the study classifies regular everyday activities. The ontology was defined in Fig. 2.2. In the study, SO1 will be considered a smart entity, and the ontology repository from the fall perception analysis is populated suitably. Another research indicated identifying signs of lameness in dairy cows in pasteurizing plants since this type of disorder is connected with the efficacy of buttermilk processing [23]. It puts cows with IoT devices to track sleeping time; exchanges per unit time to decide if the cows were active or inactive.

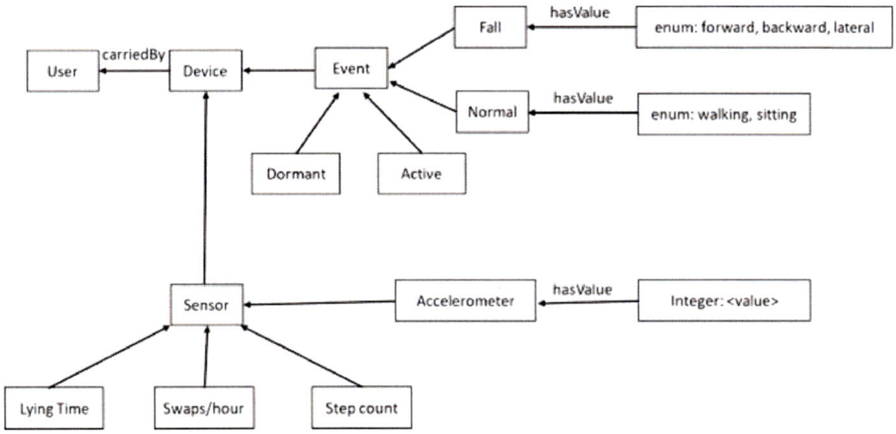

Fig. 2.2 Picture of ER internetwork for SO1 ontology repository. Gray color is mastered originating at SO2

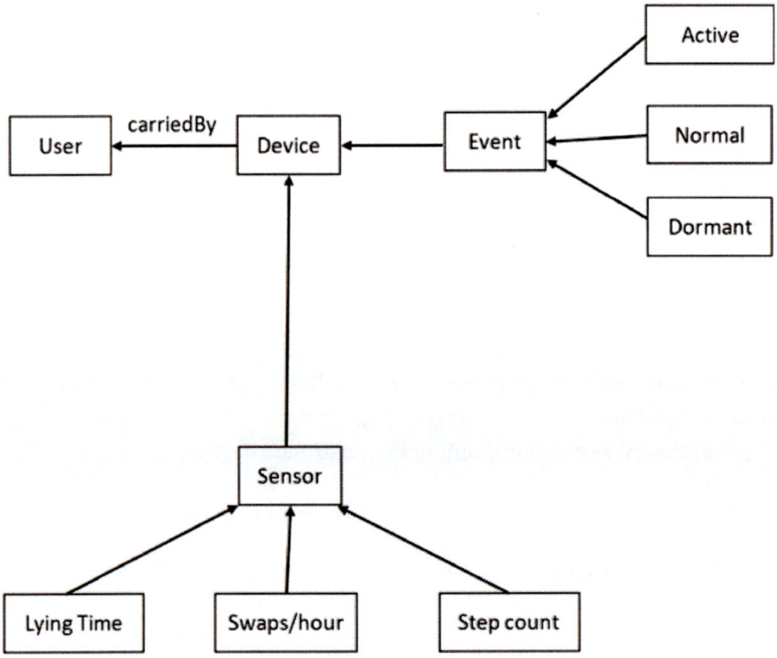

Fig. 2.3 Diagram of ER internetwork for SO2 ontology repository

Adapting this situation to the computer information system, the ontology store will have the links as seen in Fig. 2.3. The name-value combinations of the sleeping hour, interchanges at every time instant, and phase calculation will be included in the parameters database. A database of theories will be zero. The process will be named in this situation as SO2.

2.5.2 *Key Information Sharing with Other SOs*

SO1 learnt from SO2 to expand its awareness. This sends a transmitted question to show whether or not other SOs have any main episode and sensor information. SO2 responds by defining its basic information, i.e. the event element {Usual, Operative, Passive}; and the sensor component {Lying time, Swaps/hour, Phase count}. The SO1 Ontology repository is shown at this point, which is seen in Fig. 2.2, taking together the shaded agents as well as the non-shaded identities. Although such primary knowledge was accepted by SO1, SO1 asked SO2 for giving its supplementary realization [24]. Therefore, from the parameters database, SO2 transmits the name-value duet. However, since these ideas have been learnt from cows, the values taught could not be automatically adaptable to SO1. In addition, to reflect their regular, active, or inactive state, there will be various measures of human lying time and stage counting. Similarly, for cows but not humans, swaps/hour might be a valid finding.

2.5.3 Getting Key Knowledge from Supplementary Knowledge

The system teaches the way to embrace or deny the information gained from supplementary information that becomes primary knowledge. It becomes primary knowledge as secondary knowledge is generalized by induction. In this case, if SO1 lying time values can be checked to represent an SO1 episode (Usual, Operative, Passive, Fall), then the sleeping time is recognized in accordance with the SO1 sensor. Let the SO1 gather ample information after some time and changed its human sleeping time quantities, it would select a set of quantities that have been utilized to identify various incidents [25, 26]. The sleeping time quantities would then be recognized as supplementary information while sleeping time is expressed in the Ontology database as an aspect of the sensor which swaps every hour, on the other hand, are omitted from the Ontology repository as their quantities have been aborted to identify the case [27].

2.5.4 Pioneered Knowledge from Principle Knowledge

Dismissing an object will cause the system for executing inferences of abduction. Both laws in the Ontology database are comprehensively checked. An example of one direction is given here: interchanges after every time instant were determined with the help of a sensor; the sensor is a component for an appliance. SO1 speculates, by abductive logic, that the "user" is a "person" (not a tiger). SO1 went through two processes to have the following reasoning result. Next, NLP was used to detect the equivalence for the term "user" that occurred in several newer terms, like "customer" and "client" [28].

Second, SO1 shared basic information among all other SOs in order to acquire the framework of ontology with fresh terms. It carried out the processes to extend information from other SOs as previously defined and acquired the interactions as shown in Fig. 2.4 (the overshadowed portion has been derived via a smart city vehicle

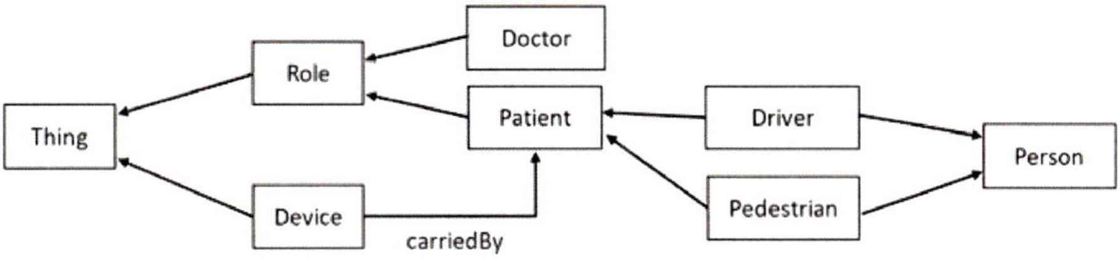

Fig. 2.4 Ontology mastered in realizing the connections a "patient" possesses

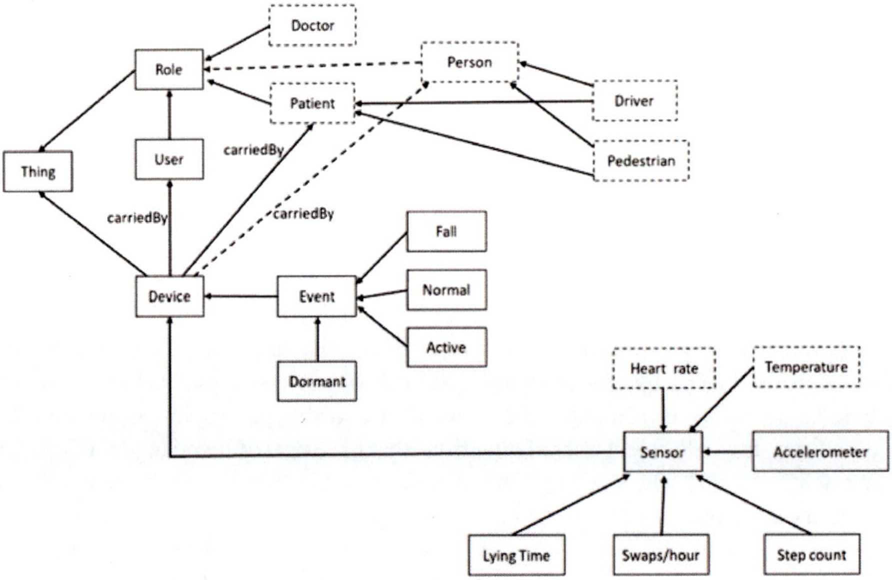

Fig. 2.5 SO1 understands granting a user is an individual related to the aspects in a sensor

management study while the connected nodes (established by non-shaded quantities) have been derived from a health domain research).

Therefore, the Ontology database has the following relationships: a user carries a device; a patient carries a device; a patient must be a chauffeur; an individual must be a driver; a person is a synonym with a user. SO1 hypothesized that the SO1 consumer is an individual by abduction inference, and a person is an aspect of a position. In the Hypotheses database, this relationship was carried out [29–31]. SO1 information will, therefore, be represented as seen in Fig. 2.5. Via the above method, the dashed entities were added; and in the Hypotheses database, the dashed arrows reflect the abduction inferences. More inferences would be drawn that will generate connected nodes; still, the diagram indicates just that is necessary to the debate that follows.

2.5.5 Being Secondary Knowledge from Fabricated Information

In technical approaches, information is obtained via experiments. If statistics from the samples indicate an appropriate confidence interval, then the conclusion can be believed. Thus, SO1 will consist of adequate data specimens to cause the statistical analysis. SO1 must be implemented with the help of different IoT solutions to obtain appropriate quantities in order to provide enough samples [32].

To forecast private warmth convenience depending on heartbeat including skin temperatures procured by IoT sensors, presume SO1 has been embraced by research.

The SO1 ontology illustrated in Fig. 2.4 was followed by the human programmer and developed a connection between "a computer is connected to a stroller" and "pleasure is an episode". Information measurements were taken according to the pulse rate and temperature of the body of the individual upon deployment. This shows that the following path was triggered (as a reference, only one path was shown): the heart rate is a sensor unit; sensor is a computer unit; an individual holds an appliance; and a person will be a pedestrian. There was a sample from this application demonstrating that "A Pedestrian is a Person".

Interestingly, the constituents utilized by different research to dispatch targeted promotional information were heart rate, position, and acceleration values [33]. The human programmer then followed the study solution and introduced a relationship that "Location is a Sensor unit". Thus, to call its user, this application activated two separate paths:

Heartbeat measure—Sensor–Appliance–Individual (mastered from temperature comfort analysis).
Accelerometer—Sensor–Appliance–User (mastered from the intelligent home analysis).

When data specimens whose amounts clarified the different related interconnections (e.g. drops, usual, comfort) were obtained by SO1, then the relationships that were enabled were proclaimed. The concept that the program uninvolved called "Person" and "User" in executing a process, in this case assert what was historically hypothetical, was that the User was an individual Human [34].

2.6 Analysis

This discussion illustrates the ways to adapt the suggested smart system to different IoT realms (i.e. intelligent house, agriculture, intelligent community, and healthcare) in sharing and developing information autonomously. Moreover, the suggested architecture would not discuss the ways in which IoT appliances might learn adaptively in restricted settings where there are very small computational and network resources [35]. The focus of our research is not how improved computation and network efficiency can be achieved; moreover, the researchers demonstrated the ways adaptive training could be done in the existing IoT frameworks. The paradigm, therefore, supports the idea that studying may be applied within the cloud domain (as in Methodology 2) or using an efficient computing approach at the edge, i.e. converting data to information (as in Model 3).

2.6.1 Latency

Choosing either model will require deciding how important the application is. For example, Model 2 (i.e. providing services in the cloud) can be followed when selecting the right methodology for a distant, task-specific approach, given that the criteria for network latency and network compatibility required in a distant application have been configured. The benefit of this methodology is that, nevertheless, for the internetwork lag that connects to the distant setups, the SO into the cloud will study from distant SOs related to the context [36, 37]. The downside is that as the need for real-time decisions rises, the mesh latency may reach the bottleneck. As another consideration, Model 3 can be implemented (i.e. getting all the services near the customer). The SO may provide time-specific information for the user in this model, but it depends on the communications network's capacity and availability to start wisdom sharing with distant SOs.

2.6.2 Machine-to-Machine Correspondence in NLP

The system tackles the present void in the reuse of ontology by ordering the usage of human speech for labeling of attributes and interactions in separate domains. The branch of artificial intelligence, i.e. NLP, is suggested to adjust the multiple concepts denoted by ontologies intelligently. Therefore, the contribution of this section, in addition to the above, is to extend the usage of NLP in node-to-node interactions [38].

Possibly the nearest comparison to the job is that defined in which computer repositories acquire human wisdom by NLP parsing, translating semantic portrayal into analytical syntax. The study reported customers as for humans and systems that produce mastery from the knowledge base and retrieve information. Moreover, the research suggested NLP-parsed data in creating an information base, enabling machines to build human speech knowledge [39, 40]. This research varies from other related researches in the process that three repositories were suggested in this method, i.e. the database of Ontology, Parameters, and Hypotheses which permits communication from node to node. In addition, the proposed study shows an innovative approach in which computers would extend their intelligence autonomously by the process of scientific abduction [41].

2.6.3 Inconveniences

While the present problem of reusing ontologies is tackled by the paradigm, it applies a poor concept of smart machines. In the case study, the Smart Entities presented (viz. SO1, SO2) are attentive to and acknowledge alterations in the surroundings, build a constructive judgment, demonstrate friendliness, and assist others with various intelligent appliances. In addition to these, when introduced to a variety of situations, powerful AI will include expressing passion and desire, creating a personal character. There is, however, no debate about whether a powerful AI [42] character can be exhibited by IoT systems or whether it could be counterproductive. Therefore, in offering new insights into intelligent IoT systems, the structure is sound [43].

2.7 Prospective Study

Huge prospects have been generated by the integration of IoT and huge-scale data analysis. System intelligence depending on IoT data has combined the virtual and physical realms altogether which dramatically advanced from a cyber-physical [44] viewpoint to investigate real-world problems. The procedures and systems have increased dramatically in their performance and reliability. System managers now have better oversight and analysis over their systems and procedures, and individuals with strategic intelligence have better insights into how to understand their problems and make rational choices. While many opportunities have been opened up by the integration of artificial intelligence and IoT, there are a few challenges that have restricted their development. The integrated incorporation of IoT with data analytics will be made possible by these potential testing opportunities. Any of the potential future paths are discussed in the following section [45].

2.8 Improved Cyber Security

ML approaches rely deeply on IoT data produced and transferred from the IoT appliances for enhanced decision-making. Various IoT levels, e.g., vision level, transport level, and application level, are endangered to cyber attacks within an IoT system. Such cases of cyber attacks within an IoT device framework are node manipulation, malicious code infiltration, routing attacks [46], DoS attack, along with data transit attack (sniffing) [47]. It is necessary to maintain a proper trust protection mechanism to protect the IoT device in case of cyber threats. Since most devices lack adequate protection mechanisms, IoT devices themselves need proper care. The complexities of maintaining IoT security, as outlined in [48], are distinct from conventional IT security, as discussed below.

First, in a conventional IT situation, users can install security fixes at any instance; but, most IoT systems undersupply security measures and some install integrated protection measures, and almost all systems do not accept added safety improvements and improvements or upgrades at a scheduled level.

Second, only lightweight algorithms are used due to low memory and processor limitations. It is still difficult, as pointed out in [49], to find the perfect stability between lesser capabilities and greater stability. Third, a large range of devices are used in an IoT environment. Because of its heterogeneous existence, due to the convergence of devices from multiple styles, platforms, and suppliers, the security risk is increased. Fourth, IoT's framework layer suffers from difficulties with encryption [50]. Possible repercussions may be data loss and eavesdropping. Fifth, IoT communicating protocols are even susceptible to cyber attacks and risks, consisting of attacks on DoS [51] attacks and routing, lack of privacy control by users, and key management challenges. The sixth dimension for tackling cyber security issues is our recommended architecture for ML and information finding in IoT. Intelligent machines that speak with human language can misunderstand signals, such as when reading homonyms (i.e. similar terms which have various connotations, like a "file" that can imply either information or a queue). Lexical-semantic analysis [52] is the latest active research in this field to claim that "April in Paris lyrics" indicates the name for an album, and "Vacation April in Paris" indicates a location's enjoyment details. Various malicious nodes or smart entities, however, may purposely spread false news in the sense of collaborating IoT devices exchanging information. This is true since, in order to trick others, homonyms and differing lexical semantics [53] will distort the content of a message. Cyber security problems are now expanding to incorporate methods of node-to-node deceit.

Upcoming IoT computers, communicating protocols, advancements, including the whole network, thus need enhanced security solutions by design. Inside the applications, system vendors must have comprehensive in-built security solutions. It is important to develop cryptographic algorithms, and key management must be made successful. Further analysis, based on the different IoT technologies and implementations, is required for validation techniques and public key infrastructure [54]. It is important to establish lightweight but robust techniques of intrusion detection at the level of the system, the edge, or the infrastructure cloud.

2.9 At the Edge, Machine Learning

Faster analysis and decision-making would be needed for IoT implementations, which will bring data processing closer to the consumer. It takes time and high bandwidth to transfer data to the cloud. Analytics at the IoT edge node has now opened the way for potential opportunities.

One driver behind this development is that in various fields of daily activities and industry, like cars, manufacture, and healthcare, the use of sensors [55] is proliferating, generating continuous data streams. By using machine learning methods, such a vast volume of information creates the raw data for an organization and policymakers for obtaining perceptivity and innovative ideas. The reasons include competitiveness or the development of improved policies when data is plentiful, giving rise to the importance of drawing information from data.

Because of their necessity in mission-centric examples, another push involves the integration of the IoT and paramount framework. As checked in the next section when low latency [56] is important, data is stored closer to the user. The new trend is that, or maybe remodeled, to serve critical involvements, trivial applications appear to become critical. The authors of [57] found out that those consumers of e-commerce [58] require quicker time to list the content of their content.

Shopping carts: it is possible to deploy urban cameras to identify a lost child; self-driving cars and airplanes produce a vast volume of information that involve speedy conclusion-making. Moreover, the researchers of [59] found that mutual education connecting the edge appliances must improve in this situation as host-to-host transmissions do not rely according to the sharing policies of cloud information.

The confrontation of the inclination needs to have edge computers appear to have smaller processing capacities than a cloud data center [60] (e.g. handheld devices). Machine learning data analysis, moreover, needs high computation power and storage. The problem can be addressed in this sense by the suggested architecture for ML regarding the IoT area. Its potential job can involve the concepts of edge appliances that share their expertise. The data processing activity can be done by an edge computer fitted with the highest computing performance. In order to offload their processing activities, an edge computer with the maximum bandwidth [61] will connect with the cloud. In [62], on behalf of a low-resource device, a group of IoT devices with appropriate resources has been charged with determining if access permission can be given. In other words, a combined methodology consisting of Methodologies 2 and 3 may be further explored (as shown in Fig. 9) whereby a community of edge appliances interact to poll on a system that is accounting for translating information into expertise.

2.10 Scalability

IoT applications make it easier in collaborating between a vast number of linked peers on the network. Whereas a large number of interconnections are needed by sensitive applications and end-users, scalability becomes a challenge that needs to be solved. For example, a vast volume of data needs to be spread to many terminal machines, where computational problems are addressed concurrently by the devices. Therefore, a possible approach is distributed machine learning algorithms for edge computing. It requires computational settlements by placing them at the edge of the IoT computers, which are closer to them. Context-aware processing is one job in this context, where scalability [63] has been accomplished by sharing information rather than any improvements in threshold quantities (as considered in Sect. 3.4, conventional IoT appliances interchange data in changing state or time). Information is shared in context-analysis, enabling the word "morning" for being supposedly identified being "8 am to 12 pm" or highway congestion is observed as "130 vehicles/hour". The approach provides the flexible answer in an internetwork of coordinating appliances since the needed data is only exchanged in accordance with the circumstances, preferred to transmitting a number. The researchers find that success in natural language processing [64] research would promote output in ML activities in a dispersed environment with respect to the approach for ML provided in this study. NLP positions meaning behind data values, empowering linked IoT appliances to attach tags to the information collaboratively, learning information from various appliances, reflecting distributed ML to address computational hazards.

2.11 Hyperconvergence

Repository provisions were spread by a huge quantity of disseminated computers within a hyperconvergence [65, 66] environment and their cumulative output aids in rebounding related to the issue of resource allocation. This model was seen as the optimal architecture for a system for IoT data analytics. The door to this pathway opens our foundation for ML in accordance with the IoT world. The databases seen in the current section (viz., the database of Ontology, Criteria, and Hypotheses) are intended in exchanging the information related to various IoT appliances in the surrounding internetwork, while the integrated information facilitates to cope with multidisciplinary-domain convergence, as stated in the next section. The problem, moreover, as shown in [64], is that modern networks are configured in individual implementations. Computers are interconnected with different physical layer technology and bandwidths in a group network, including various nodes to be sufficiently efficient than others (e.g. routing particulars and access control). It has not been thoroughly discussed if a newer node may be smoothly connected to an existent group internetwork for the case of any malfunctions. In addition, it is important to explore how it is possible to share a huge (and increasing) volume of data through paramount repository computers like data centers. Therefore, for the hyperconvergence setting, there is a further need to develop smart solutions.

In addition, not only does the convergence of intelligent IoT devices overcome technological problems but also fix regulatory problems. Instead of only satisfying breakthrough fans, it becomes important to explain how smart machines may be helpful to mankind. An instance of a contemporary challenge is that dispensed machine technologies use a great deal of resources that are starting to clash with simple personal requirements. Therefore, further works on controlling the convergence of intelligent devices involve potential paths.

2.12 Reaching the Inference

An important part of our everyday lives has been the IoT model. However, computational and connectivity capabilities that are bottlenecks in the creation of scalable, smart appliances using ML approaches are limited by IoT systems. Although advancements in technology and policy upgrades facilitate the path to a future that involves accelerated IoT expansion, the rollout of applications, and heavy profuse IoT data analytics [67, 68], it is stated that it has proved difficult to combine intelligent technologies from various realms [69, 70]. We also justified in this paper that our proposed architecture for IoT ML and information exploration facilitates the process for adaptive learning approaches to be integrated globally, in an edge, over a fog environment, or to a cloud network. Subsequently, in a broader sense of things, the ability of ML may be completely utilized in delivering utility and advantages to IoT technology users.

2.13 Conclusion

In this study, architecture brings up several new challenges in machine-to-machine interactions for future work. Research of cyber security may involve the analysis of the effect of malicious computers on other systems that could lead to vulnerability in the framework. Machines need to be designed in distributed systems to spread the resources seamlessly and permit the expandability of associated IoT appliances. The concurrent developments for ML technologies are thereby realizable in resource-dependent IoT networks as a federation of edge devices converges, and the destiny of IoT-constrained humanized lives is thereby realized.

References

1. Szilagyi I, Wira P (2016) Ontologies and semantic web for the Internet of Things—a survey. In: IECON 2016—42nd annual conference of the IEEE industrial electronics society, Florence, 2016, pp 6949–6954. https://doi.org/10.1109/IECON.2016.7793744
2. Raptis TP, Passarella A (2017) A distributed data management scheme for industrial IoT environments. In: IEEE 13th international conference on wireless and mobile computing, networking and communications (WiMob), pp 196–203. https://doi.org/10.1109/WiMOB.2017.8115846
3. Uy NQ, Nam VH (2019) A comparison of AMQP and MQTT protocols for Internet of Things. In: 6th NAFOSTED conference on information and computer science (NICS), Hanoi, Vietnam, pp 292–297. https://doi.org/10.1109/NICS48868.2019.9023812
4. Wang X, Ellul J, Azzopardi G (2020) Elderly fall detection systems: a literature survey. Front Robot AI. https://doi.org/10.3389/frobt.2020.00071
5. Wukkadada B, Wankhede K, Nambiar R, Nair A (2018) Comparison with HTTP and MQTT In Internet of Things (IoT). In: International conference on inventive research in computing applications (ICIRCA), Coimbatore, pp 249–253. https://doi.org/10.1109/ICIRCA.2018.8597401
6. Xiao S, Liu T, Wang X, Liu X, Zhou C (2020) Tailoring the absorption bandwidth of graphene at critical coupling. Phys Rev B. https://doi.org/10.1103/PhysRevB.102.085410
7. Xingyuan W, Suo G (2020) Image encryption algorithm for synchronously updating Boolean networks based on matrix semi-tensor product theory. Inf Sci 507:16–36. https://doi.org/10.1016/j.ins.2019.08.041
8. Xu X, Zhong M, Wan J et al (2016) Health monitoring and management for manufacturing workers in adverse working conditions. J Med Syst 40:222 (2016). https://doi.org/10.1007/s10916-016-0584-4
9. Yacchirema DC, Sarabia-Jáiescome D, Palau CE, Esteve M (2018) A smart system for sleep monitoring by integrating iot with big data analytics. IEEE Access 6:35988–36001

10. Yahaya AS, Javaid N, Fahad A, Rehman A, Ullah I, Shahid A, Shafiq M (2020) Blockchain based sustainable local energy trading considering home energy management and demurrage mechanism. Sustainability 12:3385. https://doi.org/10.3390/su12083385
11. Yang C (2020) The inequity of conscientious objection: refusal of emergency contraception. Nurs Ethics 27(6). https://doi.org/10.1177/0969733020918926
12. Yuan X, Wang Y, Liu J, Xu X, Yuan X (2018) Experimental and numerical study of airflow distribution optimization in high-density data center with flexible baffles 140:128–139. https://doi.org/10.1016/j.buildenv.2018.05.043
13. Zhang C, Liu Z (2019) Application of big data technology in agricultural Internet of Things. Int J Distrib Sensor Netw 15(10). https://doi.org/10.1177/1550147719881610
14. Zhang P, Yin ZY, Jin FY, Chan THT (2020) A novel hybrid surrogate intelligent model for creep index prediction based on particle swarm optimization and random forest. Eng Geol 265. https://doi.org/10.1016/j.enggeo.2019.105328
15. Jalasri M, Lakshmanan L (2018) A survey: integration of IoT and fog computing. In: 2018 second international conference on green computing and Internet of Things (ICGCIoT), Bangalore, India, pp 235–239. https://doi.org/10.1109/ICGCIoT.2018.8753010
16. Jerald F, Anand M, Deepika N (2019) Design of an industrial IoT architecture based on MQTT protocol for end device to cloud communication. Int J Recent Technol Eng 7(6S2):552–554
17. Karthigha M, Latha L, Sripriyan K (2020) A comprehensive survey of routing attacks in wireless mobile Ad hoc networks. In: 2020 international conference on inventive computation technologies (ICICT), Coimbatore, India, pp 396–402. https://doi.org/10.1109/ICICT48043.2020.9112588
18. Kavitha D, Ravikumar S (2020) Designing an IoT based autonomous vehicle meant for detecting speed bumps and lanes on road. J Ambient Intell Humaniz Comput. https://doi.org/10.1007/s12652-020-02419-8
19. Khanra S, Dhir A, Mantymaki M (2020) Big data analytics and enterprises: a bibliometric synthesis of the literature. Enterprise Inf Syst 14(6):737–768. https://doi.org/10.1080/17517575.2020.1734241
20. Kim J, Kim J, Kim H, Shim M, Choi E (2020) CNN-based network intrusion detection against denial-of-service attacks 9(6):916. https://doi.org/10.3390/electronics9060916
21. Kong XTR, Xu SX, Cheng M, Huang GQ (2018) Iot-enabled parking space sharing and allocation mechanisms. IEEE Trans Autom Sci Eng 15(4):1654–1664. https://doi.org/10.1109/TASE.2017.2785241
22. Li Y, Barthelemy J, Sun S, Perez P, Moran B (2020) A case study of WiFi sniffing performance evaluation. IEEE Access 8:129224–129235. https://doi.org/10.1109/ACCESS.2020.3008533
23. Liu Z, Li Z (2020) A blockchain based framework of cross-border E-commerce supply chain. Int J Inf Manage 52. https://doi.org/10.1016/j.ijinfomgt.2019.102059
24. Mehta G, Mitra G, Yadav VK (2018) Application of IoT to optimize data center operations. In: International conference on computing, power and communication technologies (GUCON), pp 732–742
25. Mehta R, Sahni J, Khanna K (2018) Internet of Things: vision, applications and challenges. Procedia Comput Sci 132:1263–1269. https://doi.org/10.1016/j.procs.2018.05.042
26. Muzammal M, Talat R, Sodhro AH, Pirbhulal S (2020) A multi-sensor data fusion enabled ensemble approach for medical data from body sensor networks. Inf Fusion 53:155–164. https://doi.org/10.1016/j.inffus.2019.06.021
27. Neto AJV, Zhao Z, Rodrigues JJPC, Camboim HB, Braun T (2018) Fog-based crime-assistance in smart iot transportation system. IEEE Access 6:11101–11111. https://doi.org/10.1109/ACCESS.2018.2803439
28. Nguyen H, Drebenstedt C, Bui XN et al (2020) Prediction of blast-induced ground vibration in an open-pit mine by a novel hybrid model based on clustering and artificial neural network. Nat Resour Res 29:691–709. https://doi.org/10.1007/s11053-019-09470-z
29. Obitade PO (2019) Big data analytics: a link between knowledge management capabilities and superior cyber protection. J Big Data 6:71. https://doi.org/10.1186/s40537-019-0229-9

30. Ouadghiri ME, Aghoutane B, Farissi NE (2020) Communication model in the Internet of Things. Procedia Comput Sci 177:71–77. https://doi.org/10.1016/j.procs.2020.10.013
31. Pong PWT, Annaswamy A, Kroposki B, Zhang Y, Rajagopal R, Zussman G, Poor HV (2021) Cyber-enabled grids: shaping future energy systems 1. https://doi.org/10.1016/j.adapen.2020.100003
32. Priyashman V, Ismail W (2019) Signal strength and read rate prediction modeling using machine learning algorithms for vehicular access control and identification. IEEE Sensors J 19(4):1400–1411. https://doi.org/10.1109/JSEN.2018.2880736
33. Qiu X, Sun T, Xu Y et al (2020) Pre-trained models for natural language processing: a survey. Sci China Technol Sci 63:1872–1897. https://doi.org/10.1007/s11431-020-1647-3
34. Rafei A, Carol A, Flannagan C, Elliott MR (2020) Big data for finite population inference: applying quasi-random approaches to naturalistic driving data using Bayesian additive regression trees. J Survey Stat Methodol 8(1):148–180. https://doi.org/10.1093/jssam/smz060
35. Biswal AK, Singh D, Pattanayak BK, Samanta D, Yang M-H (2021) IoT-based smart alert system for drowsy driver detection. Wireless Commun Mobile Comput 2021:13. Article ID 6627217. https://doi.org/10.1155/2021/6627217
36. Pramanik S, Samanta D, Dutta S, Ghosh R, Ghonge M, Pandey D (2020) Steganography using improved LSB approach and asymmetric cryptography. In: 2020 IEEE international conference on advent trends in multidisciplinary research and innovation (ICATMRI), Buldhana, India, 2020, pp 1–5. https://doi.org/10.1109/ICATMRI51801.2020.9398408
37. Maheswari M, Geetha S, Kumar SS, Karuppiah M, Samanta D, Park Y, PEVRM: probabilistic evolution based version recommendation model for mobile applications. IEEE Access. https://doi.org/10.1109/ACCESS.2021.3053583
38. Kumar R, Kumar R, Samanta D, Paul M, Kumar V (2017) A combining approach using DFT and FIR filter to enhance impulse response. In: 2017 international conference on computing methodologies and communication (ICCMC), Erode, India, 2017, pp 134–137. https://doi.org/10.1109/ICCMC.2017.8282660
39. Gomathy V, Padhy N, Samanta D et al (2020) Malicious node detection using heterogeneous cluster based secure routing protocol (HCBS) in wireless adhoc sensor networks. J Ambient Intell Human Comput 11:4995–5001. https://doi.org/10.1007/s12652-020-01797-3
40. Ghosh G, Samanta D, Paul M, Janghel NK (2017) Hiding based message communication techniques depends on divide and conquer approach. In: 2017 international conference on computing methodologies and communication (ICCMC), Erode, 2017, pp 123–128. https://doi.org/10.1109/ICCMC.2017.8282658
41. Sivakumar P, Nagaraju R, Samanta D et al (2020) A novel free space communication system using nonlinear InGaAsP microsystem resonators for enabling power-control toward smart cities. Wireless Netw 26:2317–2328. https://doi.org/10.1007/s11276-019-02075-7
42. Samanta D, Sanyal G (2012) A novel approach of SAR image classification using color space clustering and watersheds. In: 2012 fourth international conference on computational intelligence and communication networks, Mathura, India, 2012, pp 237–240. https://doi.org/10.1109/CICN.2012.27
43. Khamparia A, Singh PK, Rani P, Samanta D, Khanna A, Bhushan B (2020) An internet of health things-driven deep learning framework for detection and classification of skin cancer using transfer learning. Trans Emerging Tel Tech e3963. https://doi.org/10.1002/ett.3963
44. Hossain MA, Samanta D, Sanyal G (2012) Statistical approach for extraction of panic expression. In: 2012 fourth international conference on computational intelligence and communication networks, Mathura, India, 2012, pp 420–424. https://doi.org/10.1109/CICN.2012.189
45. Althar RR, Samanta D (2021) The realist approach for evaluation of computational intelligence in software engineering. Innov Syst Softw Eng. https://doi.org/10.1007/s11334-020-00383-2
46. Singh RK, Begum T, Borah L, Samanta D (2017) Text encryption: character jumbling. In: 2017 international conference on inventive systems and control (ICISC), Coimbatore, India, 2017, pp 1–3. https://doi.org/10.1109/ICISC.2017.8068691

47. Guha A, Samanta D (2021) Hybrid approach to document anomaly detection: an application to facilitate RPA in title insurance. Int J Autom Comput 18:55–72. https://doi.org/10.1007/s11633-020-1247-y
48. Agarwal M, Sarkhel D, Samanta D (2018) Architecture of 'loop' without 'for' & 'while'. In: 2018 2nd international conference on inventive systems and control (ICISC), Coimbatore, India, 2018, pp 491–494. https://doi.org/10.1109/ICISC.2018.8399121
49. Samanta D, Sivaram M, Rashed A, Boopathi CS, Amiri IS, Yupapin P (2020) Distributed Feedback Laser (DFB) for signal power amplitude level improvement in long spectral band. J Opt Commun. https://doi.org/10.1515/joc-2019-0252
50. Chakrabarti S, Samanta D (2015) Notice of removal: a novel approach to digital image steganography of key-based encrypted text. In: 2015 international conference on electrical, electronics, signals, communication and optimization (EESCO), Visakhapatnam, India, 2015, pp 1–6. https://doi.org/10.1109/EESCO.2015.7254009
51. Pramanik S, Samanta D, Bandyopadhyay S, Ghosh R, A new combinational technique in image steganography. Int J Inf Secur Privacy (IJISP) 15(3). ISSN: 1930-1650|EISSN: 1930-1669
52. Rao KR, Samanta D, Somashekara MT, Gurunath R, Paul A (2019) Automatic segmentation based graphical interface for recognition of tomography image analysis of damage cell. In: 2019 third international conference on inventive systems and control (ICISC), Coimbatore, India, 2019, pp 52–55. https://doi.org/10.1109/ICISC44355.2019.9036343
53. Gurunath R, Agarwal M, Nandi A, Samanta D (2018) An overview: security issue in IoT network. In: 2018 2nd international conference on I-SMAC (IoT in Social, Mobile, Analytics and Cloud) (I-SMAC), 2018 2nd international conference on I-SMAC (IoT in Social, Mobile, Analytics and Cloud) (I-SMAC), Palladam, India, 2018, pp 104–107. https://doi.org/10.1109/I-SMAC.2018.8653728
54. Ghosh G, Samanta D, Paul M (2016) Approach of message communication based on twisty "Zig-Zag". In: 2016 international conference on emerging technological trends (ICETT), Kollam, 2016, pp 1–5. https://doi.org/10.1109/ICETT.2016.7873676
55. Dhanush V, Mahendra AR, Kumudavalli MV, Samanta D (2017) Application of deep learning technique for automatic data exchange with air-gapped systems and its security concerns. In: 2017 international conference on computing methodologies and communication (ICCMC), Erode, India, 2017, pp 324–328. https://doi.org/10.1109/ICCMC.2017.8282701
56. Hossain MA, Samanta D, Sanyal G (2012) Extraction of panic expression depending on lip detection. In: 2012 international conference on computing sciences, Phagwara, India, 2012, pp 137–141. https://doi.org/10.1109/ICCS.2012.35
57. Hossain MA, Samanta D, Sanyal G (2012) A novel approach for panic-face extraction based on mutation. In: 2012 IEEE international conference on advanced communication control and computing technologies (ICACCCT), Ramanathapuram, India, 2012, pp 473–477. https://doi.org/10.1109/ICACCCT.2012.6320825
58. Saha AK et al, IOT-based drone for improvement of crop quality in agricultural field. In: IEEE 8th annual computing and communication workshop and conference (CCWC), pp 612–615. https://doi.org/10.1109/CCWC.2018.8301662
59. Sai PY, Harika P (2017) Illustration of IoT with big data analytics. Global J Comput Sci Technol 17(3)
60. Salloum SA, Khan R, Shaalan K (2020) A survey of semantic analysis approaches. In Hassanien AE, Azar A, Gaber T, Oliva D, Tolba F (eds) Proceedings of the international conference on artificial intelligence and computer vision (AICV2020). AICV 2020. Advances in intelligent systems and computing, vol 1153. Springer, Cham. https://doi.org/10.1007/978-3-030-44289-7_6
61. Sanchez-Huertas W, Víctor Gómez V, Hernández C (2018) Machine learning techniques and smart grid applications: a review. Int J Appl Eng Res 13(21):14876–14885
62. Saleem TJ, Chisthi MA (2019) Deep learning for Internet of Things data analytics. Procedia Comput Sci 163:381–390. https://doi.org/10.1016/j.procs.2019.12.120
63. Santamaria AF, Raimondo P, Tropea M, Rango FD, Aiello C (2019) An IoT surveillance system based on a decentralized architecture. Sensors 19:1469. https://doi.org/10.3390/s19061469

64. Shirke A, Chandane MM (2018) IoT data based predictive modeling for energy usage of appliances in smart home. Int J Eng Technol 7:931–934
65. Stergiou C, Psannis KE, Kim BG, Gupta B (2018) Secure integration of IoT and cloud computing. Futur Gener Comput Syst 78:964–975. https://doi.org/10.1016/j.future.2016.11.031
66. Sundaravadivel P, Kesavan K, Kesavan L, Mohanty SP, Kougianos E (2018) Smart-log: a deep-learning based automated nutrition monitoring system in the iot. IEEE Trans Consum Electron 64(3):390–398. https://doi.org/10.1109/TCE.2018.2867802
67. Sun S, Luo C, Chen J (2017) A review of natural language processing techniques for opinion mining systems. Inf Fusion 36:10–25. https://doi.org/10.1016/j.inffus.2016.10.004
68. Sun Y, Song H, Jara AJ, Bie R (2016) Internet of Things and big data analytics for smart and connected communities. IEEE Access 4:766–773. https://doi.org/10.1109/ACCESS.2016.2529723
69. Sun P (2020) Security and privacy protection in cloud computing: discussions and challenges. J Netw Comput Appl 160. https://doi.org/10.1016/j.jnca.2020.102642
70. Sunhare P, Chowdhary RR, Chattapadhyay MK (2020) Internet of Things and data mining: an application oriented survey. J King Saud Univ-Comput Inf Sci. https://doi.org/10.1016/j.jksuci.2020.07.002

Chapter 3
Application of Machine Intelligence and Data Science for Intelligent IoT

Abstract Applications for the Internet of Things have evolved in excessive quantities, producing a vast volume of data needed for the intelligent transformation of data. The numerous IoT frameworks (i.e. edge, fog, and cloud) and the shortcomings for the protocols of the IoT application level in the transmission/receipt of messages are, however, the obstacles to the development of acute IoT approaches. The challenges preclude existing acute IoT frameworks that learn from other IoT applications in an adaptive manner. In this article, we critically discuss how machine learning research processes the IoT-generated data and highlight the existing difficulties of fostering intelligent approaches for the IoT world. In addition, the authors suggest a foundation to allow IoT frameworks to learn appropriately from various other IoT frameworks and provide a chronology on how to apply the approach to specific literature surveys. Finally, we answer the essential variables which have an effect on potential IoT intelligent frameworks.

3.1 Introduction

The paradigm of the IoT is a combination of groundbreaking and an enabler of modern-day humans' digital and comfortable lifestyles. IoT's evolution can be traced to a confluence of developments in computation, connectivity, and device architecture that have taken place during the past decade. The subsequent IoT area of control has quickly grown to encompass the whole human race. Mobile gadgets, home aides like Google Play, self-driving cars [1], construction management frameworks including intelligent elevators, temperature adjusting frameworks, and aerial conveyances like drones [2] for surrounding surveillance [3] and recreation are all widely used IoT devices to promote our everyday activities. The enormous expansion of IoT system spreads far away from these appliances to globally distributed back-end cloud [4] facilities within data centers. As a result, IoT appliances with their assisting infrastructures produce a vast amount of data for transmission and eventual collection and retrieval at far-end cloud repository centers. IoT appliances produce a continuous rush of

D. Samanta and A. Banerjee, *Computationally Intensive Statistics for Intelligent IoT*,
Studies in Autonomic, Data-driven and Industrial Computing,
https://doi.org/10.1007/978-981-16-5936-2_3

untested data that cannot be defined as relevant information until the information is refined by the use of methods like the exploration of information and AI. The diverseness of the data produced by different IoT implementations depends on the area of operation, including intelligent healthcare, e-farming, e-health, intelligent power grids, and self-driving automobiles. For maintaining power consumption related to device functioning, IoT appliances were built with customized protocols that recognize the capability limited existence of these appliances. Message Queuing Telemetry Transfer (MQTT) [5], Constrained Application Protocol (CoAP) [6], and Advanced Message Queuing Protocol (AMQP) [7] are the various ordinary IoT application-level protocols.

The AMQP and MQTT protocols were installed over IoT appliances that have a doorway to an uninterrupted power supply. These protocols allow larger messages to be transferred and therefore are further power-hungry. CoAP protocol, on the other hand, is meant for extremely resource-mannered IoT applications, where those with very small computational power and network capacity are resource-constrained devices. The most resource-concentrated IoT networking protocol is the HTTP [8] and is better applicable for high-end IoT systems with greater connectivity, computing, and storage capacities. IoT systems generate a huge amount of data that is stored locally and transmitted to a centralized computing confluence or cloud repository provision in a restricted way, where it can be further processed or analyzed for information generation. ML [9] is described as a data analysis technique in which the technique of model establishment on tutelage knowledge is automatic, i.e. requiring almost no individual involvement. Methods of categorizing data creating separate groups are thus completely automatic. It is not necessary to understate the importance of data analytics for IoT data analysis, and ML is a very powerful donator to enable the rapid conversion of huge amounts of data from IoT appliances to produce trends of curiosity to data inquisitors.

Paradigms in present-day processing and repository include edge and cloud computing. A comprehensive data collection, storage, retrieval, and analytics architecture emerges from the convergence of these paradigms with the IoT. Such a structure has the potential to offer insights into data dynamics in real time and also enables the use of machine learning approaches for the realization of intelligent IoT data analytics. The cloud prototype is a consolidated data storage framework that centrally provides different services, like Infrastructure as a Service, Application as a Service, and Software as a Service, that facilitate IoT data transformation and scrutiny. On the other hand, edge computing [10] makes IoT data nearer to the IoT system to be stored and evaluated on regional computing nodes. As a consequence, the costs incurred with the transition to consolidated nodes of IoT data are eliminated. Fog computing [11] denotes a middle-level approach linking the paradigms of the cloud environment and edge computing, where it is not important to place IoT data collection and analysis at the border of the network or else in a centralized repository provision. Instead, of collection and analysis of IoT results, the fog model puts the idea of a distributed architecture, not solely situated at the border of the network.

3.2 The Combination of Intelligent IoT and ML

For resource-constrained IoT applications, the integration of ML and IoT creates the pathway for future progress in performance, precision, competitiveness, and all-inclusive cost reductions. We will achieve enhanced connectivity and computational efficiency, better controllability, and improved decision-making when ML algorithms and IoT function jointly. IoT has a tremendous success to increase the value of human life and future advancements for organizational development because of the updated tracking of billions of omnipresent sensing instruments and enhanced connectivity achievements (toward Industry 4.0). Due to the integration of DL [12] and AI, the ability of IoT has increased greatly. In order to provide further perceptions to a variety of real-entity concerns, and the potential to take crucial tactical commitments, sophisticated ML methods have facilitated in unearthing the vast amount in IoT sensory analysis. Therefore, IoT and ML must accompany each other in order to calculate complex real-life complications and thus effectively satisfy computational and connectivity demands. For the following factors, IoT data analysis has achieved considerable momentum and popularity in recent years.

A huge quantity of data produced by dispersion of IoT appliances in accordance with the Ericsson mobile survey says that it would be 20 billion globally connected IoT devices projected by 2022. Owing to the varied promotion of IoT appliances in a variety of vital implementations, this amount would keep growing over time. Intelligent data analysis can play a major part in detecting and forecasting the potential situation of an operation or device by effectively and intelligently unearthing the vast volume of data.

The characteristics and types of the data are distinct due to the variability of the data. Also, the data sources may vary depending on different IoT device domains. The IoT systems used for medical purposes, for example, would vary from the IoT of a smart home. In addition, because of its heterogeneity, the quality, distribution, and storing of data has often been a difficult job. In [13], some main problems emerging due to the variability of data sources are illustrated by the authors. It contains queries to crucial interrogations like how to cope up with the varied data sampling process, noise reduction and data filtering, processing and mixing of data from various origins, understanding and operability of data, logic, and perception of the situation and data development of information, collection and storing of data from heterogeneous data sources. In improving precision for decision-producing, it is necessary to warrant the right estimate, dissemination of uncertainty, and to construct models and strategies which can cope with these variables.

3.3 Overview of Different Approaches for IoT Analytics

In the section, we consider various categories of data analysis procedures. In Fig. 3.1, the key variants of the analysis groups are shown.

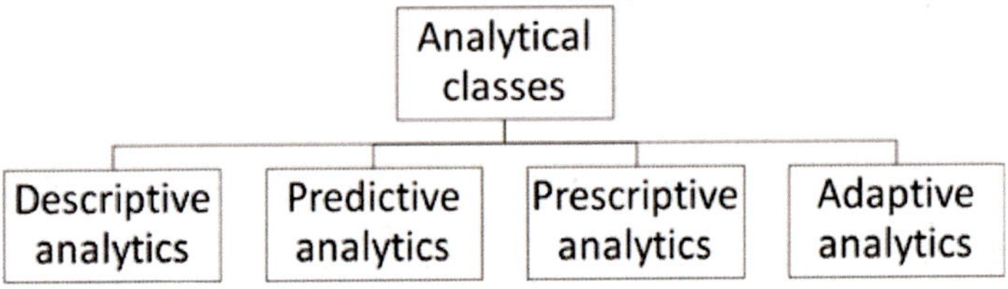

Fig. 3.1 Popular analytical categories

3.3.1 Descriptive Analysis

IoT platforms are able to store and transfer information from various intelligent devices to a cloud platform. Through the use of sophisticated machine learning methods, it is also possible to produce useful insights into historical events based on analytical evidence. The area of research called descriptive analytics is essentially made up of these classes of ML-based approaches that transform raw data and furnish better apprehension. Such examples of descriptive analytics are data analysis, data summarization, and logical processes and data manipulation. High-volume data is needed for descriptive analytics. Recent technical achievements have shown that cloud repository is competent in depositing large IoT data reserves, and cloud servers could use high-performance computers to apply IoT cloud [14] analytics to process complex activities.

3.3.2 Predictive Analysis

Predictive analysis is focused on empirical information which employs sophisticated techniques to predict mathematical or machine learning behavior or activities so that potential future innovations can be modeled. By analyzing the historical trends and data associations of current data, it estimates what can occur in the coming years. For different reasons, such as predictive maintenance, market prediction, supply–demand pattern, or risk assessment of some consequence, predictive analysis has been commonly used. One of the emerging analysis agencies SAS concluded that there are two categories of predictive frameworks: i) classification-dependent replica running class participation forecast analyses and (ii) regression-based replica prediction dependent on previous analysis and ability. Innovative methods of predictive analysis consist of models based on different regression techniques, decision trees, and approaches based on a deep neural network. Ensemble model-based analysis, Bayesian analysis [15], and so on are based on many other commonly used algorithms. These approaches to predictive analytics rely on information for conclusion-building. The IoT model will boost simplifying the phase of data collection from intelligent IoT appliances and can use the cloud or the network edge to provide an explanatory context.

3.3.3 Prescriptive Analysis

Prescriptive analysis advises when for reacting to a possible incident depending on data analysis. The research outcome not just models upcoming states, it further offers instructions for the result to be reached. In risk assessment, it is something like a possible methodology that optimizes all the advantages of predictive analysis. Although predictive analysis demonstrates how and the time the occurrence may start on the basis of upcoming forecasts, prescriptive analysis expands the ability in supplying insight into potential predictions through impact analysis. Prescriptive analytics is commonly used to maximize the market result. In an industrial IoT (IIoT) framework where enterprise intellectual ability actions are made while using the tools of cloud technology, business analytics, and deep learning, prescriptive analytics is important. Resources within the IoT network can actually make an effective decision related to the application of organizational smart tools and analysis.

3.3.4 IoT Adaptive Analysis

Throughout genuine execution, the result acquired by predictive analysis requires to be amended by concrete knowledge. In the function, adaptive analysis can be utilized in modifying or maximize a structured study, given the recent past corresponding to the data and thereby gazing at the similarities. The method for analyzing leads to the enhancement of framework efficiency, thus eliminating mistakes. The privilege for adaptive analysis is that it will change the result for an approach when a newer collection of incoming data is obtained. Adaptive analytics, particularly in an IoT context, is a better match in real-time information processing. Real-time measurement for emerging information sources, which can be constituent in malware, may be dependent on adaptive analytics in order to perform data analytics.

3.4 Information Analysis Grouping in IoT Established on Technical Foundation

3.4.1 Computation in the Cloud

Distantly situated storage resources are used in a cloud computing paradigm to store, capture, handle, and process data using the internet. Due to the newer resources and the advancing frameworks that are offered in handling various functions, including Platform as a Service, Infrastructure as a Service, and Software as a Service, cloud computing has gained much attention in recent decades, particularly more recently. The cloud provides a range of internet-based services, and the idea of all as a facility has evolved. Cloud computing can have several benefits in an IoT-based environment.

The IoT interconnects intelligent computers. A large amount of produced information is needed in processing and analyzing within an IoT paradigm.

3.4.2 Edge Computing

Edge computation is relating the logical capacity of IoT devices to the border of the network. By understanding the threats and drawbacks of cloud computation, the significance of edge computing may be preferably acknowledged. Cloud computing is a centralized data processing system that can increase the overhead of large data processing. Supplying the crude IoT data flow in the cloud will lift the expenditure and demand higher bandwidth and strength of communication. Moreover, edge computation requires the computation for the root of the data within a "local" network. Figure 3.2 presents the union of IoT framework and data analytics. The bandwidth dilemma of transmitting bulk volumes of information in the central repository is then solved. Also, as opposed to edge computation, cloud computing requires fairly complicated implementations. The architecture of a combined edge-cloud framework in IoT architectures is shown in Fig. 3.3. Uncertainty for the data sources of the IoT in functional data processing is very common. Because of the malfunction for any IoT system or connecting path throughout data transmission, these can occur in the IoT data stream. In IoT data sources, cumulative faults and lost information

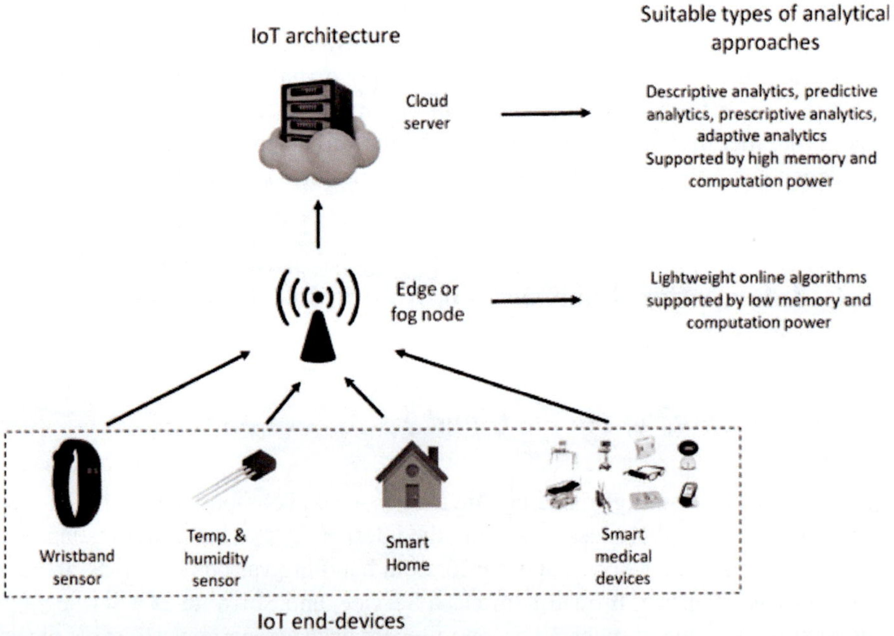

Fig. 3.2 Union of IoT framework and data analytics

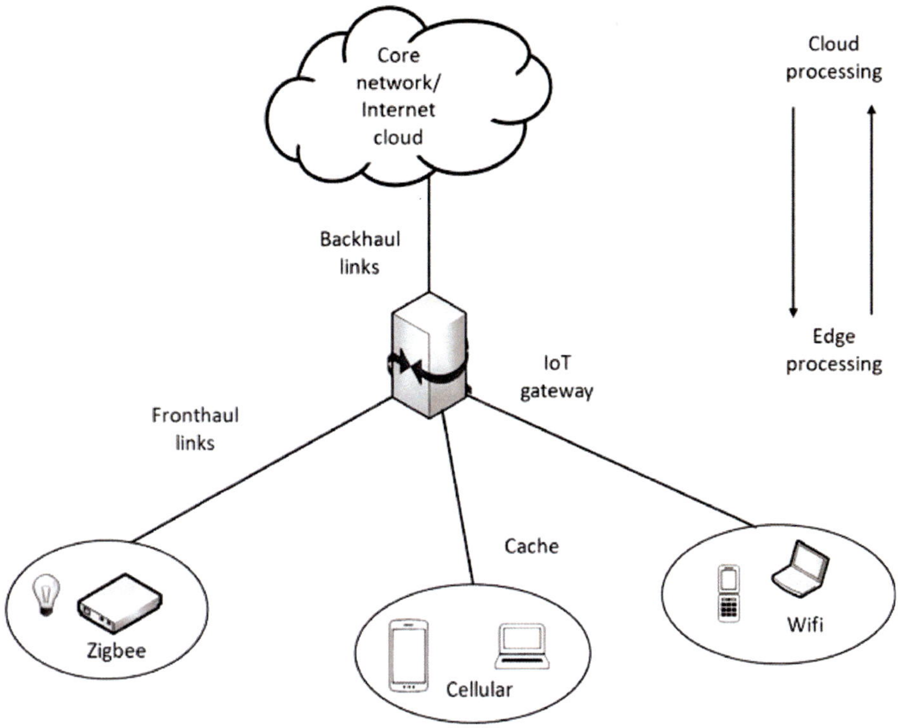

Fig. 3.3 In heterogeneous IoT networks, a simplified device architecture for collaborative edge-cloud processing

are predominant, requiring sophisticated analytics to preprocess the information. Also, cyber attack [16] may constitute the legitimate cause of data uncertainty. An important fact is in ensuring the correct estimation, dissemination, and depiction of uncertainty in building frameworks and strategies which may cope with the variables in order to increase precision during decision-making. Figure 3.4 shows the e-health cloud multi-layer architecture.

3.5 Utilizations of Data in IoT Analysis

3.5.1 Analysis in IoT in Intelligent Transportation

For crime diagnosis on bus facilities, an autonomous and real-time approach was proposed in [17, 18]. The authors illustrate the benefits of IoT technology in a fog computing environment and show the advantage of data analytics. Intelligent public safety in a connected vehicle setting has been developed as a system. The main focus

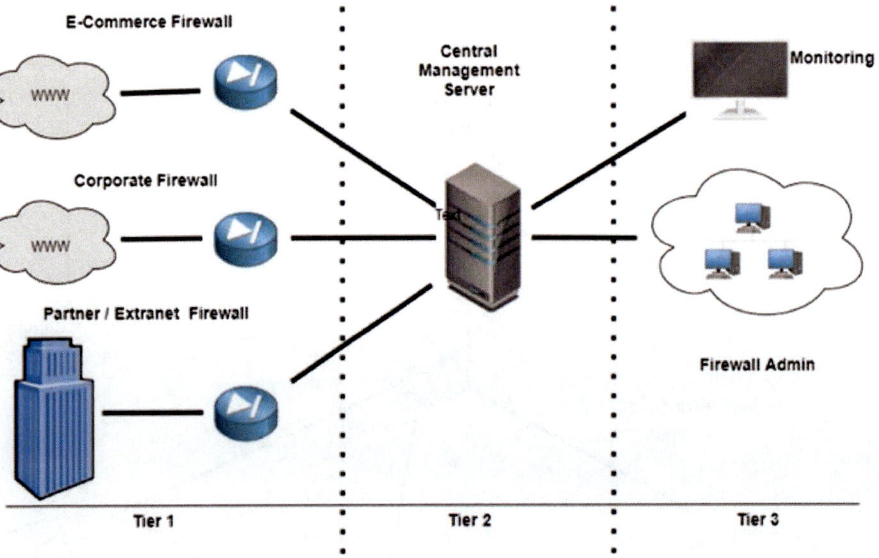

Fig. 3.4 IoT-based system's three-tier architecture for multiple applications in a linked system

of this research has been innovative data analytical capabilities for crime identification, analysis, and stoppage. The proposed architecture illustrates a major increase in efficiency and system survival over conventional usage cases for smart transport safety.

Apart from offense prevention, vehicular data analysis linked to IoT can benefit further important implementations. For instance, Luo et al. suggested a three-tier structure for efficient traffic management of the linked public transportation system. Here, in an IoT-connected world, the authors recommend creative strategies for the efficient scheduling of subways, buses, and shared taxis. For evaluating passenger and road movements, a periodic pattern mining-based algorithm is implemented. Finally, to build a theoretical model for dynamic bus scheduling, the functionality of evolutionary-based algorithms is used. Figure 4 illustrates the IoT-based system's three-tier architecture for multiple applications in a linked system.

Data is obtained from different IoT sensors and instruments in the first layer (perception layer). A traveler's mobile phone, for example, can facilitate the passenger with location details, while a smart travel card may include passenger identity and financial transaction information. The second level, i.e., the network level for the system is accountable for using both wired and wireless connectivity to transfer the original data to the final application layer. Standard networking systems such as GPRS, CDMA, fourth-generation communication (4G), fifth-generation communication (5G), etc., are used in general wireless transmissions and for private wireless transmissions like Bluetooth and Wi-Fi. In the application layer, advanced analytics make use of IoT info. For settlement-making of diverse implementations implemented for bus and shared cab networks, optimization and ML techniques are utilized here.

The subject of research discussed in [19, 20, 21] was the intelligent allocation of parking space. A systemic solution using IoT and cloud computing was developed by Kong et al. to address the issue of parking allocation. To resolve the parking allotment dilemma, the approach utilizes sale-related schemes. The primary focus of their study has been the recognition of two main explanatory components: communication quality and tag fixtures. ML techniques such as linear classification and clustering analysis will have an appropriate output for the recognition of these important parameters, as the authors in [22] demonstrate.

3.5.2 *Smart Healthcare IoT Data Analytics*

Different use fields, including healthcare, have benefited from the fast growth of IoT. Along with data processing, IoT technologies will aid to attain further detailed and better fitness diagnoses. Collecting knowledge, forecasting, and making decisions in real time are crucial prerequisites. The authors illustrate in [23] the importance of applications of synchronous feature extraction techniques in the development of patient models dependent on genomics. A complex intelligence processing framework needs to be built. Under the smart healthcare paradigm, these revolutionary models must be capable of collecting the data generated by various IoT-associated terminals. Innovative analysis and collaboration in a related medical care framework can have several advantages, together with increased durability, a smooth fusion of varied technology, collection and analytics of big data, customized patient condition forecasting, patient health tracking for life, ease of usage with wearable devices, reduction of total medical health costs, physician supervision with re-oversight. Also, it is emphasized that the framework-dependent methodology that is commonly utilized in the industry will not be an acceptable match for the medical sector as the health evidence is rapidly evolving and very vulnerable to confusion. Therefore, a data-driven approach could be a safer alternative rather than a prototype-related policy. The e-healthcare cloud multi-layer design is seen in this section. Although information processing and interaction occurs in Zone 1, in Zone 2 the important computing phase is carried out; real-time analytics and data streaming are based in zone 2. Finally, the findings are shown or enabled on the basis of the specifications of the Zone 2 program or services. In [24], an intelligent sleep management framework is suggested.

The researchers suggest a preprocessing method related to fog computation deployed on the smart computer. First, when doing batch data analysis, the power of big data over the cloud environment is used. The findings of the study are presented using the online user interface to support health practitioners, regardless of their place of activity, in real time.

In [25, 26] an IoT-enabled automatic tracking system for nutrition is proposed. Using a thorough study of Bayesian networks, the authors suggest a meal-prediction algorithm. Another algorithm that utilizes perceptron neural network-related DL framework is proposed to analyze the diet balance. The smart IoT platform for tracking and communicating is included in this computational model. Early diagnosis of dyslexia, which is a learning impairment that affects an individual's daily activities, is achievable within an IoT system with the use of ledger-based technology. The suggested solution collects information over intelligent IoT appliances like tabs, laptops, and smart-phones and uses blockchain-dependent dispersed ledger technologies for storing the details. Because of the usage of blockchains, it is open for examination by the medical practitioner irrespective of the place, and it also offers information security. In [27], a representative-dependent IoT implementation testbed was made to analyze the sleeping behavior of a patient. The simulator analyzes the sensor knowledge in the sense of a smart bed to detect posture at sleep time. In [28, 29], an emotion recognition model is proposed. Voice and picture communications from IoT appliances are processed by the suggested solution. In order to make decisions, these signals can be processed in the peripheral cloud and distant cloud. The identification uses SVMs, Fourier transform, and other filtering techniques. The suggested architecture is sufficient for implementation in a broad data setting.

3.5.3 IoT in Agriculture

Utilizing the state-of-the-art analysis of the data got from intelligent end appliances, IoT-dependent approaches may be implemented in increasing the performance and precision in service. In [30], many problems and advantages for IoT and data analysis-related intelligent farming approaches will be addressed. The opportunities, possibilities, and viability of WSN in farming are extensively designed in recent years. Environment inspection, accuracy, and automation and time stamping are included in the implementation of WSN in agriculture. Recently, because of the simplicity of the implementation of multiple wired and wireless systems and the potential to combine with advanced data collection frameworks, the importance of IoT has been highlighted. Agricultural IoT empowers agriculturalists in innovative processes for judgment-making. Moreover, it makes it possible to combine agricultural goods, resources, and expertise seamlessly, in order to boost efficiency.

The IoT is dispatched in controlling and managing agricultural properties. Inside an IoT system, going with cloud/edge data analysis, GPS can also be used for the same purpose. For productive farming, wind velocity, warmth, clouds, precipitation, and weather metrics are usually very crucial. Machine intelligence IoT can aid in forecasting the localized meteorology of farming companies.

In addition, aiding the clever utilization of IoT with the big data framework, the performance of industrial waste and water storage can be increased. The problem of storage control can be overcome by the use of intelligent scheduling algorithms. In order to monitor the storage facilities, IoT sensors can be strategically located and cloud technology will install ML along with optimization techniques to create conclusions.

The main constituent of IoT-dependent intelligent agriculture is seen in Fig. 3.5. Three of the four main components contribute to the data (marked in the darkened

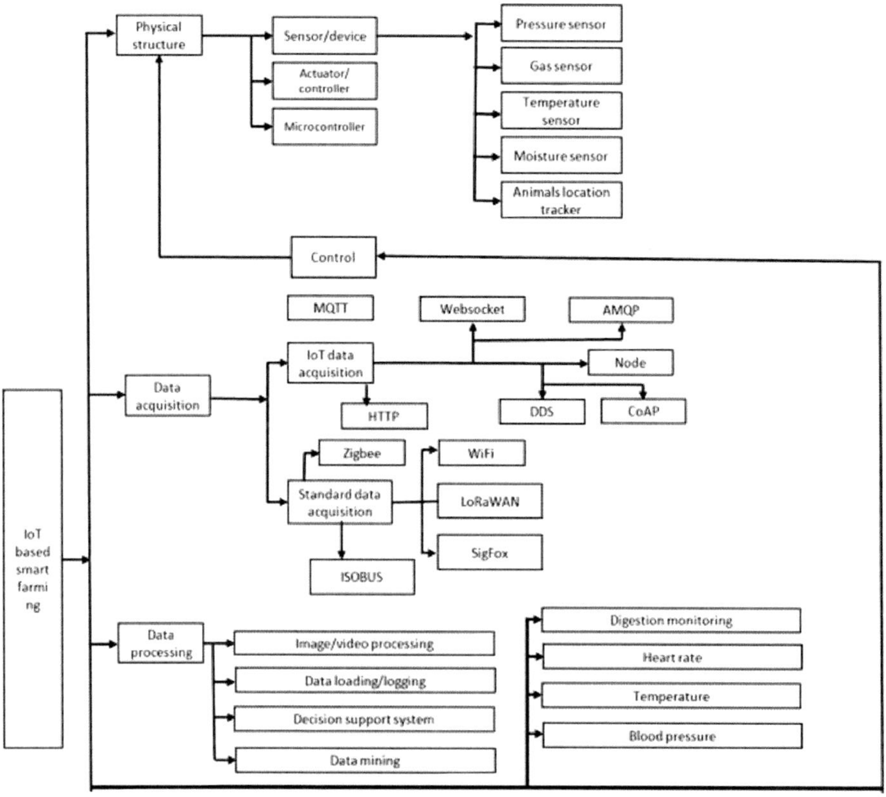

Fig. 3.5 IoT-based smart farming elements

box). Sensors, actuators, and devices are operated by the physical system and are responsible for the ultimate accuracy of data processing. Based on state-of-the-art IoT protocols, procurement of records and data analysis are close to those used in typical IoT requirements. Many techniques and frameworks for data analytics are utilized in the data analysis portion. Many IoT and data analytical-related intelligent farming resources involve tracking of animal wellbeing, training of pressure levels, detection of human movements, rumination, heart rate monitoring, monitoring of livestock locations, monitoring of climate conditions, identification of pests, control of irrigation, monitoring of greenhouse gases, and so on.

3.5.4 Analysis of Data in IoT for Energy Applications

Owing to the incorporation of photovoltaic solar cells, hybrid cars, and batteries with a low-voltage delivery network, the electricity grid has dramatically improved in recent years. There is a need to organize and manage these dispersed energy networks efficiently. Using the functionality of smart meters is one viable alternative. Smart meters are interconnected and linked with each other within an IoT environment. To increase the efficacy and efficiency of energy operations, advanced analytical decisions are required. Consequently, the authors found out in [31] that the combination of big data and IoT may be utilized to handle resources effectively. The authors are designing a framework for energy storage that can be used in a smart home. In a home area network, a centralized server is used where data is captured, saved, and analyzed. One value is that the approach suggested is capable of leveraging business analytics resources that are off-the-shelf. The design of the solution will dramatically increase the performance of applications with high energy usage, such as air conditioning. In a laboratory setting, this has been validated. In view of the smart home architecture, a peer-to-peer energy trading framework focused on IoT and sensor data optimization is suggested in [32, 33].

In [34], the analysts surveyed the opportunities and possibilities for the smart grid with big data and cloud analytics. Once data is obtained from smart meters, automated analytics can be carried out through tools on a cloud network. Such instances of cloud-related computing applications in data analysis are Google BigQuery.

Predictive research was introduced in [35] for decision assistant frameworks of an intelligent meter IoT infrastructure. Moreover, the researchers utilize a cost prediction method depending on machine learning and to boost network service efficiency. In this work, three classifiers, including decision trees, naïve Bayes, and random forest are compared with a Bayesian network model. The suggested approach in [36] is tested using data obtained from commercial settings on network coverage.

The machine learning-integrated IoT-connected smart grid will have many advantages, including consumption forecasts, cost, power creation, potential optimized schedule, error identification, regulation, scaling, and detection of invasion. Communication and data sharing creates a major part in such applications. To this end, the IoT is commonly deployed. The authors have presented the security problems in IoT data analytics in [37]

A multi-stage theft identification methodology based on ML is suggested in [38]. Multi-faceted prognosis is utilized in the estimation of intake behavior in the first step. Machine learning models depending on long short-term memory (LSTM), recurrent neural network (RNN), and multi-layer perceptron (MLP) are utilized in this step. In the second step, choices are made. Here, to classify the deviations, a daily average template is utilized. The historical uses of energy are used in the final stage to determine whether or not the phenomenon dependent on stage 2 will be a power robbery.

In [39, 40], a lightweight IoT intrusion detection system (IDS) depending on ML emerged. The suggested IDS are competent in the effective detection of denial of service intrusions. The researchers utilize classification techniques depending on SVM for establishing IDS. Apart from other books, in order to model the classifier, the suggested technique consists of a single attribute. This theory made the paradigm effective in programming and helped to achieve quicker remedies. The relative findings reported in this manuscript indicate that in precision, the SVM-related IDS beats the innovative techniques.

3.6 An Essential Analysis for IoT for Data Mining with an Exploration of Information

3.6.1 Translating Information to Data

To generate meaningful information, IoT devices must process data. The design seen in Fig. 7 shows how knowledge becomes important to its consumers. The user may be a computer or person in this architecture. The information transformation block comprises AI techniques, like ML approaches, if customers intend to obtain useful information. Relevant processed data is often referred to in this article as "knowledge".

Prescriptive, predictive, and adaptive IoT analysis will in a better way be represented by how data is interpreted by applications to produce information. Throughout this portion, the above architecture is used to structure the assessment in which recent learning applies AI for IoT prototype. This segment underlines the problems of adoption, explores how studies resolve them, and examines potential prospects for the study.

3.7 The Protocol of the Application Layer

An application layer protocol is needed in host-to-host transmissions to transmit data in a form that may be summarized by lower layer protocols. CoAP, MQTT, AMQP, and HTTP are the commonly used IoT application layer protocols, as mentioned earlier (HTTP). For abstraction from the lower levels, all these protocols allow. Figure 3.6 shows information development architecture in the IoT. Figure 3.7 expresses the protocols for the IoT program, viz., CoAP, MQTT, AMQP, and HTTP.

Constrained computers also constrain the capacity for computation, connectivity, and storage. Because various IoT devices have different resource specifications, to satisfy these necessities, the protocols vary in potentials. Through the data volumes,

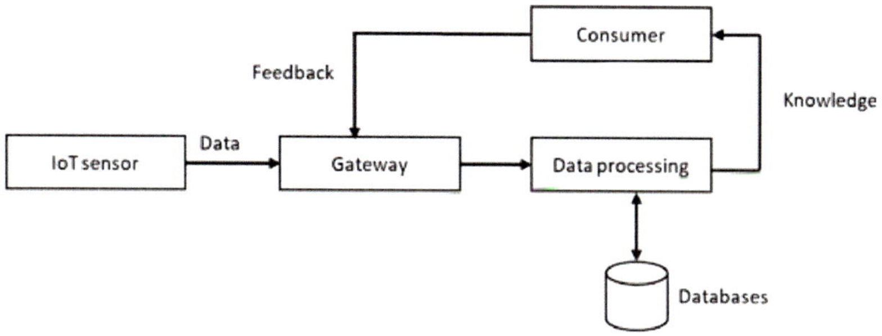

Fig. 3.6 Information development architecture in the IoT, remodeled [41]

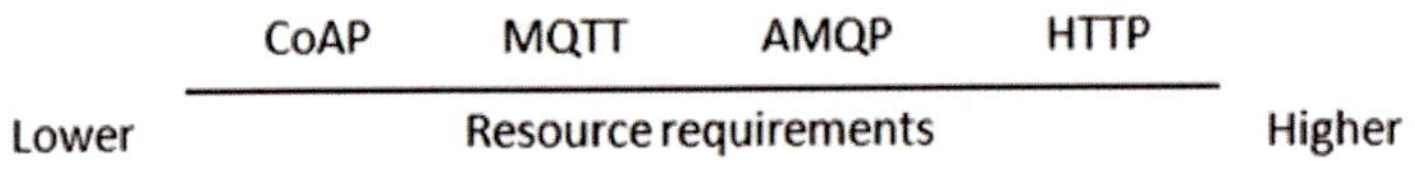

Fig. 3.7 Protocols for the IoT program, viz., CoAP, MQTT, AMQP, and HTTP remodeled by [42]

latency, and over-head, resource specifications were extracted. As highlighted in Fig. 3.8, CoAP indicates the lightest, while the preferred resource-consuming is HTTP. In approaches wherever IoT data is obtained through restricted appliances in the edge, CoAP is used. Usually, these systems are small in weight, having portable devices or lower maintained sensors that are remote. They possess lesser computational schemes, electricity, and the capacity to wirelessly transfer data. Therefore, those implementations do not give information back to IoT computers. Devices that use CoAP are also ideal, but not adaptive, for prescriptive and predictive AI applications [43, 44].

When implementations can afford higher-end IoT computers, MQTT and AMQP are employed. IoT systems are eligible in power charging or attached straightaway with the power source. In the systems, information may be transmitted over the internet to other computers or users, even back to IoT computers. Hence, for predictive prescriptive and adaptive AI implementations, this scenario can be used.

On the one side, how restricted devices can send data has been discussed by the framework protocols [45]. Machine learning research, on the other hand, involves high computational power and a vast volume of information to process the data gathered in order to translate it to practical knowledge. Therefore, the architecture of information creation differs with IoT applications (Fig. 7) in turning information into knowledge depending on the structure and internetwork resources required in information communication. Three frameworks of how the framework of information exploration may be implemented are seen in Fig. 3.8.

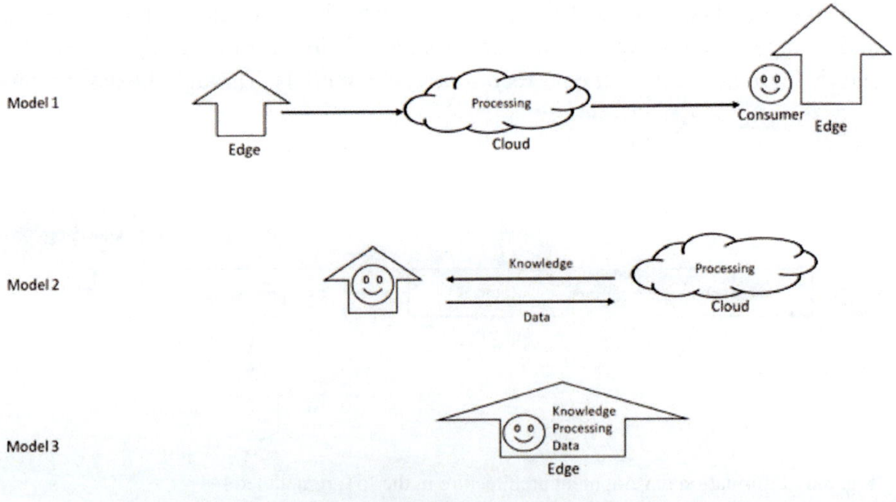

Fig. 3.8 Where data is translated to information

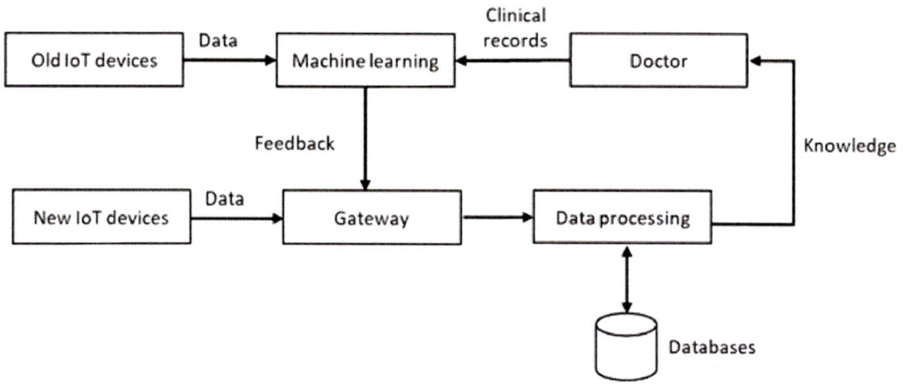

Fig. 3.9 Gateways alter diverse data through various devices

The first model is where a restricted computer transfers data in a clear way to a remote machine. It is the occurrence in data mining, and various applications can be utilized or exchanged along with the data. Every distant occurrence may undergo a convincing way of translating information into knowledge. In the cloud, adaptive learning takes place, as input cannot be returned toward IoT appliances. The IoT computer, on the other hand, is inadequate to learn adjustably [46, 47].

Compelled appliances may convey/accept information in duplex transmissions in the second model. The distant host, e.g. cloud, transforms the information and takes the computer back with the information. In several mobile apps, this model can be used. It is possible to process adaptive learning on a data processor within a cloud or within an IoT computer [48].

Smart devices have ample computational power in the third model to translate information toward knowledge regionally, else at the edge. In accordance with hindrance-dependent systems, this may be ideal. Thus, adaptive learning, maybe due to the information transforming unit or onto the IoT appliance, is processed at the edge [49].

Figure 3.9 shows gateways that alter diverse data through various devices. The comparative study shows the studies' implementations and the form of data deriving out of the sensors for demonstrating the appropriateness for the data transfer protocols. The table, moreover, indicates the category of methodology that the studies are following. The table provides the details to explain the effects of the data analysis conducted by the techniques of machine learning implemented in the research work.

The methodologies demonstrate that while framework protocols discuss to some degree how IoT applications can accept AI, there may be few restrictions on what way IoT appliances learn appropriately.

A contemporary research [50] has demonstrated the way a mixture of the application-level protocols may be used in the IoT context to share information. According to their degree of restriction, different protocols were chosen. CoAP was utilized to authorize regional contact connecting a wearable appliance with an IoT gateway; HTTP was utilized in sharing information linking the IoT gateway with the cloud environment; and MQTT was utilized in giving users, like urgent responders and members of the family, updates from the IoT gateway. Integrating protocols were widely utilized to bolster differing resources needed in various categories of approaches.

Current experiments using IoT data for ML concentrate on the way how IoT technology may help users by proposing where the data can be stored and how it is possible to explain the selection of an application layer protocol to serve its purpose.

Reviews of the literature [51] differentiated the way application-level protocols share information depending on the client–server framework, the mechanism for resource exploration like service-oriented architecture and representational state transfer, the transport layer protocol like user datagram protocol and transport control protocol, and the system for data query like organized query language. However, few studies have contrasted how information of machine-to-machine communications is adaptively learned through existing application layer protocols. While Table 1 exhibits that information for the researches is created, autonomous host-to-host learning hasn't been completely surveyed. The development of data awareness is known to be the feature of a multi-purpose box in which all the necessary information is believed to have been accessible prior to the processing of data using AI or ML techniques.

3.8 The Gateway

Merely, to execute the required operation, a gateway is a multi-purpose device at the edge. Convert, path, or even process data from a gateway. It can be used as a buffer that picks and lowers noise data of interest, moreover for a hub that collects data from various IoT appliances. Although collected information can be too wide at the edge to be distributed over the internet, gateways may be built to generate and relay low bandwidth messages as a data processor. A gateway may not be required, depending on the system specification, or may be compatible with the computers [52, 53].

The problem with the analysis of IoT sensor data stems from the diverseness in the data for finding a health management scheme that uses wearable sensors for medical device data generation. The problem of data heterogeneity will emerge as the amount of newer wearable IoT sensors that expand at a much quicker rate related to how medical gadgets will respond in accordance with the diversification of produced data. The information is unlabeled and ranges in scale. Accordingly, in supervised machine learning techniques, preprocessing of the data is necessary for its use. The research [54] has adapted the information from older IoT appliances in managing data deriving out of newer devices via a gateway. Health reports of a doctor have been utilized to teach ML algorithms in creating information that may synchronize older and modern wearable devices. The gateway here serves as an adaptor for results [55].

Data may be expressed in raw format from IoT devices. Gateways are also structured in converting raw information into a functional structure, like ways in the configuration of trademarks that may be used in analyzing ML. Altered information will exist to envelop within an internetwork packet alongside a header in the packet and various meta-data for transmission to other users, such as sensor information and labels [56].

Gateways will, thus, function like an adapter that translates one protocol to a different one. At the application level, all conform to the one utilized by the cloud on the basis of protocol used at the edge. For instance, from restricted CoAP-using IoT devices to a cloud resource which transmits via AMQP or MQTT. Lower-layer wireless protocols can also be converted from local, restricted devices to facilitate internet-based transmission to the cloud. Gateways can be used at the network layer to refine routing, viz., by judiciously prioritizing packets in vehicle-connected networks that are overflowing in characteristic. A gateway may be positioned in this case for minimizing the amount in detained packets [57].

As gateways conduct several functions, evaluating the computational resources necessary to deploy one is difficult. Studies demonstrate, thus, how their use of energy can be measured. Related assessment for implementation involves how efficiency and latency operate under various loads, such as which customers while operating a mix of services. They were built for and tested only under each particular case study, despite making gateways perform the required behavior. The latest research on the use of IoT information for ML highlights the way by which data complexity originating at various sensors can be adapted, data preprocessed, and cloud communications coordinated. However, in order to adapt heterogeneous data for multiple studies, the approach was not specifically implemented. In other words, not only altering information through newer technologies, yet further through new information, viz., significant information created by AI hosts, are the current challenges. Although a gateway is a system for executing the appropriate action, it needs to be combined with the requisite steps to discover information [58, 59].

3.9 Knowledge Derivation from Data

A stream of raw data is produced by IoT sensors, most of which is illogical for a user. Raw information is a mixture of noise and perspective. It may not reflect a shift through occurrences, quantization, or major features and associations utilized by customers. In IoT, the difficulty of deriving useful data from sensors is obvious as the ubiquitous sensor systems have different circumstances. Here, IoT information processing obeys the technique defined in the complex event processing (CEP) methodology that draws occurrence to process data from incoming sources, irrespective of the mechanization or protocol used. Figure 3.10 projects complex event processing frameworks listens for occurrences through incoming data to operate the information.

The detainment of occurrences involves the production of processed information from the raw data. Information is transmitted as incoming flows; occurrences, like an alteration in state or time in accordance to data, are derived from certain patterns. A

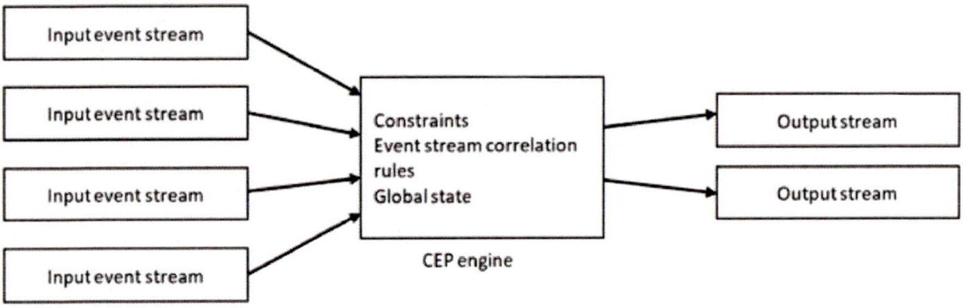

Fig. 3.10 Complex event processing frameworks listens for occurrences through incoming data to operate the information

pattern of interest may be generated by a variety of states. However, where a machine stalls to exercise them in a certain schedule, meaningful patterns will become stale. Thus, event listeners are introduced by structures that extract meaning from input patterns.

In several programming languages, event listeners are introduced, including Java providing a refined execution in pipelining, including the one which may incorporate low-stage incidents into occurrences at the application layer. The expertise obtained is this management-level material. Information is then implemented in CEP as a portrayal linking event tiers. For instance, as a link between different levels of events like news line across the planet, short message service (SMS) communications through qualified entities in certain specified regions, and e-reports through healthcare officials, a universal pandemic watch scheme called knowledge was executed [60].

A knowledge base is necessary when correlating events to define what the associations are. Although the meanings of relationships are historically given by professionals, development in machine learning techniques enables the production of self-assigned rules from input streams. The knowledge base is created in this case as regulations developed from a collection of algorithms for supervised learning. The issue with supervised ML approaches is that expert inputs are still needed for the labeling phase in the development of training datasets instead of relying on host-to-host transmissions [61].

Ontologies have been used instead of manual interaction to fix how machines mark records. Ontology is an internetwork of entities defining the relationships along with the properties. Labels may expose their significance within the domain, provided the ontology of a domain. One way to explain the context is to present the entity characteristics in a duo of mark values. For the case of cars, for example, activities such as velocity may be categorized in accordance with low, medium, and high-velocity values, apiece alongside a set of estimates. Current research demonstrated how nodes, given speed, would self-allocate their tags [62].

Although ontologies discuss how data can be classified and linked, a comprehensive structure that can exchange outcomes between various systems is still needed for the current work. The latest CEP reports, however, are distressed with how the solution can be applied and how the different applications impact the entire performance, the price of processor time, and the price of communication. As a result, diverse optimization techniques like query fetching, memory control, and concurrency have been suggested by more recent research, with every approach contrasted related to time complexities [63, 64].

3.10 Interchange of Node-to-Node Information

Semantic Web was suggested to describe the way by which nodes can interact with different nodes in a semantic manner. The definition of ontology is a central component of the Semantic Web. Ontology is a taxonomy, as previously defined, which describes a collection of objects and their relationships. Therefore, in AI, it may describe a set of inference rules [65].

The ontology of an individual in terms of a graph is seen in Fig. 3.11a. The nodes denote objects, and relationships are represented by the edges. "If an object has an email, it may be a person" these relationships will draw an inference rule.

To exchange information describing graphs, the Semantic Web uses HTTP. This is exemplified in Fig. 3.11b. There is a special standard resource identifier (URI) for each node and edge, described as a web address. The graph then enables node to track the "sent" to locate data related to a particular entity. This shows the process of how the HTTP protocol offers a means for machine-to-machine communication to share information. A gateway may be positioned at the periphery of the network as a hub in its deployment to interchange ontology data with the cloud by the use

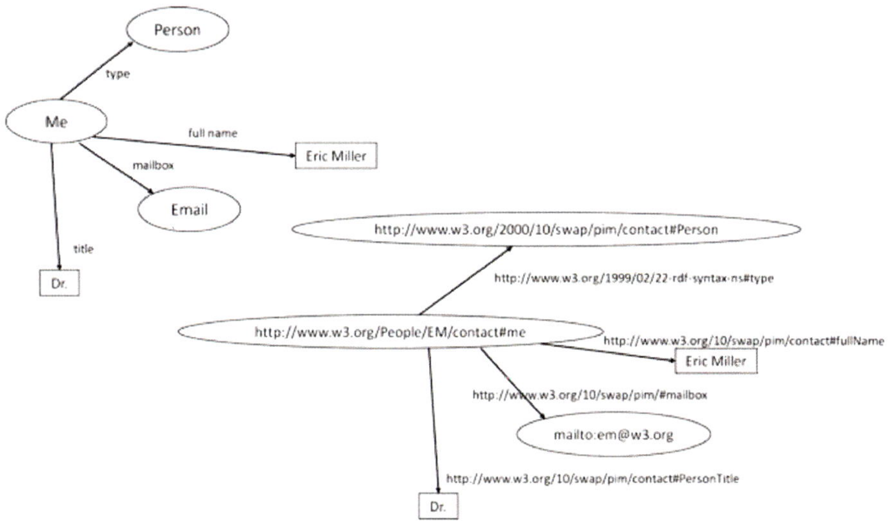

Fig. 3.11 Ontology modified from [66]. **a** Ontology for an individual. **b** Indulging an implementation-level protocol for expressing ontology

of HTTP, during enhancing localized IoT device transmissions under CoAP. An investigation to aware distant useful assistance while aged persons need help, like while a fall is noticed, may be deployed [67, 68]. The system required to identify a "fall" involves understanding how computer sensors will identify an anomalous occurrence. Knowledge between the gateway and a distant repository was exchanged in this study to narrate what usual/irregular day-to-day activity characteristics are. The repository has an ontology which "a User carries a Device" and that "a Device has Events". The gateway can differentiate anomaly from usual everyday occurrences upon receiving a meaningful input event [69, 70].

3.11 Intelligent Artifacts

While they independently share information to resolve complications, physical or software entities are known as wise. These intelligent entities are cautious of the changes in their world and respond to them and consider certain opportunities to make a decision proactively. To achieve a goal, they must demonstrate sociability with other smart items or individuals and help various implementations [71, 72, 73].

Major implementations of intelligent objects utilize ontologies, or any solution involving a structure of wisdom centered comprising of entities, their characteristics, and connections. For instance, such a knowledge base in a task analysis domain may comprise a grading of activity degradation [74].

Various simulations have information bases that are local rather than shared. A building information model [75, 76], that is basically a software interface used to handle the construction of a building for cost-effectivity and preparation, is an instance of an enriched digital knowledge base structure. The model breaks down a building's details, from room configurations to necessary building materials, creating a hierarchy of properties and ship relationships. BIM applications have progressed with the advent of IoT to create green constructions by forecasting and implementing energy frameworks and encouraging protection by speculating toxic vapors at the place where construction employees are located. BIM implementations don't consist of a widely specified ontology to get rid of information compatibility problems, despite providing state-of-the-art methods for building information bases [77].

How to discover and find shared information bases requires difficulties in integrating smart objects. Therefore, in the literature, the architecture structures introduced an exploration model to figure out the way a framework applies to different intelligent entities related to their ontologies. A framework like that is similar to a portal [78, 79]. The module helps intelligent entities to categorically decompose the way a job is represented by a knowledge base, where a job comprises a set of activities, and interactions convey laws of deduction when learning how other structures achieve an aim. It is exemplified in Fig. 3.12. The choice to process these occurrences and laws reflects the resources which can be advertised to different entities by a smart object. In the knowledge base, recently found services may be modified, ontology expanded, and new knowledge generated in return.

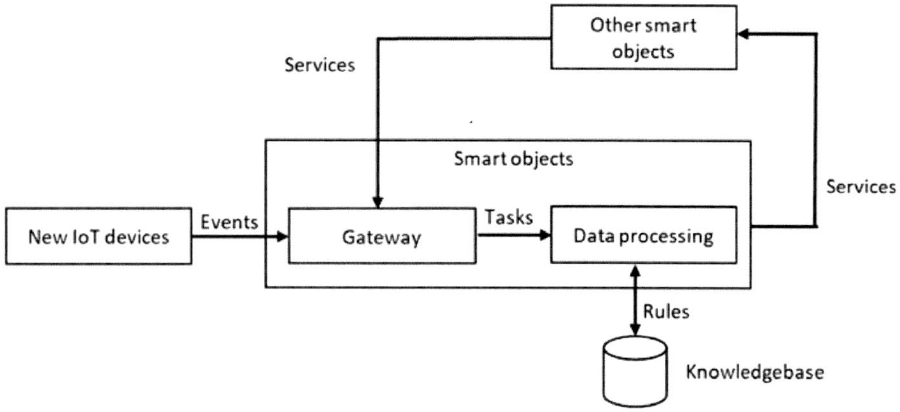

Fig. 3.12 Intelligent entities divide their assistances, authorizing them in learning the malfunction in regulations to a bunch of jobs and episodes

The use of built ontology is not commonly practiced, despite smart artifacts that have demonstrated the potential to exchange and transfer information. Instead of using built ontologies, the present work focuses on the creation and assessment of ontologies. While ontology allows objects to describe and exchange a domain's properties and relationships, as ontology is used in other domains, the ability to semantically classify services disintegrates. For example, in the different BIM ontologies, various circumstances allow meanings to be divided into whether such data is compulsory or optional.

3.12 Conclusion

Their processing capacity and network bandwidth limit message sharing between IoT devices. For machine learning-based research, intelligent technologies need a huge amount of information and vast computational power. Therefore, by offering deep learning research at the portal or in the cloud, modern smart apps respond to those constraints. These applications produce prescriptive and predictive analysis, but in a restricted computational environment, the design of adaptive applications has proved to be difficult. Adaptive applications, which involve a duplex communication channel, require input from either person or other smart machines. Furthermore, input is handled by evolutionary algorithms that need more energy than can be accomplished by constrained computers. IoT systems are thus constrained in their ability to understand, develop, and exchange information autonomously. IoT implementations use ontologies, i.e., repositories that define a connection of entities by their assets and contacts, to overcome its limitations. This makes it possible for IoT remedies to find reasoning laws or information installed on different systems or the cloud, enabling smart application frameworks. While ontologies are commonly used to construct smart applications, it has proven difficult to adopt one ontology to a miscellaneous state. While requesting ontology from a separate domain, the capacity for an IoT program to contextually define the concept of data reduces.

References

1. Al-Musawi AA, Alwanas AAH, Salih SQ et al (2020) Shear strength of SFRCB without stirrups simulation: implementation of hybrid artificial intelligence model. Eng Comput 36:1–11 (2020). https://doi.org/10.1007/s00366-018-0681-8
2. Adhikari S, Ray S, Obaidat MS, Biswas GP (2020) Efficient and secure content dissemination architecture for content centric network using ECC-based public key infrastructure, vol 157, pp 187–203. https://doi.org/10.1016/j.comcom.2020.04.024
3. Adi E, Anwar A, Baig Z et al (2020) Machine learning and data analytics for the IoT. Neural Comput Appl 32:16205–16233. https://doi.org/10.1007/s00521-020-04874-y
4. Ahmed T, Srivastava A (2016) Predicting human interest: an application of artificial intelligence and uncertainty quantification. J Uncertain Anal Appl 4:9. https://doi.org/10.1186/s40467-016-0051-2
5. Akasiadis C, Pitsilis V, Spyroupoulus CD (2019) A multi-protocol IoT platform based on open-source frameworks. Sensors 19:4217. https://doi.org/10.3390/s19194217
6. Alrowaily M, Lu Z (2018) Secure edge computing in IoT systems: review and case studies. In: IEEE/ACM Symposium on Edge Computing (SEC), Seattle, WA, pp 440–444. https://doi.org/10.1109/SEC.2018.00060
7. Arafah Y, Winarso H (2017) Refining smart city concept with resilience approach. In: 3rd international conference of planning in the era of uncertainty. https://doi.org/10.1088/1755-1315/70/1/012065
8. Aswini R, Keerthihaa V (2019) IoT based smart energy theft detection and monitoring system for smart home. In: 2020 International Conference on System, Computation, Automation and Networking (ICSCAN), Pondicherry, India, pp 1–6. https://doi.org/10.1109/ICSCAN49426.2020.9262411
9. Bai T, Pan C, Deng Y, Elkashlan M, Nallanathan A, Hanzo L (2020) Latency minimization for intelligent reflecting surface aided mobile edge computing. In: IEEE journal on selected areas in communications, vol 38, no 11, pp 2666–2682. https://doi.org/10.1109/JSAC.2020.3007035
10. Bozorgi PP, Gao X, Eastman C, Self AP (2018) Planning and developing facility management-enabled building information model. Autom Constr 87:22–38. https://doi.org/10.1016/j.autcon.2017.12.004
11. Cao K, Liu Y, Meng G, Sun Q (2020) An overview on edge computing research. IEEE Access 8:85714–85728. https://doi.org/10.1109/ACCESS.2020.2991734
12. Coetzee L, Oosthuizen L, Mkhize B (2018) An analysis of CoAP as transport in an internet of things environment, IST-Africa Week Conference (IST-Africa), Gaborone
13. Choi SO, Kim J (2021) Design and implementation of open source based on IoT and robot manipulator arm training equipment. In: Lee R, Kim JB (eds) Software engineering, artificial intelligence, networking and parallel/distributed computing. studies in computational intelligence, vol 951. Springer, Cham. https://doi.org/10.1007/978-3-030-67008-5_10
14. Dash S, Shakyawar SK, Sharma M et al (2019) Big data in healthcare: management, analysis and future prospects. J Big Data 6:54. https://doi.org/10.1186/s40537-019-0217-0
15. Dong Y, Hou J, Zhang N, Zhang M (2020) Control and stability analysis of complex dynamical systems involved in finance. Ecol Eng. https://doi.org/10.1155/2020/1680845
16. Fantini P, Pinzone M, Taisch M (2020) Placing the operator at the center of the industry 4.0 Design: modelling and assessing computers and industrial engineering, vol 139. https://doi.org/10.1016/j.cie.2018.01.025

17. Fisher P, Min M et al (2020) Scalability of high performance PDE solvers. Int J High Perform Comput Appl 24(5). https://doi.org/10.1177/1094342020915762
18. Firouzi F, Farahani B, Ibrahim M, Chakrabarty K (2018) Keynote paper: from eda to iot ehealth: promises, challenges, and solutions. IEEE Trans Comput Aided Des Integr Circuits Syst 37(12):2965–2978. https://doi.org/10.1109/TCAD.2018.2801227
19. Fu Y, Yan Z, Cao J, Kone O, Cao X (2017) An automata based intrusion detection method for internet of things. Mob Inf Syst. https://doi.org/10.1155/2017/1750637
20. Gelman A, Carpenter B (2020) Bayesian analysis of tests with unknown specificity and sensitivity. 69(5):1269–1283. https://doi.org/10.1111/rssc.12435
21. Fuertes G, Afaro M, Vargas M, Gutierrez S, Ternero R, Sabattin J (2020) Conceptual framework for strategic management: a literature review—descriptive. J Eng. https://doi.org/10.1155/2020/6253013
22. Fyshe A, Sudre G, Wehbe L, Rafidi N, Mitchell TM (2019) The lexical semantics of adjective-noun phrases in the human. Brain 40(15):4457–4469. https://doi.org/10.1002/hbm.24714
23. Ghasempour A (2017) Internet of things in smart grid: architecture, applications, services, key technologies and challenges. Inventions 4:22. https://doi.org/10.3390/inventions4010022
24. Jalasri M, Lakshmanan L (2018) A survey: integration of IoT and Fog computing. In: 2018 Second International Conference on Green Computing and Internet of Things (ICGCIoT), Bangalore, India, pp 235–239. https://doi.org/10.1109/ICGCIoT.2018.8753010
25. Jerald F, Anand M, Deepika N (2019) Design of an industrial IoT architecture based on MQTT protocol for end device to cloud communication. Int J Recent Technol Eng 7(6S2):552–554
26. Karthigha M, Latha L, Sripriyan K (2020) A comprehensive survey of routing attacks in wireless mobile ad hoc networks. In: 2020 International Conference on Inventive Computation Technologies (ICICT), Coimbatore, India, pp 396–402. https://doi.org/10.1109/ICICT48043.2020.9112588
27. Kavitha D, Ravikumar S (2020) Designing an IoT based autonomous vehicle meant for detecting speed bumps and lanes on road. J Ambient Intell Humaniz Comput. https://doi.org/10.1007/s12652-020-02419-8
28. Khanra S, Dhir A, Mantymaki M (2020) Big data analytics and enterprises: a bibliometric synthesis of the literature. Enterp Inf Syst 14(6):737–768. https://doi.org/10.1080/17517575.2020.1734241
29. Kim J, Kim J, Kim H, Shim M, Choi E (2020) CNN-based network intrusion detection against denial-of-service attacks. 9(6):916. https://doi.org/10.3390/electronics9060916
30. Kong XTR, Xu SX, Cheng M, Huang GQ (2018) Iot-enabled parking space sharing and allocation mechanisms. IEEE Trans Autom Sci Eng 15(4):1654–1664. https://doi.org/10.1109/TASE.2017.2785241
31. Li Y, Barthelemy J, Sun S, Perez P, Moran B (2020) A case study of WiFi sniffing performance evaluation. IEEE Access 8:129224–129235. https://doi.org/10.1109/ACCESS.2020.3008533
32. Liu Z, Li Z (2020) A blockchain based framework of cross-border e-commerce supply chain. Int J Inf Manag 52. https://doi.org/10.1016/j.ijinfomgt.2019.102059
33. Mehta G, Mitra G, Yadav VK (2018) Application of IoT to optimize data center operations, international conference on computing, power and communication technologies (GUCON), pp 732–742
34. Mehta R, Sahni J, Khanna K (2018) Internet of things: vision, applications and challenges. Proc Comput Sci 132:1263–1269. https://doi.org/10.1016/j.procs.2018.05.042
35. Muzammal M, Talat R, Sodhro AH, Pirbhulal S (2020) A multi-sensor data fusion enabled ensemble approach for medical data from body sensor networks. Inf Fus 53:155–164. https://doi.org/10.1016/j.inffus.2019.06.021
36. Neto AJV, Zhao Z, Rodrigues JJPC, Camboim HB, Braun T (2018) Fog-based crime-assistance in Smart IoT transportation system. IEEE Access 6:11101–11111. https://doi.org/10.1109/ACCESS.2018.2803439
37. Nguyen H, Drebenstedt C, Bui XN et al (2020) Prediction of Blast-induced ground vibration in an open-pit mine by a novel hybrid model based on clustering and artificial neural network. Nat Resour Res 29:691–709. https://doi.org/10.1007/s11053-019-09470-z

38. Obitade PO (2019) Big data analytics: a link between knowledge management capabilities and superior cyber protection. J Big Data 6:71. https://doi.org/10.1186/s40537-019-0229-9
39. Ouadghiri ME, Aghoutane B, Farissi NE (2020) Communication model in the internet of things. Proc Comput Sci 177:71–77. https://doi.org/10.1016/j.procs.2020.10.013
40. Pong PWT, Annaswamy A, Kroposki B, Zhang Y, Rajagopal R, Zussman G, Poor HV (2021) Cyber-enabled grids: shaping future energy systems, vol 1. https://doi.org/10.1016/j.adapen.2020.100003
41. Priyashman V, Ismail W (2019) Signal strength and read rate prediction modeling using machine learning algorithms for vehicular access control and identification. IEEE Sensors J 19(4):1400–1411. https://doi.org/10.1109/JSEN.2018.2880736
42. Qiu X, Sun T, Xu Y et al (2020) Pre-trained models for natural language processing: a survey. Sci China Technol Sci 63 1872–1897. https://doi.org/10.1007/s11431-020-1647-3
43. Rafei A, Carol A, Flannagan C, Elliott MR (2020) Big data for finite population inference: applying quasi-random approaches to naturalistic driving data using bayesian additive regression trees. J Surv Stat Methodol 8(1):148–180. https://doi.org/10.1093/jssam/smz060
44. Biswal AK, Singh D, Pattanayak BK, Samanta D, Yang M-H (2021) IoT-based smart alert system for drowsy driver detection. Wirel Commun Mob Comput 2021, article id 6627217:13. https://doi.org/10.1155/2021/6627217
45. Pramanik S, Samanta D, Dutta S, Ghosh R, Ghonge M, Pandey D (2020) Steganography using Improved LSB approach and asymmetric cryptography. In: 2020 IEEE International Conference on Advent Trends in Multidisciplinary Research and Innovation (ICATMRI), Buldhana, India, 2020, pp 1–5. https://doi.org/10.1109/ICATMRI51801.2020.9398408
46 Maheswari M, Geetha S, Selva kumar S, Karuppiah M, Samanta D, Park Y PEVRM: Probabilistic Evolution based Version Recommendation Model for mobile applications. IEEE Access. https://doi.org/10.1109/ACCESS.2021.3053583
47. Kumar R, Kumar R, Samanta D, Paul M, Kumar V (2017)A combining approach using DFT and FIR filter to enhance impulse response. In: 2017 International Conference on Computing Methodologies and Communication (ICCMC), Erode, India, 2017, pp 134–137. https://doi.org/10.1109/ICCMC.2017.8282660
48. Gomathy V, Padhy N, Samanta D et al (2020) Malicious node detection using heterogeneous cluster based secure routing protocol (HCBS) in wireless adhoc sensor networks. J Ambient Intell Human Comput 11:4995–5001. https://doi.org/10.1007/s12652-020-01797-3
49. Ghosh G, Samanta D, Paul M, Janghel NK (2017)Hiding based message communication techniques depends on divide and conquer approach. In: 2017 International Conference on Computing Methodologies and Communication (ICCMC), Erode, 2017, pp 123–128. https://doi.org/10.1109/ICCMC.2017.8282658
50. Sivakumar P, Nagaraju R, Samanta D et al (2020) A novel free space communication system using nonlinear InGaAsP microsystem resonators for enabling power-control toward smart cities. Wireless Netw 26:2317–2328. https://doi.org/10.1007/s11276-019-02075-7
51. Samanta D, Sanyal G (2012) A novel approach of SAR image classification using color space clustering and watersheds. In: 2012 4th international conference on computational intelligence and communication networks, Mathura, India, 2012, pp 237–240. https://doi.org/10.1109/CICN.2012.27
52. Khamparia A, Singh PK, Rani P, Samanta D, Khanna A, Bhushan B (2020) An internet of health things-driven deep learning framework for detection and classification of skin cancer using transfer learning. Trans Emerg Tel Tech 2020;e3963. https://doi.org/10.1002/ett.3963
53. Hossain MA, Samanta D, Sanyal G (2012) Statistical approach for extraction of panic expression. In: 2012 4th international conference on computational intelligence and communication networks, Mathura, India, 2012, pp 420–424. https://doi.org/10.1109/CICN.2012.189
54. Althar RR, Samanta D (2021) The realist approach for evaluation of computational intelligence in software engineering. Innovat Syst Softw Eng. https://doi.org/10.1007/s11334-020-00383-2
55. Singh RK, Begum T, Borah L, Samanta D (2017) Text encryption: character jumbling. In: 2017 International Conference on Inventive Systems and Control (ICISC), Coimbatore, India, 2017, pp 1–3. https://doi.org/10.1109/ICISC.2017.8068691

56. Guha A, Samanta D (2021) Hybrid approach to document anomaly detection: an application to facilitate RPA in title insurance. Int J Autom Comput 18:55–72. https://doi.org/10.1007/s11633-020-1247-y
57. Agarwal M, Sarkhel D, Samanta D (2018) Architecture of 'loop' without 'for' & 'while'. In: 2018 2nd International Conference on Inventive Systems and Control (ICISC), Coimbatore, India, 2018, pp 491–494. https://doi.org/10.1109/ICISC.2018.8399121.
58. Samanta D, Sivaram M, Rashed A, Boopathi CS, Iraj SA, Yupapin, P (2020) Distributed Feedback Laser (DFB) for signal power amplitude level improvement in long spectral band. J Opt Commun. https://doi.org/10.1515/joc-2019-0252
59. Chakrabarti S, Samanta D (2015) Notice of removal: a novel approach to digital image steganography of key-based encrypted text. In: 2015 International Conference on Electrical, Electronics, Signals, Communication and Optimization (EESCO), Visakhapatnam, India, 2015, pp 1–6. https://doi.org/10.1109/EESCO.2015.7254009
60. Pramanik S, Samanta D, Bandyopadhyay S, Ghosh R A new combinational technique in image steganography, International Journal of Information Security and Privacy (IJISP), vol 15, Issue 3. ISSN: 1930–1650|EISSN: 1930–1669
61. Rao KR, Samanta D, Somashekara MT, Gurunath R, Paul A (2019)Automatic segmentation based graphical interface for recognition of tomography image analysis of damage cell. In: 2019 Third International Conference on Inventive Systems and Control (ICISC), Coimbatore, India, 2019, pp 52–55. https://doi.org/10.1109/ICISC44355.2019.9036343
62. Gurunath R, Agarwal M, Nandi A, Samanta D (2018) An overview: security issue in IoT network. In: 2018 2nd International Conference on I-SMAC (IoT in Social, Mobile, Analytics and Cloud) (I-SMAC) I-SMAC (IoT in Social, Mobile, Analytics and Cloud) (I-SMAC), 2018 2nd International Conference on, Palladam, India, 2018, pp 104–107. https://doi.org/10.1109/I-SMAC.2018.8653728.
63. Ghosh G, Samanta D, Paul M (2016) Approach of message communication based on twisty "Zig-Zag". In: 2016 International Conference on Emerging Technological Trends (ICETT), Kollam, 2016, pp 1–5, doi: https://doi.org/10.1109/ICETT.2016.7873676
64. Dhanush V, Mahendra AR, Kumudavalli MV, Samanta D (2017) Application of deep learning technique for automatic data exchange with air-gapped systems and its security concerns. In: 2017 International Conference on Computing Methodologies and Communication (ICCMC), Erode, India, 2017, pp 324–328. https://doi.org/10.1109/ICCMC.2017.8282701
65. Hossain MA, Samanta D, Sanyal G (2012) Extraction of panic expression depending on lip detection. In: 2012 international conference on computing sciences, Phagwara, India, 2012, pp 137–141. https://doi.org/10.1109/ICCS.2012.35
66. Hossain MA, Samanta D, Sanyal G (2012) A novel approach for panic-face extraction based on mutation. In: 2012 IEEE International Conference on Advanced Communication Control and Computing Technologies (ICACCCT), Ramanathapuram, India, 2012, pp 473–477. https://doi.org/10.1109/ICACCCT.2012.6320825
67. Saha AK et al IOT-based drone for improvement of crop quality in agricultural field. In: IEEE 8th Annual Computing and Communication Workshop and Conference (CCWC), pp 612–615. https://doi.org/10.1109/CCWC.2018.8301662
68. Sai PY, Harika P (2017) Illustration of IoT with big data analytics. Glob J Comput Sci Technol 17(3)
69. Salloum SA, Khan R, Shaalan K (2020) A survey of semantic analysis approaches. In: Hassanien AE, Azar A, Gaber T, Oliva D, Tolba F (eds) Proceedings of the international conference on Artificial Intelligence and Computer Vision (AICV2020). AICV 2020. Advances in intelligent systems and computing, vol 1153. Springer, Cham. https://doi.org/10.1007/978-3-030-44289-7_6
70. Sanchez- W, Víctor Gómez V, Hernández C (2018) Machine learning techniques and smart grid applications: a review. Int J Appl Eng Res 13(21):14876–14885
71. Saleem TJ, Chisthi MA (2019) Deep learning for internet of things data analytics. Proc Comput Sci 163:381–390. https://doi.org/10.1016/j.procs.2019.12.120

72. Santamaria AF, Raimondo P, Tropea M, Rango FD, Aiello C (2019) An IoT surveillance system based on a decentralized architecture. Sensors 19:1469. https://doi.org/10.3390/s19061469
73. Shirke A, Chandane MM (2018) IoT data based predictive modeling for energy usage of appliances in smart home. Int J Eng Technol 7:931–934
74. Stergiou C, Psannis KE, Kim BG, Gupta B (2018) Secure integration of IoT and cloud computing. Futur Gener Comput Syst 78:964–975. https://doi.org/10.1016/j.future.2016.11.031
75. Sundaravadivel P, Kesavan K, Kesavan L, Mohanty SP, Kougianos E (2018) Smart-log: a deep-learning based automated nutrition monitoring system in the IoT. IEEE Trans Consum Electron 64(3):390–398. https://doi.org/10.1109/TCE.2018.2867802
76. Sun S, Luo C, Chen J (2017) A review of natural language processing techniques for opinion mining systems. Inf Fus 36:10–25. https://doi.org/10.1016/j.inffus.2016.10.004
77. Sun Y, Song H, Jara AJ, Bie R (2016) Internet of things and big data analytics for smart and connected communities. IEEE Access 4:766–773. https://doi.org/10.1109/ACCESS.2016.2529723
78. Sun P (2020) Security and privacy protection in cloud computing: discussions and challenges. J Netw Comput Appl 160. https://doi.org/10.1016/j.jnca.2020.102642
79. Sunhare P, Chowdhary RR, Chattapadhyay MK (2020) Internet of things and data mining: an application oriented survey. J King Saud Univ-Comput Inf Sci. https://doi.org/10.1016/j.jksuci.2020.07.002

Chapter 4
Approaches of Data Analytics in Intelligent Medicare Utilizing IoT

Abstract The Intelligent Healthcare Network is a revolutionary way of collaborating the advantages in sensors, the IoT, and big data analysis for offering quality supervision care while minimizing medical expenditures. During the coming times, the medical business is facing immense hiccups in saving and processing the produced data for extracting information from it. The growing amount of health records produced by the scanning of IoT appliances, e-health, m-health, and telemedicine involves in creation of newer approaches in handling them. In this paper, in this fast-growing field of study, most of the medical issues and big data analysis advances are briefly explored with an emphasis on those tackled by remote tracking to intelligent healthcare. For tracking the circumstances of healthcare for a sensor and IoT system assistance is important for individuals. The goal of this paper is to facilitate medical assistance for the unhealthy and unstable population by remote observation with quicker analysis and expert intervention using smart algorithms, software, and techniques for good curing suggestions. With integration in technology, the distribution of healthcare services has completely advanced. This report suggests a new big data system for smart healthcare for remote control of safe and unhealthy communities' physical everyday practices. The structure is checked by a special case tracking the physical operations of an athlete having sensors on the wrist, ankle, and chest. The messages are continually sent to the human body by the recipient. On the other hand, in order to understand the operation, the signals that are processed and interpreted by big data analysis approaches and ML techniques are utilized at the receiver end. The suggested system predicts if the contestant is active or idle depending on the body's activities. Our suggested framework has given a 99.96% accuracy that can be modified by nurses in remotely tracking fitness problems in aged victims in the case of Alzheimer's disorder, recovery, obesity control, remote tracking, etc. Physical activity by athletes can also be useful for remote surveillance of chronic conditions that need essential physical, biological, and genetic knowledge.

D. Samanta and A. Banerjee, *Computationally Intensive Statistics for Intelligent IoT*, Studies in Autonomic, Data-driven and Industrial Computing,
https://doi.org/10.1007/978-981-16-5936-2_4

4.1 Introduction

Rapid advancement comprising the sphere of telecommunications and the IoT has turned human survival very sophisticated. Intelligent means neat, orderly, and intellectual presentation, according to the Cambridge dictionary [1]. Bringing cleverness for the advanced lifestyle provides existence-wise intelligence, which may be applied to households, school, power consumption, retail, agriculture, or even healthcare (Fig. 4.1), where remote control and maintenance is possible, the smart home can be linked via smart-phones. Suppose the cameras are attached to the doorway or gates of the residence, intelligent apps may only be utilized to recognize individuals and permit the allowance in unlocking as recognized individuals penetrate, thereby reckoning protection for houses. If any light or fan is turned on, the smart home can be operated remotely if it can be switched off from the office itself, thereby saving electricity. Before leaving the workplace during the hot season, one should turn on the home's air conditioner so that you can have a pleasant and relaxing feeling by the time you get home.

In any aspect of people's lives, a stable community is created by maintaining a reasonable balance. Smart health surveillance deals with both the healthy population and the sick, such as monitoring the everyday movements of older people, monitoring obesity, monitoring the workload of sportspeople, monitoring heartbeat, glucose measure, asthma, body warmth, or all related topics of interest to remote

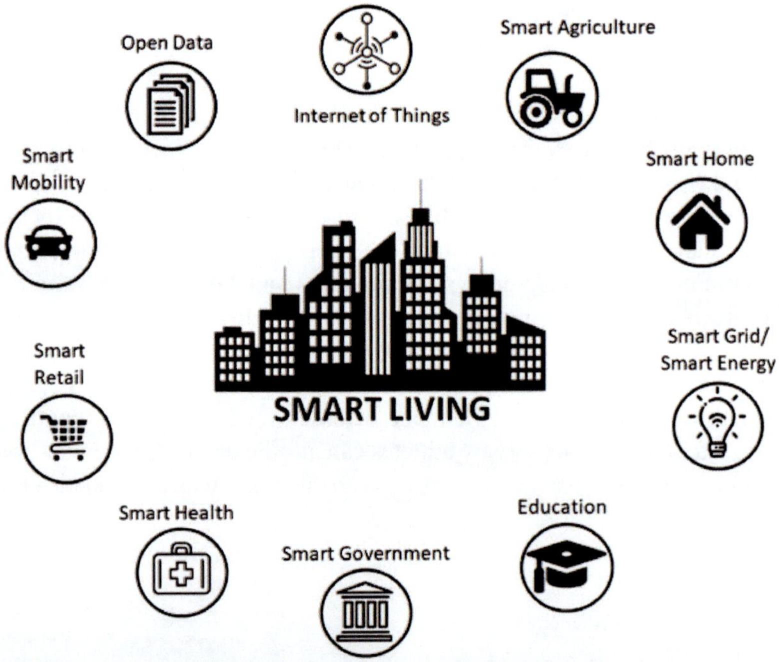

Fig. 4.1 Intelligent livelihood

physicians. In most developed countries, the healthcare industry is facing significant economic difficulties due to the growing quantity of sufferers including the quality in treatment required for the aging citizens [2, 3]. Figure 4.1 expresses intelligent livelihood. More than 200 million people worldwide are expected to suffer chronic diseases, e.g. asthma, coronary disorders, arthritis, diabetes, Alzheimer's and chronic blocking pulmonary illness that require regular detection, surveillance with specialist intervention. By 2022, some 110.3 million persons globally are dealing with dementia as well [4, 5]. The predominance of dementia is also projected to rise in every area of the globe by 2050. India and China, at about 71 million and 122 million, respectively, provide the biggest quantity of diabetes victims in the country. It is expected that this figure will increase globally ranging from the present 398 million to 726 million, by 2050 [6–8].

It places a huge pressure on the public industries. According to a recent study, a ratio of around 9.3–22.6% of the gross domestic product (GDP) [9] is consumed by most countries on medical expenditures. A healthcare sector approximate of about 625 petabytes record was obtained in 2012. It is also expected that more than 3800 petabytes data would be gathered by the medical sector by 2023. Presently, heterogeneous structures store medical, physiological, and physical information. The bulk of the materials are in unstructured, organized forms. The incorporation of all of these heterogeneous records includes a detailed review of all pertinent data for the optimal care of a single patient. Big data technologies and methods are also a major requirement. To evaluate and successfully process this immense volume of data obtains fast insights and analysis from these records for superior care decisions, high-speed processors are needed [10, 11].

Big data has many characteristics that describe it better, despite relating the big data definition mainly with the size property alone. Those characteristics are known as three Vs: volume, variety, and velocity [12]. Big data also allows for data-dependant recommendation building that is important, mainly in the medical domain. The big data domain of healthcare in the UK approaches the 60 million reports of victims who focus largely on the data-driven concept to address the frequent difficulties associated with healthcare. Consequently, developments in IoT technologies play an important part in delivering higher quality healthcare facilities [13]. The word IoT is described as a network of physical connectivity that enables the interaction between various objects by sharing captured data. IoT was described by [14]. As a method that attaches several appliances that are skillful to perceive, accumulate, and compute via internet. On the contrary, IoT pertinence depends on the quantity of information sources, which appear each time intelligent appliances are used. As a result, the scale of the data began to steadily increase [15, 16]. In the healthcare sector, wireless sensors including the quantity of attached terminals have increased drastically in 2015, to 20–40 million nodes, as seen in Fig. 4.2.

By the end of this decade, the European Delegate estimates that about 60–110 billion appliances may be wirelessly attached via IoT, indicating that about 40% of IoT-related infrastructure will be dedicated to healthcare business that makes up a 117 billion dollar market. Big data, which would result from such massive network access, must shed light on this forecast. Intelligent [17] health systems are now

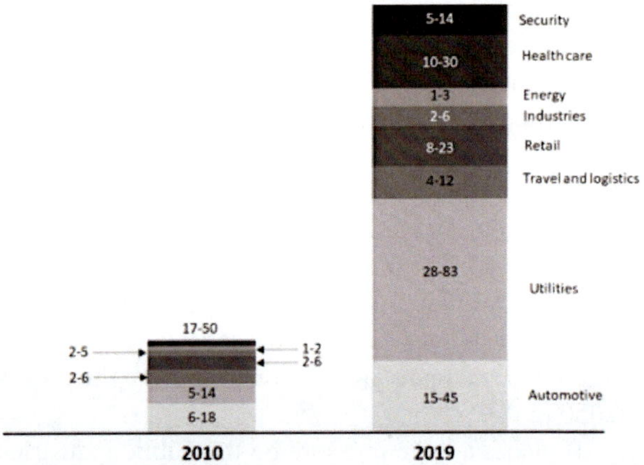

Fig. 4.2 Total of linked web nodes for each domain in 2020

possible to connect via internet, providing an opportunity for a vast provision of medical data in real time. In accordance with defining threat matters and disorder management venture, analysis in big data along with IoT in intelligent medical care will enhance the efficacy of medication facilities [18]. The inspection index criteria for hospital management can not only be fulfilled, between therapy and protection assistance, but also better extension of prices. Thus, the utilization of IoT, predictive analysis, and big data technology in the medical industry has powered a noteworthy data transition. Among the various phases, data processing is essential, i.e. ranging from information gathering and communication, their assessment, to inform and interfere [19]. There is also a requirement to exploit big data algorithms and data science strategies that lack productivity in obtaining, processing, and analyzing data produced from different origins, like digital image-related devices, lab experiments, telematics, sensors, communications, clinical notes, and sources from other parties. Currently, with advancements in medical research, successful diagnoses and solutions have been given for many ill-fated diseases [20]. The rising urban population and shifting habits, however, require an intelligent medical network that can facilitate fast and reliable therapy. Healthcare and pharmaceutical providers, healthcare practitioners, academics along with town planners were concentrating on analysis of Big Data applications along with IOT technologies that may be used to deliver improved healthcare facilities like reduced reaction time, supply distant care, provide swift catastrophe assistances, minimize hospital over congestion, and connect, exchange, and cooperate with physicians worldwide. In this chapter, the authors include a short overview of data science strategies including techniques that are highly important in the collection and overcoming of big data problems in intelligent healthcare approaches.

4.2 Literature Survey

Many clinical initiatives aim to describe a user's cardiac abnormality, but the bulk of them ignore key components. Many people are now doing e-Health studies, and many organizations have benefited from this work by building platforms that link patients with physicians all over the world. We look into two types of connected e-Health mobile apps: integrated medical appliances utilizing embedded devices along with linked electronic health mobile phone apps. Since we are designing a mobile application that connects to a smart IoT computer, our suggested solution is practically similar to attached electronic Health mobile phone apps, while other organizations concentrate on extensive medical appliances networks, which enable consumers in communicating with every individual and get aid from services [21].

Medical Care Services as a whole "PatientsLikeMe" was developed to assist patients in addressing the question, "What is the best result I can hope for, and how do I get there, considering my present situation"? Patients' questions were answered in a number of ways; including helping patients with common disorders interact with one another and sharing their perspectives. However, they neglected to address data protection or the system's usability [22].

"DailyStrength" is another similar method. It is a social network focused on peer communities, where members give moral support to one another by expressing their challenges and accomplishments. There are online forums on the web, which deal with a range of medical problems and life struggles. It is close to Developments in Human–Computer Interaction "PatientsLikeMe" in which they're together unoccupied channels where patients and doctors can communicate. The fact that "DailyStrength" aren't including R&D organizations and aren't having a smart-phone device is two big distinctions between them [23]. Furthermore, no device is based on the Internet of Things. Another research established a rigorous model that integrated several pulse parameters, EEG, and skin conductance sensors into a shirt. A different method in linking facial appearances along with voice recognition with EEG samples has been developed. Other experiments have shown that EEG alone can expose emotional characteristics. In order to better explain behaviors associated with having various emotions, facial recognition software products are linked to heartbeat rate changeability. Additionally, it is identified that particular pulse rhythms may be related to physique strain rather than emotional stress [24]. The appliances, though, may be handheld, and therefore doesn't utilize IoT as a forum.

"Omnio", an all-in-one framework for Medical Services, is another robust healthcare method. Clinical tools, medical resources, disease manuals, and prescription information are among the programs it offers. Everyday Health is an organization that owns websites and develops health and fitness content. It has better scores and publishes a vast variety of wellness reviews that can be highly useful to patients. It also consists of a smart searching feature, which helps customers to locate the particulars easily.

4.2.1 Smart-Phone eHealth

This Apps that are related despite the fact that all of the programs listed above offer healthcare, none of them have smart devices that can be used to track users' everyday habits and warn them when appropriate. Most heart sensors supply customers along with the ECG signals so that the customers may have a vigil of their status, but no one sends out an alarm warning. An Intelligent Aged House Monitoring Functionality was depicted and built over an Android-dependent smart-phone affixed with an accelerometer, and it was capable of detecting a user's fall [25, 26]. It has a mobile–user interface that shows health data obtained by the device. The biggest benefit of SEHMS is that it provides for remote control of elderly and medically aggressive patients. However, it is unable to tell the customer in case of a crisis [27].

Distant Mobile Health Tracking is a device, which uses wearable sensors to monitor a patient's health specifications like heartbeat rate. It helps nurses and loved ones to keep an eye on the patient and diagnose them remotely. The device does not have real-time tracking capabilities [28].

Predicting heart problems remains a challenging mission, and this is where our study is based. Any research group defines its own strategy for achieving its target. To detect heart irregularities, we agreed in utilizing a mixture of body warmth and ECG. Some devices use a range of techniques and hardware implementations. During the data collection, none of them addressed the power consumption rate [29, 30]. Our device utilizes a lower-power Bluetooth framework to wirelessly capture data from a smart-phone. The authors provided a study of multiple data mining methods for heart attack assumption. Instead of providing an entire system along with a data-gathering unit with a computational framework, they only offer prediction algorithms. Decision Tree, Nave Bayes, NN, and KNN are the most widely used methods for forecasting heart attacks [31]. Not only does our study involve an entire framework involving an IoT computer along with a computational network, moreover it additionally utilizes data mining strategies, namely, Decision Tree in forecasting heart attacks. It separates our framework from others in that it is a low-power smart IoT system that utilizes a data mining approach in its forecasting technique. When we tested our forecasting technique, we got high-accuracy calculations for both good and unhealthy test subjects.

Here, we suggest an intelligent IoT-dependent heart rate tracking framework to resolve the shortcomings of the discussed research and frameworks. Our framework is designed to explicitly resolve some of the shortcomings of existing solutions while still having the ability to deliver successful prediction performance [32, 33]. The most critical function of our device is the alarm, which helps the customer to stop an accident before it occurs. Our device is the initial intelligent IoT-dependent medical help that utilizes theme-dependent Physique Region Wireless Sensor signals in detecting heart-dependent accidents, to the best of our knowledge.

4.2.2 For IoT Along with Big Data Age, What Are the Problems and Open Research Issues?

The most fundamental problem with the exponential development of big data, cloud computing, and IoT is to explore vast quantities of information along with derive valuable knowledge or insight with potential measures. The below points are the main characteristics of data in the IoT period that can be called big data:

(i) Vast quantities of information for reading and writing: Volume of data may be in the TB (terabytes), PB (petabytes), along with ZB (zettabyte) levels, necessitating the development of swift and reliable implementations.
(ii) Combining miscellaneous information initiators along with data types: Within the big data age, data origin is varied; for instance, we may combine sensor information camera records, social media records, most of which are varied in forms, such as bit, binary, string, number, etc. It must be connected to having a number of appliances along with programs, as well as collect information from websites.
(iii) Extraction of dynamic information: since knowledge is profoundly buried in vast quantities of data and is not clear, we must examine data properties and identify correlations between different data.

4.2.3 Challenges

When it comes to big data and IoT, there may be several challenges: Amount of data is high, but the consistency is poor, the data are miscellaneous, like structured, semi-structured, or unstructured. Data are generated through multiple information sources, necessarily having various styles and depicted structures. The researchers look into the problems in the fields of information analysis, data mining techniques, along with data mining programs. The difficulties are described in succession [34].

(i) First, the challenge is getting entry to and collecting vast volumes of information from multiple data repository sites. The authors must tackle in accordance with the data's diversity, diverseness, and noise, and finding the fault and correcting the data are also challenging activities. In the world of data mining techniques, working out how to adapt conventional algorithms for use in a big data world is a major concern [35].
(ii) The next concern is finding out the way to use big data technologies to mine unclear and imperfect data. One major concern in a data mining environment is finding an efficient and safe way to exchange data between various applications and systems, particularly because sensitive data like financial settlements along with be an issue [36].

Research problems including data checking, parallel programming frameworks, and big data mining platform are some of the broad research concerns in the big data age.

(i) There are various studies on detecting hidden errors in records. The processes for data cleaning, filtering, and reduction are also implemented.
(ii) In data processing, a parallel programming paradigm is implemented, and certain algorithms are used to execute it. Researchers have developed current data mining techniques differently, together with improving the reliability of one-origin information finding techniques, developing a multi-source data mining approach, and researching complex data mining techniques and stream data processing. Parallel association rule mining and parallel k-means algorithms depending on the Hadoop platform, for example, are better examples of a good application. However, some algorithms are yet to be applied to parallel networks, creating an obstacle to the application of information mining technologies to big data platforms. It will be both a concern and a wonderful path for data mining researchers [37, 38].
(iii) The utmost critical challenge of the big data mining method is building an effective infrastructure to reinforce it. We must consider data protection, anonymity, data exchange mechanisms, data size development, and other factors in a big data mining technique. A well-designed big data mining platform is a crucial path and a major challenge.

Large Data Mining Method for IoT work in major corporations, like Facebook, Yahoo, and Twitter subscribe to open origin initiatives in the data mining domain. The elements below make up the infrastructure for big data mining.

(i) The Apache Mahout assignment implements a number of ML and data mining techniques.
(ii) R is a mathematical computation and visualization programming language and software environment.
(iii) The MOA project does real-time data mining and the SAMOA project combines MOA with S4.
(iv) For the Hadoop network, Pegasus denotes a graph mining library. Big data technology frameworks related to IoT have also been suggested by several IoT developers, with these solutions based on platform integration along with data mining frameworks. Figure 6 illustrates the infrastructure in promoting social networking along with cloud computing in the IoT. They implemented KDD and big data for extraction, control, along with mining levels, as well as the analysis layer. The vision layer is mapped onto the extraction layer. In comparison to conventional KDD, the proposed framework's extraction layer grants into account all actions for representatives for its appliances [39, 40].

4.2.4 IoT System Architecture Recommendations

We recommend system framework for IoT along with big data mining applications based on a research in big data mining along with IoT systems. As seen in Fig. 7, this device has five layers.

(i) Equipment: This machine can incorporate a number of IoT appliances, like sensors, RFID, cameras, along with other devices, to experience the environment and produce data on a continuous basis.
(ii) Raw data: structured, semi-structured, and unstructured data can all be mixed in a large data mining framework.
(iii) Data collection: all real-time along with group information may be collected, along with both information may be extracted.
(iv) Information calculation: Hadoop, HDFS, Hurricane, and Oozie are among the open-source solutions that have been integrated.
(v) Data mining features may be made usable as assistance.
(vi) Protection/privacy standard: In a big data mining environment, security along with privacy is essential. Unauthorized access of data and privacy exposure was protected by encryption and privacy. Data consolidation, distributing, along with mining are mostly available to the third-party developer with the Big Data Mining Framework standard.

4.3 Allied Jobs

In quick identification and actual care guidelines having specialist interference, IoT and big data play an important part. Here, for the segment, the authors plan in presenting the associated job on electronic health, mobile health, along with telemedicine utilizing IoT and big data analysis approaches because of the exponential growth in electronic health, mobile health, and telemedicine. Only various current and illustrative approaches are discussed here to illustrate the intensiveness and diversity of study in the current field [41, 42].

4.3.1 Electronic Healthcare

The IoT framework has improved the connectivity of nodes, which enables telemonitoring to be used for electronic health. Big data also enacts a major part in electronic health, converting postulate-dependant analysis through information-related research.

Massive volumes of health data are handled so easily. Thus, a trivial and non-trivial relation is made possible between different sensors and electronic health information. Likewise, ties will assist in distant medical analysis, uncovering infections, and establishing innovative healings [43].

Methodologies in Suciu et al. studied stable combinational approaches used by remote telemetry units to process big data over cloud communication (RTUs). They recommended e-health architecture constructed by building a heuristic framework also called EXALEAD CloudView.

4.3.2 Mobile Health

Tools and software can be used to construct a wellness selfie during the era of data elucidation in cognizance construction. In order to provide healthcare, several smart-phones and smart-phone apps have been created. Myo, for instance, includes a gaming motion controller, which is utilized in orthopedics for assisting people having extreme fracture exercise. Also, it helps physicians in assessing the efficiency of the patient by calculating the angle of movement. Another indication is the Zio patch, which monitors heartbeat rate and ECG and having approved by the US Drug Management for usability. In addition, Glaxo has reported that its latest investments are focused on electro pharmaceuticals and bioelectrical products that utilize nerve microstimulation. Moreover, J&J partnered with Google and Philips for building digital surgeries focused on robots including various wearable technologies like, blood pressure monitors. In addition, Novartis and Google are collaborating on sensor innovations like intelligent lens and a measurement system for wearable blood glucose levels. In addition, HeartCare+ is a smart-phone application designed to assess the risk of coronary heart disease for sufferers living in countryside regions, and to allow distant contact with city doctors [44].

Centered on a Framingham scoring model, HeartCare+ assesses the threats and allocates them as medium, average, or strong. Other mobile apps, constituting SleepBot, have recently been created. A confidential wellness initiative is revealed to experiment and rate the success of those health-centered apps and wearable by the Hacking Medicine Institute [45].

4.3.3 Telephonic Medicine

Through supporting the surrounding living and telemedicine nowadays, IoT and existing multimedia technology have a good contribution in the health sector. Telemedicine is defined as the use of telecommunication technology to offer e-medical deliberation including skilled services when necessary, such as telephone, facsimile, and distance education. Since the 1990s, the trend in using telemedicine has grown extensively, with investments of about $100 million. Currently, about 13 government departments are implementing telemedicine technologies. Any concerns emerge including the assumption, with IoT integration, standard of operation, device reliability, and growth in rapid storehouse [40, 46]. A researcher suggested a free, scalable, and reliable network which, with the support of cloud computing technologies, relies more on IoT, allowing near-by ambient connectivity for medical use. For optimization purposes, the writers have tackled some of the pitfalls discussed earlier. On the other hand introduced an m-telemedicine device which communicates an ECG wave through cellular networks to the health center [47]. Blood rate, blood sugar, glucose content, location and fall of the patient, body temperature, electrical and muscle functions of the heart by ECG and air via an android application that they created, they collected these vital signs. A portable telemedicine service tool was created by the authors to diagnose patients.

4.4 Problems of Big Data Protection and Secrecy

Hacking is a primary purpose of violations of privacy. There are different financial advantages of security threats. For different purposes, health reports can be obtained (e.g. disclosing individual fitness data unwarranted, gathering healthcare data, which is difficult to retrieve, or basically to overcome systems). Risks of privacy attacks occur mainly because of the healthcare community's lack of awareness of the application of technologies. Out of them is the big data analysis, utilized in medical industry, which has currently raised numerous safety and patient privacy issues. While records of patients are saved in data centers with varying degrees of protection, the privacy of medical information is not assured. Furthermore, healthcare data flow from multiple origins, information collection, retrieval, and communication burden [48, 49]. So, in the medical world, patient safety and the protection of health data are connected together. However, with the usage of mobile devices, it is apparent that security shortages will significantly contribute to the infringement of people's privacy in the medical field. Researchers are often finding high-grade accomplishment which, through delivery, stored and following assemblage utilize, preserves medical data. Many of the agreed-upon ones, security requirements for researchers and IT individuals during the deployment of medical applications are listed below:

Wiping confidential information from a computer until the appointment finishes with the patient.

- No interference in third-party systems (e.g. promotional ads).
- Use two-step verification to encrypt the information stored.
- End-to-end encrypted and decrypted data during communication. Transmission connecting the app and additional systems focused on SSL/TLS.

4.5 Methods and Algorithms in Computer Science

A broad specialty is data science. This works with immense datasets in different formats found on the internet or in libraries of databases. In computer science, computational and AI methods are commonly used nowadays. Speedy, analogous, and allocated approaches play an important role in applications. In terms of cloud computing technologies, Hadoop and Spark software appliances integrate the theory of distributed computation and are commonly utilized [50].

Applications correlated with data science use common approaches and frameworks. Random forests, regression, SVM, clustering, decision trees, visualization, KNN, analysis of time series, text mining, identification of anomaly detection, optimization, neural networks, consisting of the common approaches and methods utilized by data scientists currently are deep learning and SVD [51]. Government and commercial computer scientists use algorithms that are more distinct from those used by university academics and students. Data scientists from industry are found to most commonly use regression, time series, and random forests. Time sequences along with simulation are commonly utilized by various organizations. Data mining that are common and deeply interconnected fields in information technology are also entirely included. In ML, frameworks are designed in such a provision that they spontaneously recognize and comprehend the incoming information and can provide smart conclusions depending on the provided information. Recommendation, grouping, and clustering are its common techniques [52, 53].

The two most widely used methods to apply ML techniques are supervised and unsupervised approaches. In order to learn a feature, the earlier approach utilizes specified tutoring records and provides typical instances like categorizing electronic mails as spam, marking web pages in the wake of evaluating the constituents and recognizing speech in the future, using the most commonly used technique for the clustering of similar records into cohesive collections without predetermined testing samples. Any well-known supervised K-nearest neighbor system, Naive Bayes, etc. can be used [54].

Data science regulates the different methods and algorithms borrowed from the disciplines alluded to above. There are no winning algorithms since they are intended for various circumstances in the current algorithms, depending on the scale of the basic data records and repetitions. In addition to the goal of looking for the right strategies, one must know the essentials of numerous techniques, the relevance of their clarity, and even their implementations. Any common data sciences' algorithms are briefly discussed below [55].

4.5.1 Classification

A type of supervised learning is classification, also called categorization. It is an ML approach in which established information is used to assess the distribution of current techniques to newer information. Moreover, it gathers several specimens of established categorizing. Identification is based on new object types. By making use of classification, iTunes apps prepare playlists. Yahoo and Hotmail, which are e-mail assistance providers, utilization classification methods in deciding whether or not a newer e-mail is a spammed mail where all user activities are evaluated by the controlled classification algorithm to indicate those mails as spammed [56].

4.5.2 Clustering

Because of the uncertain performance to the observer, clustering or also referred to as unsupervised learning, attempts in classifying data into special, distinct clusters. Instead of specifying the output for users, the technique is not tutored on any prior incoming or outgoing data. Customer data covering 1000 rows, for example, maybe divided into altered categories depending on factors like population-related knowledge [57].

In newsgroups, separate posts are clustered by clustering strategies focused on similar topics. Google and Hotmail utilize clustering strategies in rendering classes based on common characteristics as clusters with linked data. It implements a classification engine, which handles the library of tutorials similarly that depends on its content; a new incoming tutorial is clustered into the identical related collections [58].

4.5.3 Minimizing Dimensions

To minimize the quantity in measurements or in a data record excluding a lack of data borne by the data records, dimension reduction techniques are used. Two well-known variable reduction methods are factor analysis and principal component analysis (PCA). The essence of PCA enhances evaluation in knowledge. Upon rotating the axis of various variables to the greatest eigenvector, the main components may be clarified as the largest variation axis and are un-related and orthogonal [59].

4.5.4 Identifying Irregularities

An abnormality or exception, or noise is also known as irregularities. It is all about finding the objects, or other occurrences or findings that do not fit the trend of a predicted behavior, to detect an anomaly. Sensitive information can be identified in data, and is particularly feasible in accordance with a variety of implemented realms. Irregularities are various types of issues in a text, such as cyber attacks, debit card fraud, configuration bug, medical conditions and errors. Detecting irregularities in medical reports of healthcare informatics suggests outbreaks of cancer, instrumentation failures, etc. In healthcare records, the main challenges are the scarcity of uniform labels alone with the probability of high complicated spatiotemporal information [60].

To describe a condition, various measurements are used related to a sufferer data records, like attributes such as heartbeat, cholesterol level, blood pressure. In order to separate the groups after defining the hyper plane, larger attributes are derived for these phases by Support Vector Machine. SVM-related edges are the separation of each equivalent class between the two nearest objects and the hyper plane. The nearest separation within the stick and the blue and red ball is taken as the edge in the running case. SVM attempts to optimize this margin in order to place the hyper plane as distant apart as the blue ball from the red ball [61].

Reducing the opportunity of misclassification hyper plane, therefore, resides at similar intervals ranging from a blue sphere along with a red sphere and owing to their support for hyper plane, the balls are known as information positions as support vectors. SVM and C4.5 include two first preference classifiers for exploration. Some of its drawbacks are kernel selection and interpretability. SVM implementations are various types, like MATLAB, libsvm, and scikit-learn.

4.5.5 *Ensemble Strategies*

Ensemble approaches are a combined advancement in furnishing a strong forecast for weak learners. An ensemble method called a random forest is found to be currently reliable in the current methods of classification. The basic decision tree functions as a feeble trainee, while the strong learner is a random forest. Out of a subdivision of the similar data record as a specimen, Random grows several decision trees and thereby improves the outcome to detect the favorable classification framework. We explore the ways by which data science approaches may be utilized for big data analysis in the following segment [62].

4.6 The Methods and Strategies of Big Data Analytics

Data are particulars that are structured in a particular form. Big data represents an immense dataset that may be organized or unorganized. Big data pertains in relation to databases and whose scale is over the mark of an organized information processing structure's capability in tackling. The acquisition of big data has seen enormous development, according to Forbes, from 18% in 2016 to 61% in 2018. VCloudNews study records about 3.2 quintillion bytes of information per day. In the last 2 years, 89% of the globe's records have been segregated.

Four Vs, length, velocity, variety, and veracity, are the core features of big data. Internet data volumes have grown from 48 GB per day in 1989 to 26,4265 GB per second in 2017 and are expected to hit 48,000 GB per second in 2020. Velocity is the pace at which information is generated, preserved, and evaluated. 2,32,000 Facebook posts, 30 crores of electronic mails, 2,62,000 tweets, and 13 h of video content are posted to the cyber world every minute. Complementing the rise of big data are Twitter, WhatsApp, Scopus, Study Doors, and several other outlets. Variety means big data from different sources, such as text, photographs, videos, sensor data, and keystrokes, clicks, created over the internet. According to a report by VCloudNews, 90% of the data produced is unstructured in nature. The accessible info, that has

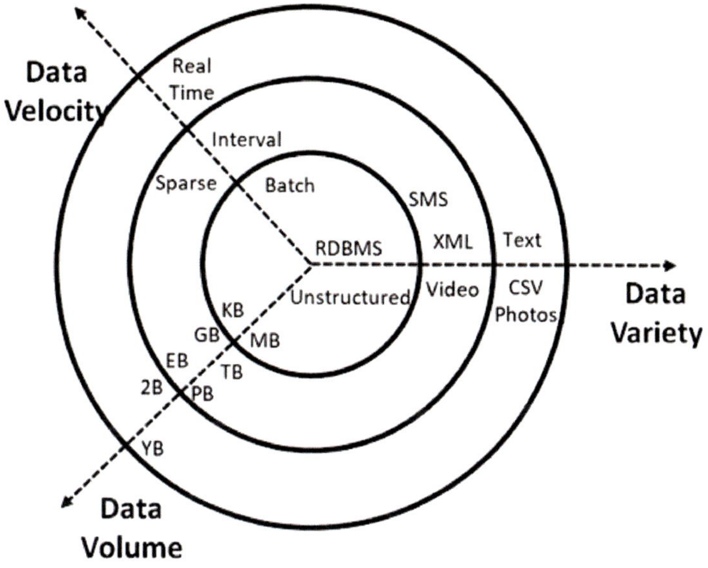

Fig. 4.3 V's in big data

rational move and form, may be semi-arrangement. It is also possible to multi-structure the files, which suggests that the information pattern is not user-beneficial [63]. Figures 4.3 and 4.4 say V's in big data.

Additional functions are introduced in addition to the 3 V's in big data analysis (Fig. 4.3). Another significant aspect of big data that the researcher usually overlooks is veracity. Veracity stands for data inconsistency, data complexity, data imprecision, and prototype estimation. Various big data examiners also incorporate three supplementary Vs, namely, functions, changeability, realization, along with meaning. Figure 4.4 displays seven Big Data vs. Self-health tracking or reporting has been growing enormously in recent years. A research shows that about 70% of the population of the US and UK were interested in self-health monitoring. More than one lakh applications linked to health tracking are hosted by the Google play store. Applications for monitoring sleep, feeding, mood and fertility cycles, and several more are available. Specific habits of physical and mental well-being are tracked [64, 65].

4.6.1 Big Data Systems

There is a generation of big data every second using an unregulated way. Big data can help analyze a person, his preferences, goals, and actions in the form of customer comments, product ratings, use of applications, or the information posted by an individual on social platform. To develop their business, the data generated can be used by the company. Here are a few apps enumerated (Fig. 4.5).

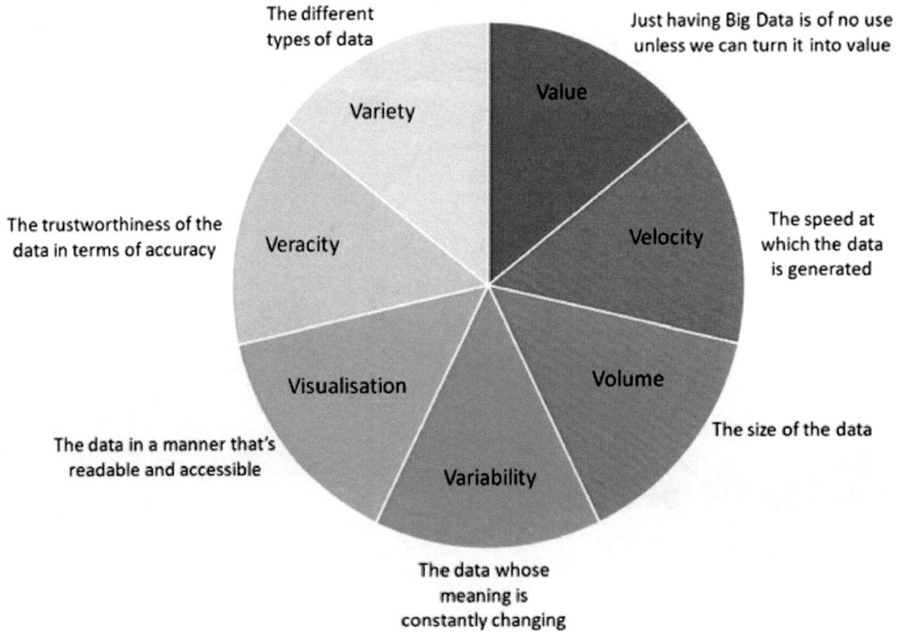

Fig. 4.4 V's in big data in different ways

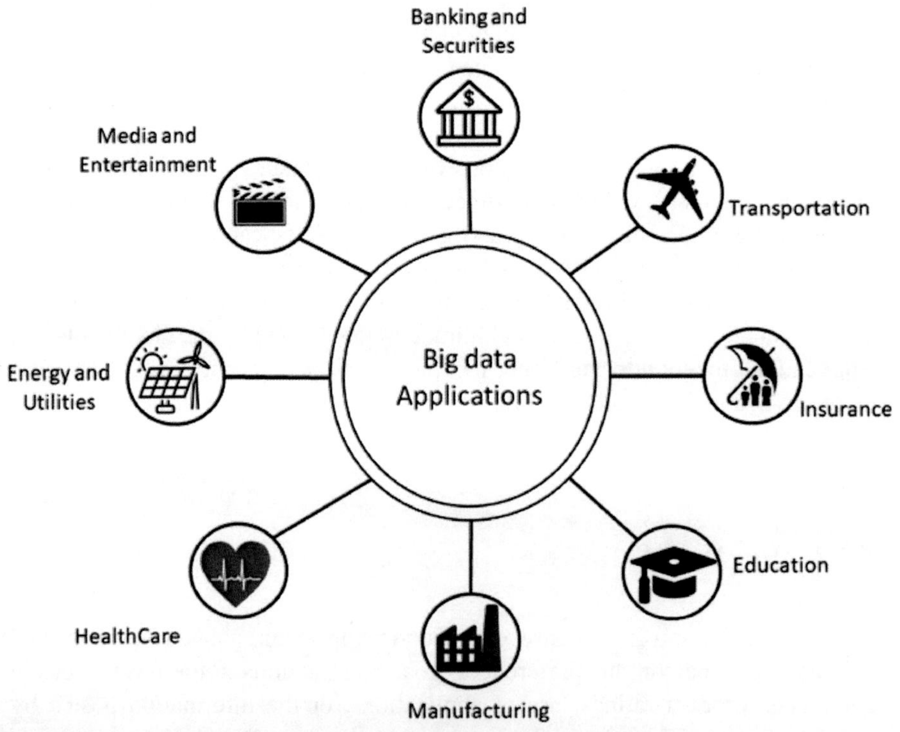

Fig. 4.5 Utilization of big data

Bank and Security: The absolute digital conversion for financial answers creates tremendous data. Scrutinizing the customer's benefits and responsibilities will allow a manager to provide different categories in loans, accept debit cards, incentive, minimize interest percentages, and tailor each individual's financial solutions as well [66, 67].

Insurance: Insurance firms often aim to evaluate an individual's lifestyle and sell the most important policies to the intended consumers, thereby increasing the company's income. If full detail is obtainable, so affirmations may be quickly resolved, that may include worthiness to the services.

Conveying: Detecting travel in recent years is a state-of-the-art technology. Product suppliers need to ensure that the goods are shipped in acceptable condition to the consumer. With the aid of RFID, the products can be constantly monitored at any given point in time to know the precise location [68, 69].

Education: It is possible to personalize the education system depending on an individual's criteria. Individuals involved in making films can only have education linked to that. Instead of a lethargic system of loading all items, schooling can be packed as per the student's need. Manufacturing: The whole production method will be enhanced if former procedures are evaluated systematically by soliciting big data methodologies.

Power and utilizations: Intelligent cities that will give birth to intelligent power meters that may be organized in any home or organization are thought of by people. These smart energy meters can analyze an individual's consumption pattern, and monetary expenditures may possibly be minimized depending on the utilized forms [70].

Health industry: Another area where an extremely large data storehouse is developed in healthcare tracking. People are health aware, and so, using many mobile applications, they self-monitor themselves. Tracking levels of glucose, blood pressure levels, study of sleeping habits, diet, and much more facilitates, healthcare awareness of a healthier lifestyle is also growing. Media and entertainment: Big data is very prevalent in the entertainment business. High-resolution audio files, HD quality video files, many TV programs, live news portal alerts, etc., have tremendous info. In order to scan and play the demonstrations of an individual interest, many applications such as voot and savan are available. In addition to the above-mentioned applications, big data applications have several dimensions. Online data will show a person's buying habits, client interests, suggestion systems, opinion mining, and study of the retail market. Online stores in the telecommunication industry will tailor the right bundle for clients depending on their use habits [71, 72].

4.6.2 Big Data Appliances and Strategies

Huge information must be collected and interpreted, and from the voluminous data, useful information must be obtained. Since the data volume is immense, it isn't feasible to reserve full records in conventional repositories, so it becomes important to utilize a repository that allows non-structured information manipulation [73]. To conduct analysis on big data, there are various instruments and approaches available. The few methods and strategies under consideration are below.

- Hadoop General: The other Hadoop modules are provided by common utilities.
- Hadoop Distributed File Structure (HDFS): A distributed file structure, which offers accessibility to utilization of records with high throughput. Hadoop belongs to a clone of MapReduce, which is open-source. HDFS indicates Hadoop Distributed File System, which operates primarily related to equipments for commodities. Hadoop belongs to a level of Apache's data storage.
- Hadoop Map Reduce: This is a YARN-dependent method to handle massive databases in parallel and is neither a database nor a database rival. MapReduce is a dispersed computing mechanism, which is applied in many applications.

It involves two methods, Map along with Reduce, which will consider all structured and non-structured data effectively (Fig. 4.6).

The incoming information is broken into several bits and applied as incoming to dispersed file frameworks to chart activities. The chunk is transformed to a set of key-estimate pairs by the Map activities. The key-value pairs are obtained and sorted by a master controller from each Map task depending on a key value. Among all the reduction tasks, the key is broken.

So, at the same reduction job, all key-concept pairs for the similar key are dissolved. The Minimize assignments run on one key at a time and incorporate in a particular way most of the quantities related to that key value. The map explores the

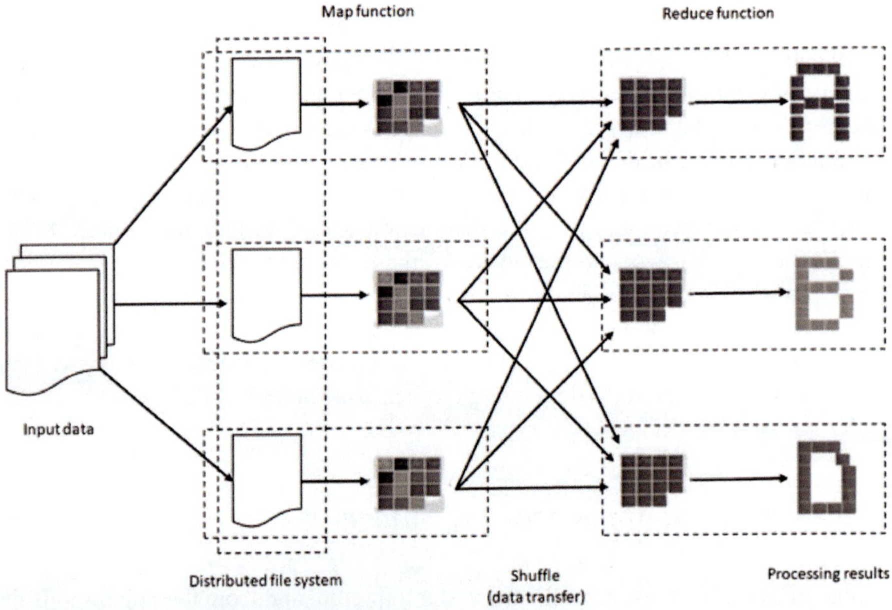

Fig. 4.6 MapReduce utilization framework

disc information and implements the concepts found in it. The final result is summed and aggregated by Minimize. The advantages for MapReduce are cost-dependent, simple to measure and extend performance, and information will be easily customized in meeting the needs. The drawbacks of Map Reduce aren't a repository; and therefore, no protection, classification, questioning, because there's no mature strategy [74].

Apache Hive: Fundamentally, it is configured to handle and execute data warehouse framework analytics developed specifically for Hadoop. Initially, Facebook began the Hive initiative, and eventually, it became an open source. A warehouse that typically includes a vast amount of archived information is done utilizing a SQL-dependent scripting language known as Hive Query Language to query the data [75].

Pig: This belongs to high-level information proceeding language including parallel processing platform in execution. Spark: For Hadoop information, it is a speedy and common computation framework. It offers an easy and expressive model of programming that facilitates a number of implementations. ETL means retrieval, modification and uploading, manipulation of streams, along with computing of diagrams.

Machine Learning: Apache involves a extension focused fundamentally along with the development of machine learning algorithms. The primary aim is to build algorithms for gathering, categorization, along with teamwork which may be expansible to manage increasing big data analysis. The approaches are constructed over Apache's MapReduce. The three common techniques of ML are applied:

- Suggestion.
- Classifying.
- Assembling.

The concept of linear algebra and computational mythologies is also the subject of Mahout. We have used the classification technique for Hadoop Map Reduce and Mahout NB in our proposed work.

4.7 Intelligent Healthcare

The integration of telephonic medicine, electronic health, and mobile health for sufferer management with ML, IoT, and big data has significantly revolutionized and customized health industry by enhancing the standard of patient attention and reducing expenditures. Mobile health technologies are known in addressing major problems in remote patient monitoring. Potential advantages include continued patient health surveillance, irrespective of the position of patients, expanded proximity to health services, decreased levels of protection, including a better grade of protection [76, 77].

As mobile medicine, electronic health, and mobile health innovations continue developing, better and better innovative newer IoT-dependent nursing requisitions are emerging for data processing, delivery, and analysis. For sufferers, the tracking framework that offers essential corporeal, hereditary, and organic knowledge, many biomedical sensors have been used.

4.7.1 Healthcare Tracking Biomedical Sensors

It is possible to identify many chronic health diseases utilizing smart bioinformatics sensors, such as:

Heart disorders: The breast strap monitor and intelligent watches are utilized to diagnose heart infection using ECG in registering the heart's electrical exercise. ECG messages related to the heartbeat may be continuously sent to the communicator utilizing Bluetooth including a attached smart-phone.

Mobile equipment

Blood sugar extent tracking: Google intelligent contact glasses are utilized to monitor patients with diabetes for glucose levels. Using a condenser, a controller, including an antenna fixed to them, information obtained from the glasses may be transmitted starting with the eye to the glasses.

Asthma: Utilizing a wristband, environmental conditions including CO, O_3, and NO_2 layers may be tracked. At the same time, it may detect heartbeat along with various critical details. A cell phone is utilized to relay data from sensors. It can also be communicated to doctors for action in the case of emergencies.

Alzheimer's, autism, or related neurological illness: For these cases, it is required to identify suspicious circumstances like sufferer roaming, intelligent apparel biological sensors like GPS Smart Soles, including movement tracking detectors, based on the Alzheimer's association, will alert neighbors, relatives, or the nearest hospital [78, 79].

In order to transmit location coordinates, GPS Smart Soles consist of a miniaturized Global Positioning System including a mobile transmitter. For position history on a map, a smart-phone or a computer may be used. Send updates via text messaging or through e-mail. Warning choices involve the junction of a regional border, signal on/off, including low battery, moving detector sensors job having a speedometer to monitor sufferer's motions with provision of real-time information using the Zigbee protocol or via GSM.

RFID readers can often be used to check the patient's incoming and outgoing; audio sensors may sense movement with an order service including illumination for checking the refrigerator perforation and track how frequently patients consume nourishment. Intelligent clothes: Here, sensors are built into fabric attire that is utilized in calculating important indications and to continuously monitor the heartbeat including our feelings. Below, numerous bioscience sensors are displayed (Fig. 4.7).

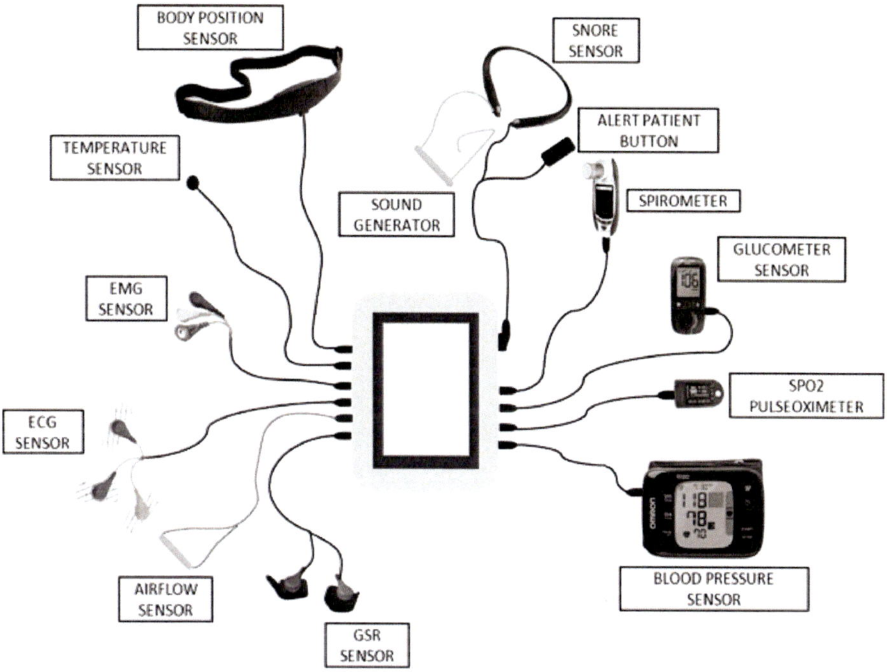

Fig. 4.7 Sensors for biomedicine

4.7.2 Big Data Platform for Intelligent Healthcare

Information processing, having sensors mounted around the physique, defines a significant problem in various medical practices utilizing biological sensors.

The present condition contributes to the introduction of newer instruments having methods comprising of the IoT, AI, big data, including software for real-time medical facility. We have suggested intelligent healthcare in order to address the above obstacles. A system that can be used by remote surveillance to forecast chronic conditions like heart disorders, obesity, blood sugar, Alzheimer's disease, dementia, blood pressure, neurological problems including various important physique and physiological signs [80]. Four main components of the proposed structure are (Fig. 4.8).

1. *Possession of information*: Data must be obtained from numerous biological sensors, like ECG, EEG, EMG, glucometer, blood pressure, physique posture, and physique motion sensors, connected with various parts of a person physique, like the abdomen, foot, and hand. These data repository formats are available in different forms, like structured, semi-structured, or non-structured formats. DICOM requirements have been taken into consideration during the transfer of clinical and non-clinical results. DICOM complies with international standards [81, 82].
2. *Cloud Storage and Internet of Things*: Information obtained from different sensors, phones, including multiple IoT appliances are migrated via the cloud

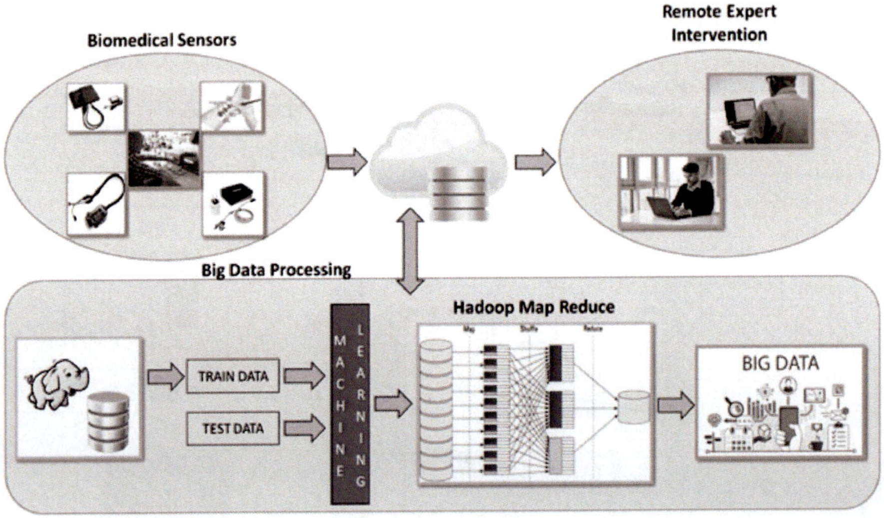

Fig. 4.8 Four main components of the proposed structure

environment to big data microprocessor for future processing using ML approaches. It can be inflexible and highly expensive to store and process data obtained by these IoT devices due to the massive increase in data on healthcare. Therefore, cloud computing can be used for vast volumes of medical records and can allow organizations to reserve expenditures.

3. *Big Data Analysis*: This is best accomplished in big data implementation including analysis due to a diversity, veracity, and amount of healthcare data. The health data obtained from numerous sensors and IoT appliances must be transferred to an ordinary Big Data Processing Network. For the processing of this massive volume of health data, we utilize the Hadoop Distributed File System. HDFS includes MapReduce, a Hadoop programming paradigm that operates vast numbers of datasets at the same time. The biological sensor input information is split into data subsets for tutoring and research. Using Apache Mahout, the machine learning algorithm can be applied to do smart analysis for the incoming information thus generating results of the study that will be used to produce data for early diagnosis of health abnormalities [81].
4. *Specialist interventions*: the findings of the study are submitted for additional recommendations on therapy to medical professionals and healthcare assistance. Notification alerts may be wirelessly delivered to patients. The initial intelligent big data healthcare platform will be altered to different medical uses, like caregiver tracking of elderly patients, remote monitoring of physical exertion of sportspersons. Heterogeneous forms of essential physical, biological, and genetic knowledge may also be tracked remotely. The end objective of our proposed smart healthcare system is the individualized management of a sufferer, having effective implementation having prompt entry to wisely conclusion making.

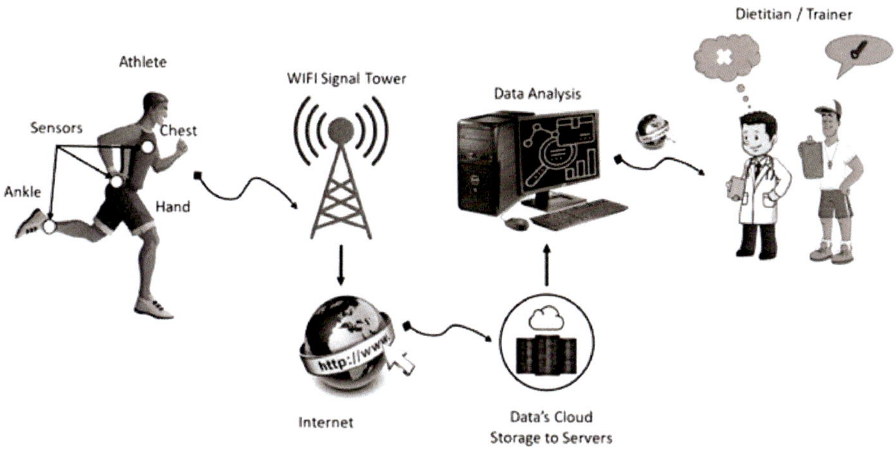

Fig. 4.9 Distant physical exercise performance case tracking for athletes

4.7.3 Case Analysis

The focus of this research is on the suggested scenario outlined in Fig. 4.9. The layout described begins by wearing biological sensors to the breast, wrist, including knee of the athlete's body to gather information relevant to activity. It then transmits this information [83, 84].

Wi-Fi signal towers are placed in cloud-depending storage web-servers utilizing IoT in a standardized form using Wi-Fi. Afterward, results must perform a proposed review in determining whether a positive physical function is expressed by the athlete. Big data processing is used on the Hadoop Distributed File System using machine learning algorithms, Map Reduce, and Mahout, where the measurements derived from biomedical sensors will be separated into datasets for preparation and research [85]. In the analytical study form, these specifics are shown to the specialists afterward, together with the nutritionist including athlete coaches in managing tracking the fitness standard. It helps professionals to remotely track and submit potential feedback on the lifestyle of the athletes. Physique activity tracking standard repository was utilized to track the physique and everyday movements of sportsperson to verify the proposed scenario that will be discussed later.

4.8 Results and Discussion

4.8.1 Gathering of Data

For the analysis, PAMAP2 Physique Venture Tracking Dataset was utilized partially in extricating the functionality, which can track a sportsperson's workout status utilizing IoT-dependent facilities, which includes linked sensors. Originally, documents were intended to identify 18 principal physical behaviors in total. These events that have been scheduled are:

1. When doing nothing, lying flat.
2. To rest comfortably on a throne.
3. When talking, standing.
4. Ironing T-shirts 1–2.
5. Vacuum sweeping in 1–2 business rooms as items is being relocated.
6. Five stories of rising stairs.
7. Five stories of descending stairs.
8. Walking (speed of 4–6 km/h).
9. The walking sticks in Nordic walking.
10. Cycling at an acceptable pace with a real bike.
11. Moving at an appropriate rate.
12. In the shape of a simple leap or the alternative foot hop, rope jumping.
13. At home, watching TV.
14. Act at the workplace on laptops.
15. Moving a vehicle between the workplace and house.
16. Collapsible washing.
17. House cleaning and shelves for dusting.
18. Play soccer ball.

In the data files, other junk behaviors were also reported, including traveling from one place to other or deferring for the preparation of appliances. Nine participants (eight males and one female having an age span of 28–32 years) who used three sensors including a heartbeat screen carried out the main 18 tasks.

4.8.2 The Configuration of Internet of Things Framework

The three wireless inactivity calculation units of Colibri were placed over the supreme forearm of the arms, the breast,

including the dominant side of the ankle. Data analysis, attribute extrication, and classification approaches can be applied to the dataset using different computational methods to classify the human behavior using big data and estimate the severity.

The raw data sensors are available in the.dat file format. Missing values were labeled as NaN due to hardware configuration problems (e.g. link failure in the sensors).

The following fields per document are found in each subject's data file:

- Stamp of time.
- The Activity ID.
- Heartbeat rate.
- Hand warmth of IMU.

- 3D acceleration IMU hand.
- 3D acceleration IMU hand (different dimension).
- 3D gyroscope IMU-hand.
- 3D magnetometer IMU that can be handheld.
- Hand inclination of IMU.
- Warmth of the IMU breast (rc).
- 3D acceleration of the IMU chest.
- 3D acceleration IMU breast.
- 3D gyroscope with IMU chest (unit: radian per second).
- 3D magnetometer for IMU chest.
- Chest orientation of IMU.
- Warmth of the IMU ankle.
- 3D acceleration of IMU ankles.
- 3D acceleration of IMU ankles.
- 3D gyroscope with IMU ankle (unit: rad/s).
- 3D magnetometer IMU ankle.
- IMU direction of ankle.

It was important to prepare the dataset for the introduction of a consistent classifier using big data survey (like Hadoop Map Reduce) for remotely tracking the scheme position of athletes by dieticians and accounted workers training. In the ensuing section, phases of information processing (e.g. data cleaning and pre-processing) would be built in deeply.

4.8.3 Information Pre-Processing Planning for Information Analysis

Above several phases, PAMAP2 data preparation was done. Conversion of the.dat file structure to the.csv file structure began with these moves. Furthermore, all dataset columns of numeric values have been assigned attribute names. Action ID (0–24) was then mapped based on the given data to the real activity name corresponding to it. Action status (e.g. active or inactive) was allocated depending on the activity name specified. Afterward, information pre-processing was applied using Weka 3.5 filters that may later be clarified. Furthermore, for each subject information file, active along with inactive occurrences were divided including every dynamic case files was conserved in an operative folder, while inert cases were rescued in an inert folder. Every lone information file was then separated into n data files, editor-based files and n denotes a quantity of successions per.csv column. Ultimately, n information folders have been transferred for processing to the Hadoop Cloudera environment.

4.8.4 The Cleaning of Evidence

Both unauthorized documents were cleared from the PAMAP2 dataset. There were different measures involved in the data cleaning process. Next, the cleanup of data from useless tasks unrelated to everyday athletic activity for athletes. The following events are involved in the deleted records:

1. Just standing.
2. Moving vehicles.
3. TV watching.
4. Work on computers.
5. Cleaning the house.
6. Cleaning from the vacuum.
7. With ironing.
8. To play soccer.
9. Collapsible laundry.

In addition, for an accurate analysis, every document including task noticeable as additional were rejected because they constitute the noise information between tasks (e.g. recess time and stand-by time tasks). Furthermore, for smoother pre-processing, every absent value having NaN quantities was restored with vacant fields. In addition, all data files have been cleaned up starting with existing ASCII values (e.g. double quotation and semicolons). Thus, the ultimate records chosen in accordance with the Hadoop analysis step were 238,623 distributed in total: (1) 238,623 functioning and (2) 8781 non-functioning occurrences. These occurrences have been allocated accordingly to the functional along with non-functioning files.

4.8.5 Pre-Processing

Prior to survey on Hadoop to pre-calculate, the records were uploaded to Weka 3.6. The succeeding unsupervised filters were approved in the pre-processing phase that are:

(1) Change misplaced quantities unattended filter: where every absent numeral quantities have been restored by training dataset means throughout every data file.
(2) Establish Unsupervised Filter: For preventing any grouping bias during the data review process, all numerical values were confined between 0 and 1.

Every record file was subsequently stored as a newer CSV folder and characteristics were removed as described before in the module of information composing. EmEditor is utilized in partitioning the folders into n information records that have been transferred to the Hadoop Cloudera processing environment.

4.8.6 Range of Characteristics

As seen before within the IoT framework configuration portion, in the reason of identifying the physique scheme which takes place, about 21 features were collated using sensors and tracking systems. However, the proper attributes have to be derived for reliable outcomes for the reason of information refining to teach the classifier on whatever the scheme label represents regarding an athlete's physical activity status. Any attributes have, however, been omitted from the elicited dataset. For example twice (one time utilizing 20 g scale and a different utilizing 10 g scale), 3D accelerometer data were collected. However, it is established that 10 g scale accelerometer wasn't correctly measured relative to another one because of some impact gestures (e.g. running) on 10 g scale sensor. Furthermore, time stamps have been separated from the actual database as they aren't required in the analysis of the model. Thus, the timestamp, 10 g scale was deleted for IMU limb, breast, and knee sensors.

Any other elements were too restored, as previously described (e.g. task id was restored by scheme label). Therefore, the ending set of characteristics included in the study includes the subsequent 17 allocations:

- Title of operation.
- Heartbeat rate.
- Palm warmth of IMU.
- 3D acceleration information from the IMU hand (unit: ms-2, 10 g size).
- 3D gyroscope information from IMU hands (unit: radian/second).
- Data from the IMU portable 3D magnetometer.
- Hand inclination of IMU.
- Breast warmth of IMU.
- 3D acceleration details for the IMU chest (unit: ms-2, 10 g scale).
- 3D gyroscope details IMU breast (unit: radian/second).
- Data from IMU breast 3D magnetometer.
- Breast alignment of IMU.
- Warmth of the IMU leg
- 3D acceleration information from the IMU ankle (unit: ms-2, 20 g size).
- 3D gyroscope data from IMU ankle (unit: radian/second).
- Data from IMU leg 3D magnetometer.
- IMU direction of leg.

Any.csv information record containing certain characteristics after cleaning and pre-processing,

Using EmEditor, the n data files were then split into n data files, and the aforesaid n information records were transferred for review for the Hadoop Distributed File System surroundings as outlined in the next module.

```
=======================================================
Summary
.......................................................
Correctly Classified Instances       :      272018        99.9669%
Incorrectly Classified Instances     :          90         0.0331%
Total Classified Instances           :      272108

=======================================================
Confusion Matrix
.......................................................
a       b         <--Classified as
31977   0         |  31977       a      = Inactive
90      240041    |  240131      b      = active

=======================================================
Statistics
.......................................................
Kappa                                      -0.2664
Accuracy                                   99.9669%
Reliability                                66.6542%
Reliability (standard deviation)            0.5772
```

Fig. 4.10 Exploratory findings for physical exercise screening

4.8.7 Big Data Collection Research

The chosen characteristics from various sensors are transferred to the virtual computer cloud, a large information microprocessor network in the study together with retrieval in healthy living physique activity tracking. The incoming information is coursed to HDFS on a large information server. MapReduce adapts the input information for parallel processing with vast quantities of data. In comparison, the input data are divided into teaching and examining data records; 70% of the input information is submitted for training and 30% stays in experimenting. Apache Mahout is utilized in the application of ML approaches that execute input data processing intelligently. We also utilized the classification of NB in our suggested technique to classify multiple physical behaviors that are additionally classified into dynamic and idle situations. In the following section, the categorization outcomes are described. Figure 4.10 shows exploratory findings for physical exercise screening, and Fig. 4.11 expresses confusion matrix with assessment of results.

4.9 Experimental Review Along with Findings

Simulations were conducted on a dataset of various records having 17 descriptors. The classifier's observations are seen in Fig. 4.10. The classifier's output is assessed by the confusion matrix created. Confusion matrix denotes a form in table, which facilitates output for classification dependent on inactive or active cases that are correctly and incorrectly expected, as seen in (Fig. 4.10).

Depending on confusion matrix, it is used to calculate the classifier's efficiency, precision, sensitivity, and specificity.

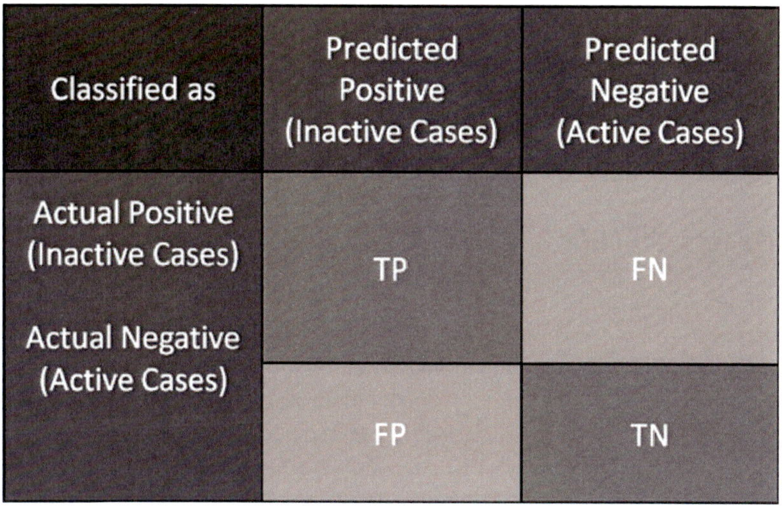

Fig. 4.11 Confusion matrix with assessment of results

Accuracy: A test's accuracy is the ability to accurately distinguish between inactive and active events. That is, in other words, the proportion of right predictions. It is determined using the Equation below depending on the confusion matrix.

$$\text{Accuracy} = (\text{TP} + \text{TN})/\text{TP} + \text{TN} + \text{FP} + \text{FN} \tag{4.1}$$

TP = True Positive.
TN = True Negative.
FP = False Positive.
FN = False Negative.

If true positive (TP) is the quantity of cases rightly recognized as inert instances; false positive (FN) is the quantity in cases falsely recognized as inert occurrences; TN is a quantity for cases rightly recognized as operative occurrences; FN is a quantity in cases wrongly associated as animated occurrences.

The confusion matrix outcomes displayed in Fig. 4.10 constitute 99.966% of the precision in the NB classifier.

Sensitivity: It is the capacity of a questionnaire to better classify people of physical behaviors that are inactive. Using Eq. 4.2, sensitivity can be measured.

Sensitivity = TP/(TP + FN)

$$\text{Sensitivity} = (33426/(33426)) * 100 \tag{4.2}$$

FN = 0.
Sensitivity = 100.
100% sensitivity means that dormant cases have been properly spotted as stagnant.

Definition of specificity: It shows test's capability in classifying people having dynamic body activity. Using Eq. 4.3, accuracy is measured.

Specificity = TN/(TN + FP)

$$\text{Specificity} = [26232/(26232 + 90)] * 100 \tag{4.3}$$

Specificity = 99.65.

99.97% sensitivity suggests that most dynamic events remain appropriately classified as dynamic.

Parameters like specificity, precision, and sensitivity show that NB classification assumes 98.932% accuracy along with 99.97% specificity, suggesting that most athletes are healthy and actively practices their athletic workouts, and the methodology shows the correctly calculated inert occurrences with 99.868% sensitivity. This proves to be very much effective in terminologies of precision, sensitivity, and specificity; the suggested methodology may be evaluated for every medical enactment.

4.10 Conclusions

This segment provides a short overview of strategies along with approaches in data science, which are particularly important for working along with also for addressing the complexities of big data in the healthcare sector. The problem of introducing technical innovations in ML along with data science is focused on smart healthcare systems to overcome the challenges posed by distant sufferer management. The hi-tech advancement related to the domains of the IoT and telecommunications has compelled us to suggest a smart healthcare application that makes it easier to move toward intelligent globe growth. The information gathered by IoT appliances is analyzed by biological sensors linked with a person's body, along with the prediction for human behavior is accomplished with very good precision through the application of machine learning algorithms.

References

1. Adi E, Anwar A, Baig Z et al (2020) Machine learning and data analytics for the IoT. Neural Comput Appl 32:16205–16233. https://doi.org/10.1007/s00521-020-04874-y
2. Aguilera-Mendoza L, Llorente-Quesada MT (2013) Modeling and simulation of hadoop distributed file system in a cluster of workstations. In: Cuzzocrea A, Maabout S (eds) Model and data engineering. MEDI 2013. Lecture notes in computer science, vol 8216. Springer, Berlin, Heidelberg. https://doi.org/10.1007/978-3-642-41366-7_1
3. Antons D, Grunwald E, Cichy P, Salge TO (2020) The application of text mining methods in innovation research: current state. Evol Parameters Dev Priorities 50(3):329–351. https://doi.org/10.1111/radm.12408

4. Ardagna D, Barbierato E, Gianniti E et al (2020) Predicting the performance of big data applications on the cloud. J Supercomput 77:1321–1353 (2021). https://doi.org/10.1007/s11227-020-03307-w
5. Azad M, Chikalov I, Moshkov M (2020) Representation of knowledge by decision trees for decision tables with multiple decisions. Procedia Comput Sci 176. https://doi.org/10.1016/j.procs.2020.09.037
6. Bol N, Helberger N, Weert JCM (2018) Differences in mobile health app use: a source of new digital inequalities? Inf Soc 183–193. https://doi.org/10.1080/01972243.2018.1438550
7. Appel G, Grewal L, Hadi R et al (2020) The future of social media in marketing. J Acad Mark Sci **48**:79–95. https://doi.org/10.1007/s11747-019-00695-1
8. Catalan HEN, Gordon D (2018) The importance of reliability and construct validity in multidimensional poverty measurement: an illustration using multidimensional poverty index for Latin America. J Dev Stud 1763–1783. https://doi.org/10.1080/00220388.2019.1663176
9. Chaudhury M, Sodani PR, Das S (2020) Effect of Covid 19 on economy in India: some reflections for policy and program. J Health Manag 22(2):169–180. https://doi.org/10.1177/0972063420935541
10. Chen Y, Xie Y, Song L, Chen F, Tang T (2020) A survey of accelelator architectures for deep neural networks. Engineering 6(3):264–274. https://doi.org/10.1016/j.eng.2020.01.007
11. Chiffelle DOJ, Loi M (2020) Ethical and unethical hacking.The ethics of cybersecurity. The international library of ethics, law and technology, vol 21. Springer, Cham. https://doi.org/10.1007/978-3-030-29053-5_9
12. Cioffi R, Travaglioni M, Piscitelli G, Petrillio A, Felice FD (2020) Artificial intelligence and machine learning applications in smart production: progress, trends, and directions. Sustainability 12:492. https://doi.org/10.3390/su12020492
13. Das S (2020) Mental health and psychosocial aspects of Covid-19 in India: the challenges and responses. J Health Manag 22(2). https://doi.org/10.1177/0972063420935544
14. Ding J, Chen Y, Wang X et al (2020) Land degradation sensitivity assessment and convergence analysis in Korla of Xinjiang, China. J. Arid Land 12:594–608. https://doi.org/10.1007/s40333-020-0057-y
15. Dolatkhah R, Somi MH, Jafarabadi MA et al (2020) Breast cancer survival and incidence: 10 years cancer registry data in the Northwest, Iran. Article ID 1963814. https://doi.org/10.1155/2020/1963814
16. Espinosa JA, Kaisler S, Armour F, Money WH (2019) Big data redux: new issues and challenges moving forward. In: Proceedings of the 52nd Hawaii international conference on system sciences. https://hdl.handle.net/10125/59546
17. Fang Z, Costas R (2020) Studying the accumulation velocity of altmetric data tracked by Altmetric.com. Scientometrics 123:1077–1101. https://doi.org/10.1007/s11192-020-03405-9
18. Flack JM, Adekola B (2020) Blood pressure and the new ACC/AHA hypertension guidelines. Trends Cardiovasc Med 30(3):160–164. https://doi.org/10.1016/j.tcm.2019.05.003
19. Faconti L, Chowienczyk P, Shah AM (2020) Cardiovascular disease, heart failure and Covid-19. J Renin Angiotensin Aldosterone Syst. https://doi.org/10.1177/1470320320926903
20. Gijrath SJH (2018) Telecommunications networks: towards smarter regulation and contracts? 18(3–4):175–197. https://doi.org/10.1177/1783591718782305
21. Guo G, Wang H, Bell D, Bi Y, Greer K (2003) KNN model-based approach in classification. In: Meersman R, Tari Z, Schmidt DC (eds) On the move to meaningful internet systems 2003: CoopIS, DOA, and ODBASE. OTM 2003. Lecture notes in computer science, vol 2888. Springer, Berlin, Heidelberg. https://doi.org/10.1007/978-3-540-39964-3_62
22. Gupta D, Rani R (2018) A study of big data evolution and research challenges. J Inf Sci 45(3):322–340. https://doi.org/10.1177/0165551518789880
23. Hermes S, Riasanow T, Clemons EK et al (2020) The digital transformation of the healthcare industry: exploring the rise of emerging platform ecosystems and their influence on the role of patients. Bus Res 13:1033–1069. https://doi.org/10.1007/s40685-020-00125-x
24. Izquierdo JL, Almonacid C, González Y, Del Rio-Bermúdez C, Ancochea J, Cárdenas R, Soriano JB (2020) The impact of Covid-19 on patients with asthma. Eur Respir J. https://doi.org/10.1183/13993003.03142-2020

25. Jumabekova A, Berger J, Foucquier (2020) An efficient sensitivity analysis for energy performance of building envelope: a continuous derivative based approach. Build Simul. https://doi.org/10.1007/s12273-020-0712-4
26. Kaur S, Kaur R, Aggarwal R (2020) E-Health and its impact on Indian healthcare: an analysis. Paradigm 23(2). https://doi.org/10.1177/0971890719859943
27. Aleya, Kanij Fatema, and D. Samanta. "AUTOMATED DAMAGED FLOWER DETECTION USING IMAGE PROCESSING." Undefined, 2013, https://www.semanticscholar.org/paper/AUTOMATED-DAMAGED-FLOWER-DETECTION-USING-IMAGE-Aleya-Samanta/11f8ebd4082acef98b7329cecc81601b6ec20bc8.
28. Kijsanayothin P, Chalumporn G, Hewett R (2020) On using MapReduce to scale algorithms for big data analytics: a case study. J Big Data 6:105. https://doi.org/10.1186/s40537-019-0269-1
29. Lanzer JD, Leuschner F, Kramann R et al (2020) Big data approaches in heart failure research. Curr Heart Fail Rep 17:213–224. https://doi.org/10.1007/s11897-020-00469-9
30. Lepenioti K, Bousdekis A, Apostoulou D, Mentzas G (2020) Predictive analytics: literature review and research challenges. Int J Inf Manage 50:57–70. https://doi.org/10.1016/j.ijinfomgt.2019.04.003
31. Khadri SKA, Samanta D, Paul M (2014) Approach of message communication using Fibonacci series: in cryptology. Lecture notes on information theory, vol 2, no 2, pp 168–171. https://doi.org/10.12720/lnit.2.2.168-171
32. Khadri SKA et al (2014) Approach of message communication using fibonacci series: in cryptology. Lecture notes on information theory. https://doi.org/10.12720/lnit.2.2.168-171
33. Samanta D, Paul M, Khadri SKA (2013) Message communication using phase shifting method (PSM). Int J Adv Res Comput Sci 4(11):9–11. https://doi.org/10.26483/ijarcs.v4i11.1936
34. Mukherjee M, Samanta D (2014) Fibonacci based text hiding using image cryptography. Lecture notes on information theory, vol 2, no 2, pp 172–176. https://doi.org/10.12720/lnit.2.2.172-176
35. Khadri SKA et al (2016) Message encryption using pascal triangle multiplication: in cryptology. Asian J Math Comput Res 262–270
36. Jaferi F, Saeid KT, Borah L, Samanta D (2016) Recognition of potential drug-drug interactions in diabetic's patients in hospital pharmacy. Int J Control Theory Appl 10(9):–487. ISSN 0974-5572
37. Kuchy SA, Ahmed SK, Khadri MM, Samanta D, Le D-N (2017) An aggregation approach based on elasticsearch. J Eng Appl Sci 12:9451–9454. https://doi.org/10.36478/jeasci.2017.9451.9454
38. Manu MK, Roy S, Samanta D (2018) Effects of liver cancer drugs on cellular energy metabolism in hepatocellular carcinoma cells. Int J Pharm Res 10(3). ISSN 0975-2366. https://doi.org/10.31838/ijpr/2018.10.03.079.
39. Sivakumar P, Nagaraju R, Samanta D et al (2020) A novel free space communication system using nonlinear InGaAsP microsystem resonators for enabling power-control toward smart cities. Wireless Netw 26:2317–2328. https://doi.org/10.1007/s11276-019-02075-7
40. Kureethara V, Biswas J, Samanta D, Eapen NG (2019) Balanced constrained partitioning of distinct objects. Int J Innov Technol Explor Eng. ISSN: 2278-3075 (Online). https://doi.org/10.35940/ijitee.K1023.09811S19
41. Anwar Z, Banerjee S, Eapen NG, Samanta D (2019) A clinical study of Hepatitis B. J Crit Rev 6(5):81–84. https://doi.org/10.22159/jcr.06.05.13
42. Samanta D et al (2020) Distributed feedback Laser (DFB) for signal power amplitude level improvement in long spectral band. J Opt Commun. www.degruyter.com. https://doi.org/10.1515/joc-2019-0252
43. Biswal AK, Singh D, Pattanayak BK, Samanta D, Yang M-H (2021) IoT-based smart alert system for drowsy driver detection. Wireless communications and mobile computing. 2021:13 pages. Article ID 6627217. https://doi.org/10.1155/2021/6627217
44. Maheswari M, Geetha S, Selva kumar S, Karuppiah M, Samanta D, Park Y (2021) PEVRM: probabilistic evolution based version recommendation model for mobile applications. IEEE Access. https://doi.org/10.1109/ACCESS.2021.3053583

45. Gomathy V, Padhy N, Samanta D et al (2020) Malicious node detection using heterogeneous cluster based secure routing protocol (HCBS) in wireless adhoc sensor networks. J Ambient Intell Human Comput 11:4995–5001. https://doi.org/10.1007/s12652-020-01797-3
46. Khamparia A, Singh PK, Rani P, Samanta D, Khanna A, Bhushan B (2020) An internet of health things-driven deep learning framework for detection and classification of skin cancer using transfer learning. Trans Emerg Tel Tech 2020:e3963. https://doi.org/10.1002/ett.3963
47. Althar RR, Samanta D (2021) The realist approach for evaluation of computational intelligence in software engineering. Innov Syst Softw Eng. https://doi.org/10.1007/s11334-020-00383-2
48. Guha A, Samanta D (2021) Hybrid approach to document anomaly detection: an application to facilitate RPA in title insurance. Int J Autom Comput 18:55–72. https://doi.org/10.1007/s11633-020-1247-y
49. Samanta D, Sivaram M, Rashed A, Boopathi CS, Sadegh Amiri I, Yupapin P (2020) Distributed Feedback Laser (DFB) for signal power amplitude level improvement in long spectral band. J Opt Commun. https://doi.org/10.1515/joc-2019-0252
50. Leung JM, Niikura M, Cheng WT, Yang CW, Sin DD (2020) Covid-19 and COPD. Eur Respir J. https://doi.org/10.1183/13993003.02108-2020
51. Li D, Lu X (2020) Parallel-batch scheduling with deterioration and rejection on a single machine. Appl Math J Chin Univ 35:141–156. https://doi.org/10.1007/s11766-020-3624-2
52. Maple C (2017) Security and privacy in internet of things. J Cyber Policy 2(2):155–184. https://doi.org/10.1080/23738871.2017.1366536
53. Mehraeen E, Alinaghi SAS, Nowroozi A, Dadros O, Alilou S, Shobeiri P, Karimi A (2020) A Systetematic review of ecg findings in patients with COVID-19. Indian Heart J 72(6):500–507. https://doi.org/10.1016/j.ihj.2020.11.007
54. Mohandas N, Thampi SM (2011) Improving hadoop performance in handling small files. In: Abraham A, Mauri JL, Buford JF, Suzuki J, Thampi SM (eds) Advances in computing and communications. ACC 2011. Communications in computer and information science, vol 193. Springer, Berlin, Heidelberg. https://doi.org/10.1007/978-3-642-22726-4_20
55. Sulaiman M, Saleh B, Saida R, Kacem RH, Abid M (2020) Wireless sensor network design methodologies: a survey. J Sens 2020:13 pages. Article ID 9592836. https://doi.org/10.1155/2020/9592836
56. Mohammadzadeh N, Gholamzadeh M, Saeedi S et al (2020) The application of wearable smart sensors for monitoring the vital signs of patients in epidemics: a systematic literature review. J Ambient Intell Human Comput. https://doi.org/10.1007/s12652-020-02656-x
57. Naicker N (2020) Linear support vector machines for prediction of student performance in school based education. Math Probl Engi 2020:7 pages. Article ID 4761468. https://doi.org/10.1155/2020/4761468
58. Zhao N, Bao J, Chen N (2020) Ranking influential nodes in complex networks with information entropy method. Complexity 2020:15 pages. Article ID 5903798. https://doi.org/10.1155/2020/5903798
59. Narayanan NH, Hegarty M (2002) Multimedia design for communication of dynamic information. 57(4):279–315. https://doi.org/10.1006/ijhc.2002.1019
60. Nascimento JR, Nunes JBS, Falcao EL, Sampiao L, Brito A (2020) On the tracking of sensitive data and confidential executions. In: DEBS '20: proceedings of the 14th ACM international conference on distributed and event-based systems. https://doi.org/10.1145/3401025.3404097
61. Nishiga M, Wang DW, Han Y, Lewis DB, Wu JC (2020) Covid-19 and cardiovascular disease: from basic mechanisms to clinical perspectives. Nat Rev Cardiol 17:543–558. https://doi.org/10.1038/s41569-020-0413-9
62. Ozturk T, Talo M, Yildirim EA, Baloglu UB, Yildirim O, Acharya UR (2020) Automated detection of Covid-19 cases using deep neural networks with X-ray images. Comput Bio Med. https://doi.org/10.1016/j.compbiomed.2020.103792
63. Paras EB (2017)Contact lens technology to 2020 and beyond: a review of recent patent literature, vol 100, issue 5, pp 529–536. https://doi.org/10.1111/cxo.12596
64. Raban DR, Gordon A (2020) The evolution of data science and big data research: a bibliometric analysis. Scientometrics 122:1563–1581. https://doi.org/10.1007/s11192-020-03371-2

65. Rampersad G (2020) Robot will take your job: innovation for an era of artificial intelligence. J Bus Res 116:68–74. https://doi.org/10.1016/j.jbusres.2020.05.019
66. Rizk A, Elragal A (2020) Data science: developing theoretical contributions in information systems via text analytics. J Big Data 7. https://doi.org/10.1186/s40537-019-0280-6
67. Rick SR, Goldberg AP, Weibel N (2019) SleepBot: encouraging sleep hygiene using an intelligent chatbot. In: IUI '19: proceedings of the 24th international conference on intelligent user interfaces: companion, pp 107–108. https://doi.org/10.1145/3308557.3308712
68. Richards CL et al (2017) Advances in public health surveillance and information dissemination at the centers for disease control and prevention. Public Health Rep 132(4):403–410
69. Salmi N, Rustam Z (2019) Naïve Bayes classifier models for predicting the colon cancer. IOP Conf Ser Mater Sci Eng 546:052068. https://doi.org/10.1088/1757-899X/546/5/052068
70. Santos BS, Silva I, Dantas MCR, Alves G, Endo PT, Lima L (2020) Covid-19: a scholarly production dataset report for research analysis. https://doi.org/10.1016/j.dib.2020.106178
71. Saura JR (2020) Using data sciences in digital marketing: framework. Methods Perform Metr J Innov Knowl. https://doi.org/10.1016/j.jik.2020.08.001
72. Schmiedl, S. R. and Raghu, G. 2020. Telemedicine — maintaining quality during times of transition. *Nat Rev Dis Primers* **6,** 45 (2020). https://doi.org/10.1038/s41572-020-0185-x
73. Scherer HU, Haupl T, BGR (2020) Etiol Rheum J Autoimmun 110. https://doi.org/10.1016/j.jaut.2019.102400
74. Schuh G, Reinhart G, Prote JP, Sauerman F, Horsthofer J, Oppolzer F, Knoll D (2019) Data mining definitions and applications for the management of production complexity. Procedia CIRP 81:874–879. https://doi.org/10.1016/j.procir.2019.03.217
75. Uddin MI, Zada N, Aziz F, Saeed Y, Zeb A, Shah SAA, Mahmoud M (2020) Prediction of future terrorist activities using deep neural networks. Complexity 2020:16 pages. Article ID 1373087. https://doi.org/10.1155/2020/1373087
76. Sharma T, Bashir M (2020) Use of apps in the COVID-19 response and the loss of privacy protection. Nat Med 26:1165–1167. https://doi.org/10.1038/s41591-020-0928-y
77. Shuja J, Alanazi E, Alasmary W et al (2020) COVID-19 open source data sets: a comprehensive survey. Appl Intell 51:1296–1325. https://doi.org/10.1007/s10489-020-01862-6
78. Sivarajah U, Kamal MM, Irani Z et al (2017) Critical analysis of big data challenges and analytical methods. J Bus Res 70:263–280. https://doi.org/10.1016/j.jbusres.2016.08.001
79. Tsuei HJ, Tsai WH, Pan FT et al (2020). Improving search engine optimization (SEO) by using hybrid modified MCDM models. Artif Intell Rev 53:1–16. https://doi.org/10.1007/s10462-018-9644-0
80. Wall ME, Rechtsteiner A, Rocha LM (2003) Singular value decomposition and principal component analysis. In: Berrar DP, Dubitzky W, Granzow M (eds) A practical approach to microarray data analysis. Springer, Boston, MA. https://doi.org/10.1007/0-306-47815-3_5
81. Wiener M, Saunders C, Marabelli M (2020) Big-data business models: a critical literature review and multiperspective research. Framework 35(1):66–91. https://doi.org/10.1177/0268396219896811
82. Yaqoob I, Hashem IAT, Inayat Z, Ali WKM, Alam M, Shiraz M, Gani A (2014) Big data: survey, technologies, opportunities and challenges. Sci World J 2014:18 pages. Article ID 712826. https://doi.org/10.1155/2014/712826
83. Yiannopoulou KG, Papageorgiou SG (2020) Current and future treatments in Alzheimer disease: an update. J Central Nervous Dis. https://doi.org/10.1177/1179573520907397
84. You J, Klein SAS, Lou E, Martin J, Zuidhorf (2020) Application of random forest classification to predict daily oviposition events in broiler breeders fed by precision feeding system. Comput Electron Agric 175. https://doi.org/10.1016/j.compag.2020.105526
85. Faizal khan Z, Refa Alotaibi S (2020) Applications of artificial intelligence and big data analytics in m-health: a healthcare system perspective. J Healthc Eng 2020:15 pages. Article ID 8894694. https://doi.org/10.1155/2020/8894694

Chapter 5
Trends and Applications of Intelligent IoT in Agriculture

Abstract The world's population is rapidly growing, necessitating a shift to more sustainable farming practices. Because of declining natural supplies, scarce arable land, and highly unpredictable weather patterns, food security is a major issue for most countries. Only as a consequence data analytics (DA) and the Internet of Things are being used to increase the agricultural sector's operational efficiency and productivity. Wireless sensor networks (WSN) have given way to IoT and DA as a main driver of smart agriculture. The Internet of Things includes wireless sensor networks, radio frequency recognition, cloud networking, middleware platforms, and end-user software. In this article, the benefits and challenges of IoT have been discussed. The IoT environment is discussed, as well as how IoT and DA work together to help intelligent agriculture. The latest technologies along with opportunities are often presented, and they are grouped into four categories: technological advancements, deployment scenarios, business, and marketability.

5.1 Introduction

IoT is being used in a variety of areas, including connected industry, smart city, intelligent-home, intelligent-energy, intelligent vehicle, intelligent-agriculture, medical care, and logistics. The Internet of Things (IoT) aims to link the physical and virtual realms by using the internet as a means of connectivity and information exchange. IoT is a framework of connected computational machines, mechanized and programmed computers, entities, organisms, or individuals with provided with unique identifiers in transferring information over an internetwork but without individual-to-individual or human-to-computer contact. This essay is mainly concerned with the use of IoT in agriculture [1, 2].

The global population is projected to exceed 10 billion people by 2060, resulting in increased food demand. Because of dwindling environmental supplies, agricultural land, and unpredictable climate conditions, food security is a big issue for various nations. The society is transitioning to IoT together with data analysis to satisfy the

D. Samanta and A. Banerjee, *Computationally Intensive Statistics for Intelligent IoT*, Studies in Autonomic, Data-driven and Industrial Computing,
https://doi.org/10.1007/978-981-16-5936-2_5

planet's edible shortages in near future. In agriculture, the number of IoT devices deployed is expected to expand from 40 million in 2021 to 10 million by 2025 [3].

The usage of IoT along with Data Analytics would allow intelligent farming that would be anticipated to grow competence along with productivity and yielding. For years, WSNs have been used in intelligent farming along with edible yield, focusing on ambient protection, accuracy farming, device and control systems automation, and traceability. Because of its ability to individual-organizing capacity, individual-configuration, individual-diagnosis, and individual-healing capacity, WSN is a great option for intelligent farming along with the food processing industry [4, 5]. The WSN includes radio waves (RF) device, sensors, microprocessors, and electrical systems. The paradigm has moved from using WSN for intelligent farming to using IoT as the primary driver for intelligent farming since the introduction of IoT. WSN, RF awareness, cloud networking, middleware networks, and end-user applications are only a few of the IoT technologies. IoT is used in agriculture to provide farming with judgment-making tools and automated techniques, which allow them to efficiently combine products, skills, and facilities with improved production, quality, and value. The disputes and drawbacks for huge-scaling pilots in the agri-food distribution supply have been the subject of current studies on the Internet of Things in farming. Figure 5.1 shows IoT habitat in agriculture. Alternative market structures, data control, and ownership solutions, and security and privacy are only a couple of the major topics explored. Other intelligent farming studies have primarily concentrated on the usage of WSNs. Though these literature review manuscripts address sensor technology and the challenges of applying IoT to the agriculture industry, communication technology is limited to conventional techniques that rely on low-range communication technologies [6–8].

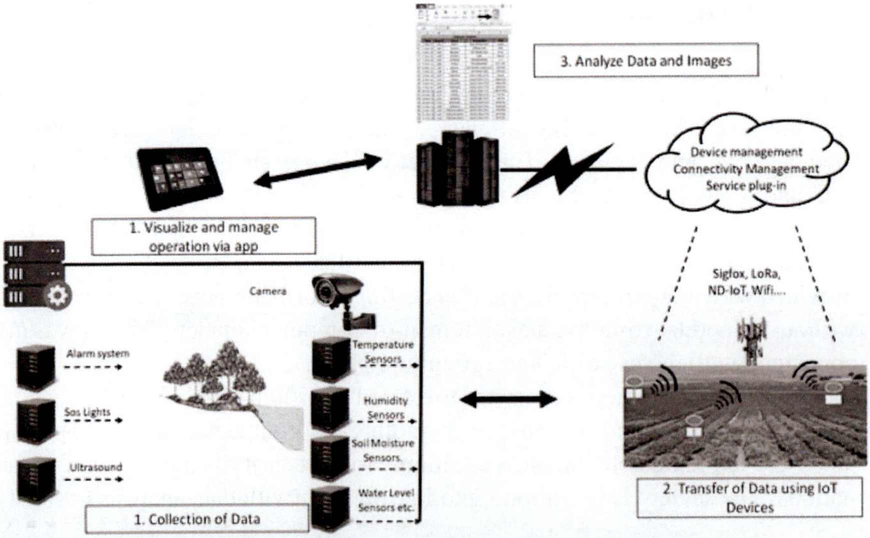

Fig. 5.1 IoT habitat in agriculture

A comprehensive study of IoT in farming is performed in this article. An overview of journal manuscripts, white papers, along with current approaches is included in the study. The agricultural IoT ecosystem is broken down into four main components: IoT computers, networking infrastructure, the web, information collection, along with transformation. The usage of IoT along with DA in agriculture is discussed, as well as how it is helping smart agriculture. Often addressed are the advantages, obstacles, open questions, future developments, and prospects [8].

The below is a schematic of the chapter's composition.

(1) The IoT environment for agriculture is discussed in Sect. 5.2, and it consists of four main components: The following topics are discussed: (a) Internet of Things appliances, (b) networking techniques, (c) the Web along with, and d) information.
(2) The description of IoT applications in agriculture is addressed in Sect. 5.3. (a) Monitoring, (b) logging and tracking, (c) farm equipments, (d) accurate farming along with, and (e) greenhouse development are all relevant areas to remember.
(3) The value of IoT and DA is discussed in Sect. 5.4. (a) Estimation, (b) Stock superintendence, (c) Conclusion building, (d) Field control, (e) accurate farming, and (f) assurance are the six main fields considered.
(4) The advantages are illustrated in Sect. 5.5. IoT can be used to encourage cooperative farming, protection and deception avoidance combative dominance, resource generation, expenditure savings, organizational performance, cognizance, and treasure superintendence, among other things.
(5) Section 5.10 addresses a variety of unanswered problems and significant roadblocks to IoT adoption in agriculture. Three key types of issues are listed and discussed: (a) professional (b) hi-tech, and (c) sector-based.
(6) The next module examines future developments and prospects.
(7) This chapter comes to a close with Sect. 5.12.

5.2 Internet of Things Ecosystem

This segment provides a description of IoT environment for farming. The Internet of Things, information infrastructure, the internet, and data collection and processing are the four main components. The IoT environment is depicted in Fig. 5.2. Any IoT implementation needs four main components. The following is a breakdown of the IoT elements as they contribute to agriculture [9].

5.2.1 Internet of Things (IoT) Devices

IoT devices are embedded systems that communicate with sensors that actuators and need to be connected to the internet. IoT sensors are another name for these

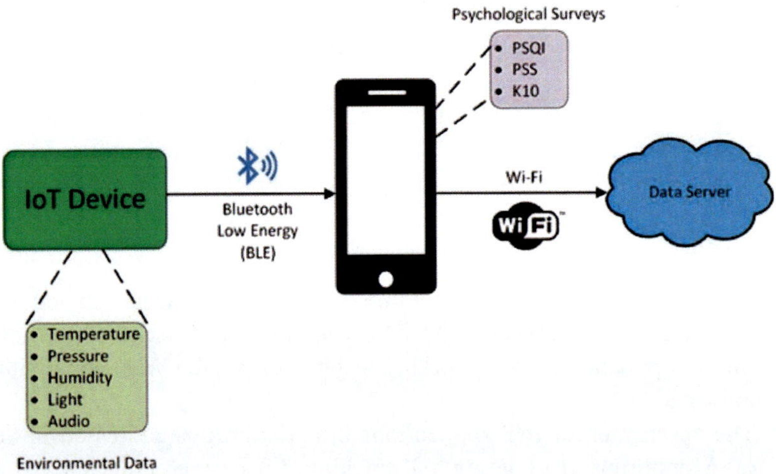

Fig. 5.2 IoT device framework

IoT products. It is referred to as an IoT system in this article. Figure 5.2 depicts the framework of a standard IoT unit for farming. FPGAs or microprocessors, transmission frameworks, memory, and I/O interfaces make up an embedded device [10, 11]. The sensors are used to monitor and quantify a variety of farming variables (e.g. soil supplements and meteorology data) as well as production-related factors. Positional sensors, vision sensors, electro-mechanical sensors, electrochemical sensors, along with gust sensors are the different types of sensors. Air warmth, soil warmth at varying depths, precipitation, leaf moisture, chlorophyll, breeze velocity, mist point warmth, wind alignment, comparative humidness, astral radiation, and environmental pressure are all collected using these instruments. Table 5.1 summarizes fewer sensors as well as their implementations. There are many main features of IoT devices, which make oneself ideal for use in farming [12]. (1) Energy planning (2) repository (3) computing power (4) flexibility (5) resilience (6) broadcasting (7) dependability along with (8) expenditure.

5.2.2 Information and Transmission Automation

Transmission infrastructure is critical to the successful deployment of IoT programs. Standards, scope, and implementation scenarios will all be used to categorize current networking technologies. Short-range transmission standards along with long-range transmission standards are two types of communication standards. Registered and unlicensed spectra are two types of contact spectrum. Sensors or backhaul networks can be seen in IoT system application scenarios, as well as implementation frameworks [13].

Table 5.1 Farming sensors description

Type of sensors	Functions	Examples of applications
Optical		Photodiodes and photodectors to determine clay, organic matter, and moisture content of the soil
Mechanical		Tensiometers to detect the force used by the roots in water absorption and useful for irrigation interventions
Electrochemical	Use of electrodes to detect specific ions in the soil	Use of ion-selective electrodes (ISE) and ion-selective field effect transistor sensors (ISEFT) for detecting nitrogen phosphorus potassium (NPK) in soils
Dielectric soil moisture	Use of electrodes to assess moisture levels by measuring the dielectric constant in the soil	Frequency domain reflectometry (FDR) or time domain reflectometry (TDR) to sense soil water content
Airflow	Measure soil air permeability	Properties such as compaction, structure, soil type, and moisturelevel of the soil can be measured
Location	Use of global positioning system (GPS) satellites to determines the latitude, longitude, and altitude	The GPS provides precise positioning for which is a corner stone for precision agriculture

(1) **The Spectrum**: The unauthorized spectrum requires the usage of the commercial, analysis, along with medical RF band. Security risks, maintenance costs, and interference are all drawbacks of using the unlicensed spectrum. ISM IoT systems cause electromagnetic interference, which disrupts radio signals on the same wavelength. The licensed spectrum that is assigned to the wireless network, on the other hand, provides customers with more effective traffic control, less congestion, improved authenticity, and enhanced QoS, higher reliability, broader exploration, along with lower configuration costs. The cost of data transfer subscriptions and transmit power use on IoT devices are all disadvantages of using licensed spectrum [14].

(2) **Standard**: There are several wireless networking protocols, some of which are specified. It is categorized into two categories: shorter-range and longer-range connectivity levels. Closer-field transmission applications, Bluetooth, and submissive and energetic RFID structures are examples of shorter-range specifications. Short-range standards are capable of reaching lengths of less than 100 m. Long-range contact protocols are capable of covering lengths of up to ten kilometers. Low power large area (LPWA) networking protocols are used for longer-range transmission. The LPWA is a low-power device that can protect a large area [15].

(3) **Scenario for Application**: The IoT device's implementations affect the networking technologies selected. IoT devices that serve as nodes or backhaul networks will also benefit from the networking technology. The nodes send small amounts of data over short distances while using relatively little fuel. High data speeds are supported by the backhaul network, which can be used over long distances. Table 5.1 shows farming sensors description. Bi-directional links are supported by several networking systems. Further error handling, handshaking for information durability, data encoding, and above-the-atmosphere firmware upgrades, along with system connectivity are all possible with the bidirectional connection. The comparison of long range and Narrow Band Internet of Things reveals that individual automation has its own set of benefits and drawbacks, so the best technology depends on the use [16, 17]. Furthermore, the type of topology to be implemented influences the communication infrastructure chosen for the IoT device. P2P/line topology, star/mesh/ring/tree/bus topologies are only a few examples.

An IoT computer executes various responsibilities along with functionalities in every topology. A personal area coordinator or a terminating computer may play this part. A full functional device or a reduced functional device will perform the functions RFD. Figure 5.3 shows two groups of topologies along with the positions they perform. The PAN acts as an FFD and initiates contact in the P2P topology, while the end devices will act as either an FFD or an RFD. The FFD-connected appliances may have several links, and the RFD terminating device may only associate to a single FFD and must not associate with other RFD. The PAN in the star network initiates correspondence and accepts connections from other devices. Only the PAN coordinator may create contacts with the end devices [18].

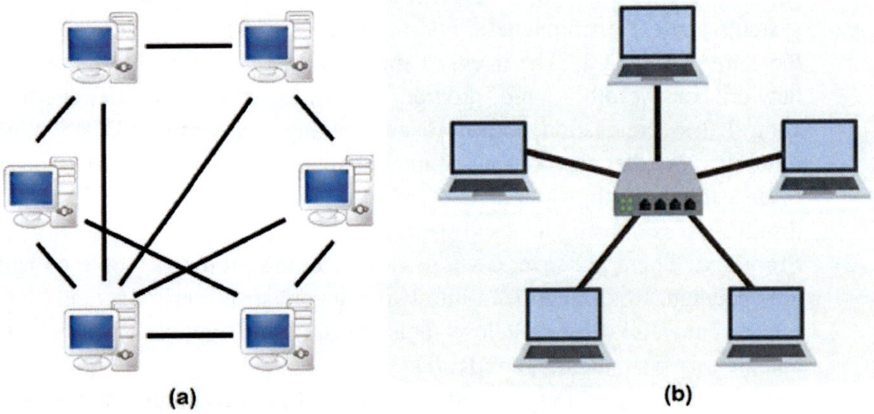

Fig. 5.3 Network topologies **a** P2P **b** Star

5.2.3 Internet

The development of wireless networking, handheld computers, along with ubiquitous roles, have facilitated the approach for widespread web approach. The quantity of linked farming appliances is forecasted to increase from 16 million during 2016 to 230 million within 2025, in accordance with Machina study. The web is the middling internetwork level, which offers routes for data and network information to be transported and shared between various internetworks [19, 20]. When IoT devices are connected to the internet, data can be viewed from anywhere and at any instant. Though, data transmission over the web necessitates enough reliability, instant-time information support, and facilitates access. Cloud computing was made possible by the internet, which allows vast amounts of data to be collected for repository and retrieval. Cloud infrastructure includes an administration of client interfaces, assistances, network node organization and collaboration, computing, and data analysis. IoT middleware and networking protocols are constructed to connect diverse systems along with appliances over the web. SOA architecture, cloud-dependent IoT middleware are examples of IoT middleware that is utilized to bolster IoT [21, 22]. Multilayer architecture is used in SOA for IoT. The following layers make up each of the proposed IoT architecture: sensing, accessing, internetworking, middleware, and appliance layers. For more knowledge on IoT architecture and technologies, the concept is well described.

5.2.4 Computer Management and Retrieval Units

Data-dependent farming necessitates the gathering of massive amounts of effective, nuanced, and conceptual records that must be stored along with processing. The information's sophistication can vary from organized to unstructured that may take the formation of text, photographs, sound, and video. Historical records, sensor records, live-streamed records, commercial, and merchandise records are all examples of data. Big data obtained from sensors may be processed within the cloud infrastructure using cloud-oriented IoT frameworks. It entails hosting essential requisitions for delivering utilities as well as managing terminal-to-terminal IoT frameworks. Edge/fog computation has currently been promoted; in which IoT devices along with gateways execute computation along with analysis in minimizing latency in sensitive applications, lower expenditures, along with improving QoS [23, 24]. To handle the different types of data, many agriculture management information systems have been created.

5.2.5 *Inference*

There are many important technological criteria to remember when installing an IoT system. The scope of transmission stretch, data rate, battery usage, portability, latency, protection along with durability, along with the expenditure of gateway modems should all be weighed when considering wireless networking. The LPWA is attracting a lot of attention among communication technologies, particularly with the advent of NB-IoT [25]. Low system power usage, ultralow appliance expenditure, easiness in deploying, framework for a large range of lower-throughput applications, longer-span reach, along with data uploading and downloading are all capabilities that the NB-IoT promises. In agriculture, there are many IoT usage cases that have embraced the IoT ecosystems mentioned in this section. Section 5.3 goes through a few of these applications [26].

5.3 Intellectual Property in Agriculture

In farming, there are many instances in IoT implementations. Reaping and flock equipments, drainage and water standard tracking, meteorology tracking, soil tracking, illness and plague management, robotization, and precision are several examples of such usage cases. Monitoring, recording, and tracing, agricultural equipment, precision agriculture, and greenhouse production are all addressed as examples of IoT applications [27].

5.3.1 *Observation*

Several aspects of agriculture can be tracked, depending on the kind of agriculture being considered. The following are some of the most important things to keep an eye on. Crop farming is the first step in the process. Several environmental conditions have an effect on farm produce in crop farming. Obtaining such information aids in understanding the farm's habits and processes.

Precipitation, leaf moisture, warmth, evaporation, soil wetness, saltiness, atmosphere, stellar emission, insect activity, personage undertakings, and so on are examples of such data. The purchase of such comprehensive evidence allows for excellent resolution-making to increase farm produce efficiency, reduce risk, and optimize profits. Solar radiation data, for example, contain the details on the plants' vulnerability to sunshine, helping the cultivator to assess whether the plants are sufficiently revealed or overexposed [28, 29]. The soil wetness constituent provides data on the soil's wetness that may aid in soil management and lower the threat of plant disease. Moreover, reliable along with timely meteorology predicting records, like climatic shifts along with precipitation, will boost production. Furthermore, this knowledge will assist cultivators in the drafting level and lower labor costs. Farmers may also use the data to take correction and prevention steps ahead of time. Pest movement records maneuver can be gathered and catered instantly to cultivators for pest checking, or it can be utilized in providing guidance to cultivators built on pest attack reports. Figure 5.3 shows Network Topologies (a) P2P and (b) Star.

(1) Aquaponics: Aquaponics relates to hybridization between aquaculture and hydroponics, in which fish waste is fed to plant farms to supply the nutrients that plants need. Water standards, water levels, warmth, fish fitness, saltiness, pH demarcations, dew, along with sunshine must all be continuously monitored in such farms. Since reliable data help nutrients to be transferred between plants and fish, it can increase fish and plant yield. With less human interference, the data can also be used for automation [30].
(2) Forestry: Forests play critical criteria in the carbon levels and are home to more than two-thirds of all recognized organisms on the planet. Dirt and air warmth and moisture, as well as various amounts of gases like CO, CO_2, toluene, O_2, H_2, methane, isobutane, NH_3, ethanol, H_2S, along with NO_2, may all be tracked in a forest. These metrics may help with quick caution along with alarm apparatus for grassland fires in the woodlands, as well as disease monitoring [31].
(3) Domestic Agriculture: The variables in controlling cattle vary depending on the beasts being studied [32]. The getting of milk from cows along with buffaloes, for example, will reveal details about the mammal's well-being. Warmth, humidity, output, insect incursion, along with water standards are all various contemplations to consider. Farmers may also use the deployment and installation solution to monitor and question the position of the cattle by marking each mammal through an RFID system, avoiding animal theft [33].

Other fields can be tracked, like repository tracking, that incorporates food, water, and animal nourishments, and the records may facilitate cultivators chalk out beforehand and retain money. Although various monitoring schemes are developed, acquisition in smaller and mid-size farms is restricted, particularly in developing nations, due to a shortage in knowledge along with implementation costs. The scope for developing expenditure-efficient farming IoT approaches remains untapped [34].

5.3.2 *Tracing and Monitoring*

Asset monitoring will also benefit from IoT to strengthen a company's supply chain along with logistics. Agricultural businesses may use dataset from IoT in making smarter decisions, schedule ahead, communicate intelligently along with business associates, and conserve time along with resources. RFID along with cloud-dependent global positioning system will detect records such as position and resource detection. The ability to track and trace agricultural product chains helps consumers to learn about the product's entire history, increasing customer trust in product quality and health-related concerns. While monitoring refers to the ability to record, compile, and store data from upstream to downstream in the supply chain, tracing enables the commodity in separating from down-level to upper-level [35, 36]. Monitoring along with finding facilitates multiple data points to be gathered along the supply chain, ensuring that the sources, position, along with survival records for a commodity are known to the customer and other stakeholders. The growing climate, manufacturing circumstances, pest components, administration constituents, repository positions, conveyance, along with time to market are the various elements that may be tracked. Consumers may be exposed to overt or indirect health risks as a result of these causes. Soil, climate, and water are three major factors that influence the rising world [37].

Herbicides, fertilizers, and pesticides all have an effect on the production conditions. Moreover, the types of nourishments and boosters are given to animals should be monitored because they can cause health problems. Pests can impact agricultural goods in the process, affecting the aggregate and attributes of the crop. Monitoring the commodities may indulge cultivators increase their productivity and supply chain [38].

Knowledge input, storage, transition, operation, and output should all be used in a monitoring and tracing system. The input data contain data from the product's entire life cycle, its geographical origin, current location, and destination, as well as the collaborators engaged in the complete supply chain. Memory must be used in the devices to allow for long-term storage of data for research and development. The method of unifying and standardizing all information is referred to as information transfer [39, 40]. The monitoring and tracing device should also be able to process the information obtained and then transmit it to all stakeholders participating in the supply chain stresses the utilization of RFID for monitoring originating at the manufacturing level to packaging, conveyance, repository, delivery, sales, and after-sales facilities. It allows the processing, retrieval, and review of information for a lengthy interval at a high pace [41].

5.3.3 Farming Equipments

IoT-enabled farming equipments may aid in reaping along with grain loss reduction. The equipments may be run in auto driver mechanism by using proper positioning, GPS, along with worldwide way finding satellite system vehicles, unmanned aerial vehicles along with robotics, among other devices, may be distantly administered depending on data collected from the IoT system for precise and productive resource deployment to the necessary farming locations [42, 43]. The equipments may also accumulate data, which can assist cultivators in designing the fields in order to schedule plans like fertilization, drainage, and nourishment. CLAAS, an agricultural equipment maker, for example, has incorporated IoT on its machinery, allowing it to run in autopilot mode. The Precisionhawk's UAV sensors are another choice, as they may facilitate cultivators with data like wind velocity along with air pressure, including other aspects. The approach may, moreover, be utilized for agricultural plot imagination and imaging [44].

5.3.4 *Farming Precision*

Precision farming is known as the accumulation of instant-time records from farm variables along with the application of predictive analysis to make intelligent settlements for optimization. Climate, earth along with air quality, crop maturation along with even machinery, as well as labor costs and supply, are examples of farm variables, which yield, reduce expense, and reduce environmental impact. Precision agriculture uses a variety of technologies to increase crop production, including sensor connections, Global Positioning System, and big data analysis. The DA's wise judgment also means less loss of energy like water in irrigation schemes, manure, pesticides, and so on. Researchers in automation, image analysis, meteorological data sensing, and other fields will face new obstacles as a result of precision agriculture [45, 46].

Farmers may use GPS and GNSS to pinpoint specific locations and map locations with various information variables that are then utilized by varying technology to dispense farming tools like planting, sprinkling, along with various assistances more efficiently. While precision farming automation may increase harvesting, it is critical to furnish farmers with capabilities, which are simple to utilize and to facilitate teaching so that smaller and mid-scale cultivators can profit from the frameworks [47].

Green technology, also called glasshouse high tech, is a process for growing vegetation in a regulated climate. By having appropriate environmental conditions, it allows you to grow any plant at any location at any time. Several researches with the utilization of Wireless Sensor Networks in greenhouses to track ambient situations have been conducted. Recent studies have shown how IoT can be used in greenhouses to minimize human resources, save electricity, improve greenhouse-site monitoring performance, and bind greenhouse cultivators directly to clients [48].

5.4 Internet of Things and Big Data Analysis in Farming

In farming, precise information processing is critical for optimizing operating performance and increasing productivity. Depending on the specifications in IoT implementations, Data Analytics has been classified into categories. Spontaneous-time analysis, memory-level analysis, business intelligence-level analysis, and mega analytics are all examples of this. Sensor records, sound, pictures, along with video make up the data. Picture alteration is widely utilized in farming in a variety of applications, including disease identification in leaves, stems, and fruits, fruit consistency, and weed perception along with drainage. In agriculture, image processing and IoT have recently been combined to deliver high-standard production and minimize crop production [49, 50]. It entails the utilization of drones in collecting above-ground photographs at frequent intervals, and the utilization of IoT sensors to detect environmental conditions. There are a number of DA processes, which are explored in depth. Classification, clustering, estimation, and correlation law are the different types of processes. The content of this paper does not provide a description of these approaches. We chat about how Data Analysis may assist with assurance, forecasting, stock administration, settlement making, farming administration, along with precision agriculture [51].

5.4.1 Forecasting

The Internet of Things (IoT) offers large amounts of records, which may be analyzed within time in predicting current environmental conditions. The information gathered by Data Analysis may be used to investigate sensors in a number of networks. To forecast ambient alterations along with providing data-driven answers, a smart algorithm may be built. While IoT data can be used to monitor different facets of a plantation, like drainage systems, it may be utilized to forecast and alert cultivators about illness or severe weather events, like floods or droughts. For example in forest management, sensors can be utilized to detect fire outbreaks or forecast which areas of a plantation are at threat of catching fire. The detail will aid firefighters in taking preventative steps at the precise site. Early alert of natural hazards to boost emergency response is another field of prediction [52].

5.4.2 Storage Administration

Weak storage control systems typically result in the loss of a significant amount of agricultural items. Although temperature, moisture, and other environmental factors have a significant impact on food product toxicity, insects, microorganisms, rodents, and other factors may have an impact on the quality and quantity of food. Storage control systems that incorporate IoT and DA will help boost agricultural commodity storage. Sensors may be used to keep an eye on storage warehouses and the surrounding area. The data are uploaded to the cloud and processed there. To change the environmental conditions, a oneself-mechanized forecasting mechanism based on scrutinized records may be utilized. Furthermore, when adverse situations are outreached or pests are detected in the repository provisions, a warning signal can be sent to farmers. According to reports from India, 35–40% of fresh produce is wasted after harvesting due to a variety of factors such as pest [53].

A cold storage organization facility depending on IoT technologies is built in, and the storage provision is run at a stable hotness condition. While the Internet of Things will boost agricultural storage facilities, protection should be built into the infrastructure to prevent commodity theft in the event of a power failure.

5.4.3 Determination

Making decisions necessitates accurate data, which can be derived from sensor data. The vast amount of data collected by sensors provides opportunities for learning to enhance decision-making in continuously changing environmental environments, which can be done in the short, medium, or long term. When those requirements are met, the IoT device will make automatic decisions, requiring little to no human interference [54]. Such automatic decisions could include anything from temperature management to irrigation system water supply control. For example, in greenhouses, machine learning can be used to evaluate the best conditions for growing a specific crop by analyzing data from sensors that measure nourishments, productivity, enhancement, water loss, color, and flavor as well as illumination, hotness, pest extents, and air aspects. The amount of information gathered from DA will also help the government and other stakeholders make better policy decisions, so it's critical that the data are reliable, succinct, full, and timely. A number of farming conclusion-making mechanisms are built to help cultivators make well-knowledgeable decisions about their plantation and cattle. The Data Analytics makes decisions on technological advice for farmers, pest and disease control, and distant specialist counseling system guidelines [55, 56].

5.4.4 Farming Administration

A consolidated farming administering framework facilitates the monitoring of a whole farm. The data are gathered using an internetwork of sensors, having on-body sensors in cattle, having the only goal of increasing efficiency. Risk organization, expenditure, and production yield are three main variables that must be handled along with spontaneous-time data along with better configuration to improve the yield. Data Analysis plays a key role in providing cultivators and other stakeholders with vast amounts of data that can be closely examined in order to reduce undue risk or introduce mitigation steps to boost production. DA also enables many farms to be linked and operated on a single site, where knowledge on technological advancements, development, vending, farm organization, advice, along with various other relevant subjects can be distributed in order to improve efficiency, yield, and revenue [57].

5.4.5 Accurate Implementation

DA The use of sensor data to allow correct requisition of chemicals and manures to particular regions of the farmland will increase productivity while lowering farming costs. While advanced countries have implemented precision farming systems in their farms, developed nations are starting to embrace the framework, particularly in the science of farming. But, in developed countries, implementation costs, infrastructure, and knowledge continue to hinder the utilization of IoT-dependent precision agriculture systems. Furthermore, since the majority of farms in developed countries are small-scale; most farmers do not see the need to introduce such technologies. Researchers and designers are now focusing on designing effective precision farming technologies for small farms. Another benefit of DA in precision farming is its use of directing machinery to specific positions in the farm using GPS and position data, which improves farming productivity as opposed to human-driven machines. This will save time, gasoline, and money in the long run [58].

5.4.6 *Insurance*

Farmers are often subject to adverse conditions, which may result in a bad harvest. Farmers, on the other hand, may be certain of their crops and animals if IoT technology is implemented. An internetwork of sensors may be established, and distant unmanned terminals can track the situation.

Information may be uploaded to the cloud infrastructure and processed there. The insurance scheme will have an alarm device that predicts adverse weather events and sends text messages to the covered farmers. Farmers would be able to take precautionary measures to secure their farms as a result of this. When severe conditions are detected, an additional benefit to Data Analytics in insurance is that assurance providers have accessibility to records from distant farmlands and may trigger an automatic payout via IoT mobile billing system networks. This may remove the need for a long claim period in which the insurance agent visits the farms to assess the extent of the loss [59, 60].

5.5 Benefits

This may remove the need for a long claim period in which the insurance agent visits the farms to assess the extent of the loss. The use of IoT in agriculture will have a number of advantages. Any of the advantages were discussed in next sections when discussing IoT applications. However, some of the advantages are re-iterated and summarized below.

(1) *Community Farming*: The Internet of Things will aid in the promotion of group farming, specifically in rural locations. The Internet of Things may be used in encouraging facilities that enable the population to exchange information along with knowledge, as well as increase contact between farmers and agriculture experts. Mobile applications and IoT facilities can also be used to share equipment within the city for free or for a fee [61, 62].

(2) *Food Safety and Fraud Prevention*: The agricultural industry faces a number of challenges, including not only ensuring adequate productivity but also ensuring a healthy and nutritious food supply. Adulteration, counterfeiting, and artificial enhancement have all been documented in the sense of food theft. This form of fraud is dangerous to one's well-being and may have a negative economic effect. Product honesty, operation integrity, person's integrity, and data integrity are some of the components of food theft discussed and they can all be solved with IoT technology. The Internet of Things should be used to have logistical and qualitative food traceability.

(3) *Technological Advantages*: With the food demand and the use of cutting-edge technologies, the agriculture market is projected to become extremely competitive. In addition, the use of IoT to allow data-driven agriculture would open up new opportunities in trading, tracking, and marketing. Productivity is improved as prices are decreased and misuse in the solicitation of agricultural inputs like manures and weed killer is reduced. Farmers who follow the IoT environment would achieve a strategic edge by leveraging spontaneous-time information in conclusion making [63].

(4) *Treasury building and Distribution*: The implementation of IoT would open up new market methodologies for individual cultivators, allowing them to circumvent the manipulation of "middle men" and establish direct relationships with customers, resulting in higher profits.

(5) *Cost-cutting and waste reduction*: Main ostensible benefits of IoT are the capability to distantly track instruments along with appliances. When opposed to workers manually inspecting the field using cars or walking, the use of IoT in farming can facilitate reduce time and costs when checking vast farmlands. The ability in using IoT to decide when and where pesticides or insecticides can be added will minimize costs and pollution [64].

(6) *Organizational Efficiency*: This applies in addition to producers, and also to conclusion creators in the farming field, like governmental and non-government organizations. Agriculture surveillance information obtained through IoT can be used as a reference for agricultural interventions. Disease avoidance, vend fire outbreaks, reimbursement programs, and capital distributions are examples of such measures. Furthermore, farmers may use IoT and Data Analysis to make correct including suitable conclusions related to farming organization and procedures. The capability to inevitably log the well-being status of crops would encourage veterinary or agriculture officers to diagnose and administer medication to farmers in a timely and efficient manner [65]. This will result in the elimination of damage. Agri-food supply chains may also be streamlined by the use of IoT. The usage of IoT in the supply chain would assist in real-time demand and supply balancing.

(7) *Awareness*: In the agriculture industry, IoT is projected in accelerating lower-price applications and connectivity to wireless internetwork facilities. Mobile applications may be used to obtain information on stocks, sales, and utilities. Government programs and regulatory guidelines for various agricultural goods can also be made conveniently accessible. Furthermore, customers captivated

in biological along with fresh food may quickly find producers or receive notifications when fresh goods become obtainable [66].

(8) Asset organization: Internet of Things can allow for spontaneous-time surveillance of farming equipment and equipment in order to avoid theft, repair components, and conduct scheduled maintenance on time.

5.6 Research Methodology

5.6.1 Data Collection Using Sensors for Different Parameters

The sensors are set up in an area that resembles a farming ecosystem. There are two kinds of sensors: inland sensors and overland sensors. A soil moisture measurement sensor and a pH sensor are among the inland sensors. A temperature thermostat and a humidity sensor will be used as overland sensors. For data feeding, all of these sensors will be attached to an Arduino microcontroller. Soil content will assist a farmer in estimating important factors like scheduling and quantitative specifications when applying fertilizers or pesticides to the soil, as well as other important parameters like measuring the percentage of fertility. A pH sensor may be used to determine whether the soil is basic, acidic, or neutral. Using acceptable constants, the pH sensor's measurements can be translated to the normal pH scale measurement of 0–14. These findings would be useful since some crops can only grow in specific types of soil. An alarm is activated by the moisture sensor in order to irrigate the soil with a submersible pump. The pump starts automatically when the soil moisture falls below a certain amount. The air temperature and humidity sensors will aid in regulating the type of crop being planted, the total number of crops to be planted, and determining whether or not a greenhouse system is needed [67].

5.6.2 Monitoring the Data Process on a Regular Basis

The data obtained by the sensors will be stored in an Arduino IDE program. This is where the primary selection will take place. In addition, the output values will be displayed on the LCD screen in the appropriate manner. The device and NodeMCU are both connected to the same network, and sensor values are imported wirelessly using the NodeMCU ESP8266, a Wi-Fi-enabled Arduino Module. With the support, you should be able to post this [68].

The sensor values are collected in real time using Python code and stored in a database. This database is made in Microsoft Excel (CSV format) and contains the names of the variables. Following this, real-time values are automatically updated to the database whenever the Python code is executed. Using distinct variables and imported source code, all of the sensor values will be fed into the Firebase server. This will serve as a backup data storage network. The Firebase framework can be used to upload all of the values for a specific frequency. Temperature values, for example, can be registered at regular intervals since the Firebase server is an always-on network [69].

5.7 Data Visualization and Analysis

After the values have been set in the Excel files, there are two ways to evaluate patterns and relationships between the variables. First, upload the conditional source code to the PHP environment of the host website and use internal libraries and variables to represent graphical analysis. Regression patterns can also be used to make predictions, and thus dependencies can be determined. The second method is to create a server-side application using Python and libraries to plot some variations and perform Singular and Multivariate analysis, after which it is possible to directly access the plots and understand the variations in the Arduino results. After that, a range of items can be shown and showcased. Implementing the latter approach will eliminate a time-consuming portion of PHP coding for each and every graph, as well as the same for mobile platforms. XAMPP servers running masked Apache engines on PCs or laptops are usually used to host the pages. It would be very time-consuming and exhausting to do the same for the mobile-end app [70, 71]. Figure 5.4 shows system layout execution.

Following the completion of the database with real-time values, Python code with specific libraries and functions to design graphs is executed. Graphs such as

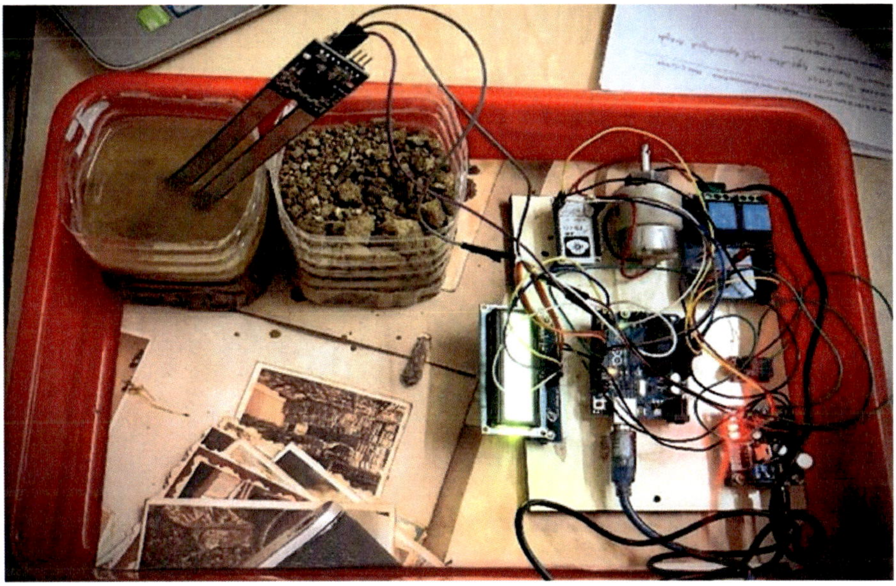

Fig. 5.4 System layout execution

bar and line graphs can be generated using NumPy, Pandas, and Matplotlib. On a daily/weekly/monthly basis, these graphs display the fluctuations in temperature, humidity, soil moisture, and pH. The dataset will be read by Pandas, and the numerical values will be read by NumPy. The graphs will be plotted with the aid of Matplotlib. Temperature is just one element to consider; other factors may also be considered. As a consequence, after a careful examination of the plotted graphs, definitive results that will increase crop quality can be predicted. The results will then be seen on the Firebase website. This will be the Precision Agriculture Application's Front-End, showing to farmers all of the relevant findings, analytical inferences, and conclusions. Firebase can be used for just about any internet connection [72, 73].

5.8 Hosting and Connection

Upon completed, the two Python files, one for displaying the results and analyzing the data, and the other for running the plot application code, will be the primary source of project outcome and understanding. An effective internet hosting platform for displaying the results is developed using Firebase [74]. The Firebase platform can be mapped to the headings in the csv sheet, and the import command will fetch the results in the Firebase console window. This will be the Precision Agriculture Application's Front-End, showing to farmers all of the relevant findings, analytical inferences, and conclusions. Firebase can be used for just about any internet connection. Finally, using the ESP8266, a Wi-Fi-enabled module, wirelessly import the sensor values. Figure 5.5 expresses the design framework.

5.9 System Architecture Proposed

Temperature and Humidity Sensor—The DHT11 is a low-cost sensor that measures temperature and humidity and provides greater reliability and stability.

Moisture Sensor—This will measure the amount of moisture in the soil by changing the resistance between the two leading plates. The resistance between these varies according to the amount of moisture in the soil at the time. Arduino is an open-source electronics platform that relies on a user-friendly program and equipment. Inputs such as ultrasound, light, and even infrared can be detected by Arduino microcontrollers, which can then be converted into outputs such as starting a pump, turning on a light, and so on. A series of instructions can be sent to the board, resulting in outputs [75].

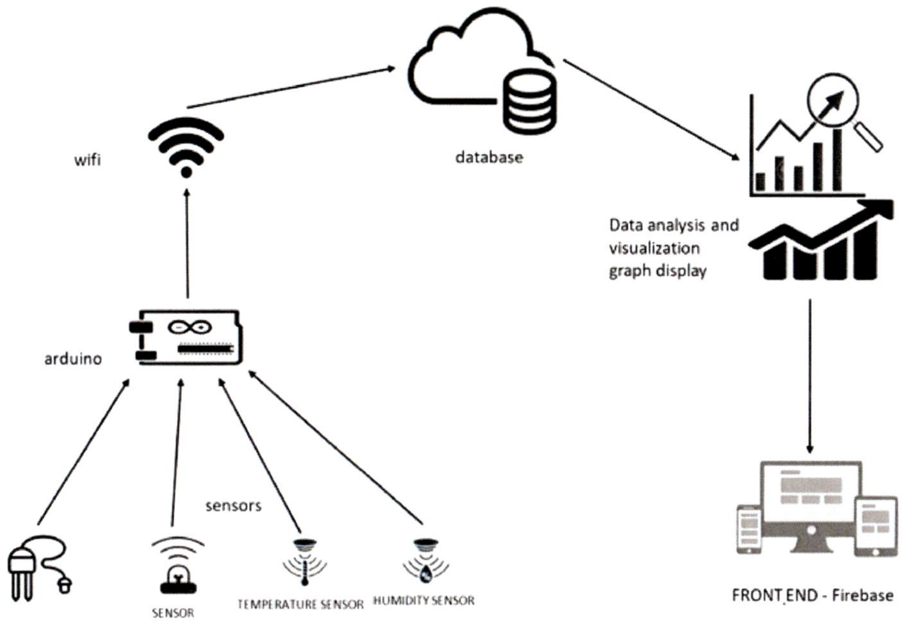

Fig. 5.5 Design framework

The Arduino Uno is a microcontroller board that evolved from the ATmega328P. It has 6 analog inputs, 14 input/output digital pins, a USB port, a power jack, a 16 MHz ceramic resonator, a reset button, and an ICSP header. It includes everything needed to make the microcontroller's functions easier. NodeMCU—This package includes a Wi-Fi-enabled ESP8266 chip. This is a low-cost Wi-Fi chip built by Espressif Systems, which uses the TCP/IP protocol. GPIOpins, 17 of them, are integrated into the chip. Relay Module—A relay module is an electrically powered switch that can be turned on or off, allowing current to flow, and it can be controlled with small voltages, similar to the voltage supplied by the Arduino pins. A Liquid Crystal Display, or LCD for short, is a flat-paneled display that uses liquid crystals as the primary mode of operation [76].

The plotting of various graphs with real-time values obtained from the sensors is done with the aid of Python code. The plot of the number of times the pump was turned on is shown below. The graph shows how many times the pump was turned on that specific day. It can be used to determine which day the soil water level was the lowest, as well as what caused it. Figure 5.6 shows pump use as a frequency plot. Figure 5.7 expresses the plot for pump use. Figure 5.8 represents the average moisture content plot.

The average time the pump was held on those specific days is plotted in the Average time of Pump Consumption Analysis. The soil conditions are depicted in the pie chart above. The soil can be subjected to a variety of conditions. Just a few types of crops can be grown in the soil depending on the conditions. This graph can be used to forecast the same. Daily temperature averages (in Celsius) can be plotted

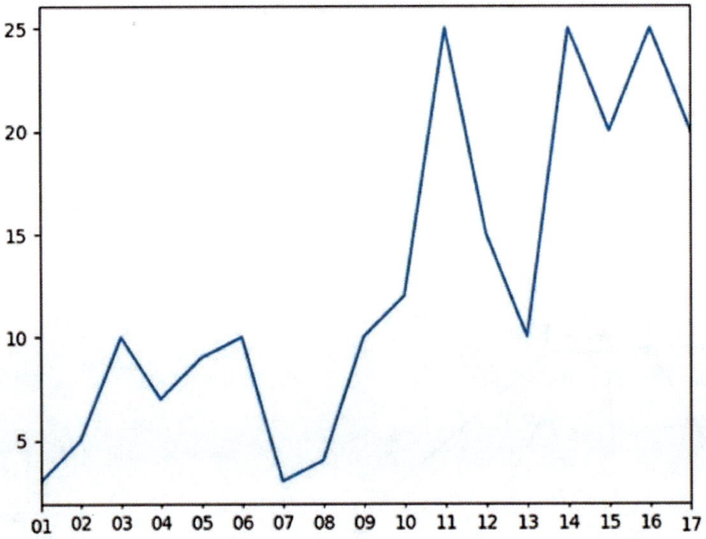

Fig. 5.6 Pump use as a frequency plot

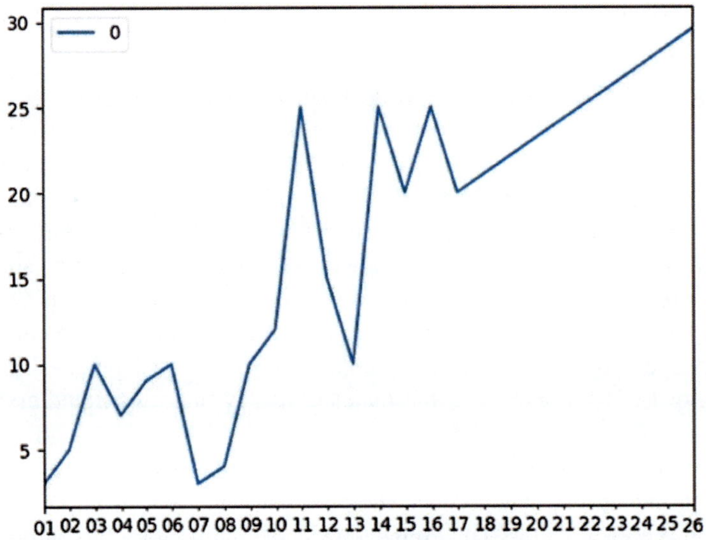

Fig. 5.7 Plot for pump use

against the number of days in a line chart to display the closer difference over time. The sensor values, as well as the real-time values, can be uploaded to the Firebase real-time database and accessed at any time.

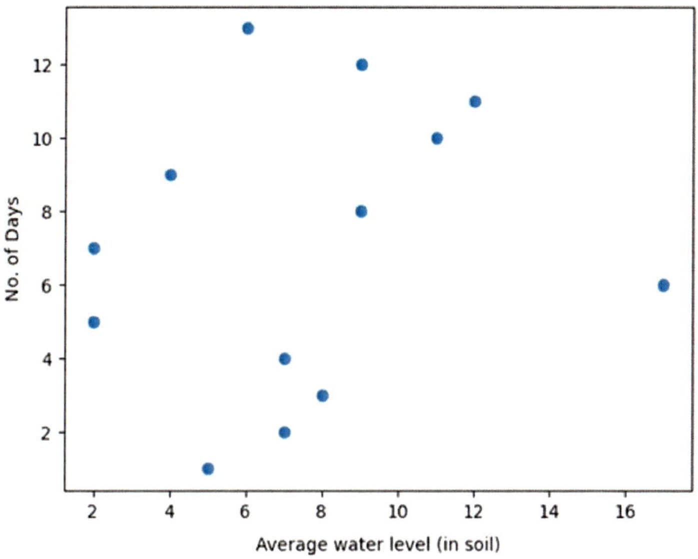

Fig. 5.8 Average moisture content plot

5.10 Main Challenges and Open Issues

There are a variety of problems involved with IoT implementation and application. Privacy and security, information integration and proprietorship, need for compatibility [77], diverseness of IoT appliances, and complexity in commercial frameworks are some of the problems found in the company, technological, and sectored topics are the three major categories in which we address issues.

5.10.1 Commercial Concerns

Since the gain limit in agriculture is so thin, there is a need to find a balance between the distribution of IoT warranting technologies and the future gains. As a consequence, our own selves consider cost and market models when addressing business problems relevant to IoT rollout [78].

(1) Price: There are two types of costs associated with IoT implementation in agriculture: configuration and operating costs. The cost of configuration requires the procurement of hardware (IoT appliances, base terminals frameworks).

Continuous subscriptions for centralized networks or IoT systems, that offer information gathering, maintenance of IoT appliances, and knowledge allocation, among various aids, are included in the operating expense. Costs associated with data sharing between IoT computers, gateways, and cloud servers, as well as energy and upkeep, are all added operating costs. According to [79], the Internet of Things must meet two criteria: (1) users must be convinced that the IoT appliances have a benefit that outweighs the physical and privacy costs and (2) IoT companies must be able to earn funds. The initial circumstances may be indicated

$$\left(W_s - D_{pri} - D_h^{user} - D_{pay}\right) > 0 \tag{5.1}$$

where W_s is the user's perceived value, D_{pri} is the cost of privacy loss, $D_h{}^{user}$ involves the expenditure of hardware peripherals along with related assistances, and D_{pay} denotes the amount for servicing cost, while the second state may be denoted as

$$\left(W_{info} + S_{pay} - D_h^{business}\right) > 0 \tag{5.2}$$

where W_{info} denotes the value for record obtained, S_{pay} denotes the cost of hardware along with associated services, and $D_h{}^{business}$ denotes the organization's quota for hardware peripherals along with maintaining expenditure.

Although the usefulness of the information collected is intended to provide the customer with the services they need, it may be economically abused by service providers during procurement of such services. While few IoT network suppliers facilitate free of charge premium packages with restricted availability, such as a restricted quantity in IoT appliances, which may be linked along with a restricted quantity of data, which may be stored, others charge for their services. Higher subscription fees are attracted by more functionality and facilities.

(2) Models of Business: Farmers are interested in business models that enable them to generate revenue from the records collected on their farmland utilizing IoT frameworks. The majority of current IoT platform resource suppliers facilitate free restricted assistances as well as full assistances in various subscription levels. The data generated is abused by IoT service providers, and farmers' management and possession of their data remain a point of contention [80].

(3) Inadequate Awareness: A crucial constituent delaying the acquisition of IoT for farming is a shortage of enough expertise of IoT along with its applications, especially among cultivators in rural locations. It is typical in developed nations, where the vast maximum cultivators live in village locations and are generally uneducated. If human interference is not available, the cultivator's incompetence to utilize knowledge may be a big hindrance [81].

5.10.2 Technical Concerns

(1) Interference: Widespread implementation for IoT appliances in farming along with various motives would create interference, mainly with IoT appliances that use the unapproved spectrum. (Look Table 2). The resulting intrusion may result in data losing along with reducing the IoT ecosystem's dependability. The

technologies required to make IoT devices that operate on unlicensed spectrum interference-free would increase the device's cost. The use of IoT systems that operate on approved bandwidth, on the other hand, is intended to minimize unwanted interference. Due to the restricted pilot task in the cellular spectrum, however, reutilization for non-orthogonal numerous communication schemes along with frequency reuse may moreover produce interference among IoT appliances utilizing cellular authorized spectrum [82].

(2) Privacy along with Security: At various levels of the IoT ecosystem, there are many security concerns that must be resolved. Inadequate protection may result in data loss, breach of privacy, along with access to raw data regarding on-field criteria along with other important intelligent characteristics. It will jeopardize private farm owners' competitive advantages. The topics of IoT stability (Park, D.S. 2018) and privacy have been thoroughly explored in ref. [83]. Security was deemed a significant challenge in the implementation of IoT, according to Asplund and Nadjm [84] Tehrani's interview-based research on attitudes and perceptions of IoT. At various levels of the IoT ecosystem, there are many security concerns that must be resolved.

Physical malpractices, like burglary or assaults by carnivores along with animals, as well as a change of physical address or connection, render IoT devices vulnerable in agriculture. Furthermore, because of restricted memory, networking capacities, along with lower energy utilization, complex and sophisticated algorithms are difficult to incorporate in IoT devices. Congestion, DoS, along with forwarding assaults will all affect the gateway. Device capture attacks expose the confidentiality and location of data and IoT allowed location-dependent services utilized for accuracy agriculture to assaults. An intruder arrests an IoT appliance and steals encrypted executions, as well as having unlimited privilege to the data contained in the appliance's database, in a device capture attack. DoS threats and man-in-the-middle attacks will all affect higher connectivity layers. Furthermore, cloud servers are vulnerable to information meddling and unwarranted assistances that can disrupt farm automation. Session hijacking, server accession supremacy and repository problems, hijacking intrusions, login assault, along with Denial of Services are various other security threats that may harm cloud framework [85].

(3) Technology Selection: Many IoT technologies have recently been introduced, several of which are still undergoing pilot testing. Since emerging developments need a lot of money, making the best IoT technology option is a huge challenge. It's impossible to foresee the current IoT innovations would control the scenario at this time. Various considerations must be weighed, including roaming service, infrastructure suitability for small-, medium-, and large-scale applications, and suitability for various geographical locations, soil categories, and climatic situations [86].

(4) Accuracy: IoT appliances would most likely be used in an outdoor ambience. It would subject the instruments to extreme environments, potentially resulting in sensor loss and connectivity errors over time. To safeguard the expensive tools from adverse weather situations including flooding and cyclones, the

physical protection for the stationed IoT sensors along with infrastructures will be assured.

(5) Scalability: The agriculture sector is expected to install billions of IoT units. Existing gateways and protocols would need to be able to handle a huge number of IoT appliances and systems.

(6) Localization: When it comes to IoT system rollout, there are many things to consider. The ability of the IoT system to help position and play features, i.e. the ability to be put anywhere and linked to the internet, is one of these considerations, the remaining planet with minimum supplementary system implementation. Various considerations include the optimal location for the IoT system to have acceptable data and stability without risking minimal interference. Furthermore, the potential in enabling IoT system roaming for roaming IoT appliances as well as the implementation of fixed IoT appliances in a region excluding previous understanding of mobile IoT framework must be taken into granted [87].

(7) Resource Management: Cultivators require a resource accession process in deciding the number of gateways; IoT computers, communicated record volumes, and cloud repository capacity are required in achieving a development in gain extents. It is made more difficult by various farmland dimensions along with types of sensors used in tracking farm parameters for unique crops. To evaluate optimum resource allocation while reducing costs and optimizing agricultural produce and income, complex algorithms [88] and mathematical models will be needed.

5.10.3 Sectoral Issues

(1) Policy Issues: Farmers and data providers must iron out their discrepancies in regulation and ownership of farm data. In terminology of asset distribution (viz. spectrum of cellular IoT), technological issues, competitiveness, information protection, and privacy, rules can vary from country to country. Different laws in different regions or countries can have an effect on the use of IoT in applications like monitoring and agricultural food supply [89].

(2) Exchangeability: Protocols and standards are currently being established to allow billions of IoT devices to communicate with one another. Functional, syntactic, semantic, and organizational interoperability are all involved. Scientific exchangeability entails the burgeoning of protocols along with infrastructure, which enable IoT appliances in connecting with one another. It's normally aligned with the IoT ecosystem's hardware and device elements. Information forms like XML, JSON, CSVs, along with digital information exchange as normal syntax for data transmission are synonymous with syntactical interoperability. Semantic interoperability is concerned with the representation of knowledge shared through humans. The ability to efficiently connect and

transmit data through diverse infrastructure, geographic regions, and communities is referred to as organizational interoperability. As a result, all systems must have transport facilities or API access, which gives back common forms, like JSON/XML that must be supplied with suitable exchange gateways where possible.

Exchangeability may be accomplished in three ways, according to (1) collaborations between software along with solution formulators; (2) open along with closed levels; and (3) negotiator assistances. Interoperability in IoT is being promoted by organizations such as open networking in order to achieve it. In addition, adapter services, such as if this then that, are currently being used to enable clients in constructing robust relations along with bonds of easy dependent announcements. Due to scalability, most of the techniques could not be able to facilitate broadly authorized exchangeability across IoT appliances. For achieving better feasibility for various IoT appliances along with facilities, further job is needed in the advancements of open levels.

5.10.4 Conclusion

If not tackled properly, the open topics and threats mentioned in the section may lead to the steady acquisition of IoT for the farming sector. More studies related to the financial advantages of IoT adoption in farming are required. Farmers will continue to emphasize privacy and security considerations, though this is likely to change as people get more used to IoT and its services. Small to mid-scale cultivators must install IoT frameworks as the expenditure of IoT appliances along with information collection, filtering, and transport decreases over time.

5.11 Future Opportunities and Trends

We portray upcoming developments depending on the succeeding regions, based on our education along with reviews of existing patterns for the implementation of IoT in farming:

(1) Technical breakthroughs, (2) implementation scenarios, and (3) commercial viability and marketability.

5.11.1 Scientific Progress

More IoT solutions will appear in the future, bringing with them new and revolutionary innovations, mainly in the farming domain. Below are most of the places that were found.

(1) LPWA Technology Deployment: The LPWA is projected to command the farming domain due to its numerous benefits, including lower power and longer-span connectivity. The delivery in the 3GPP NB-IoT specification along with widespread acceptance by telcos would pique interest in research into the utilization of NB-IoT networking frameworks. It would make heavy-scale IoT pilot tests in farming possible.

(2) Common policies: The creation of IoT platforms in farming would step away from particular crops and toward a common framework (called general objectives), which will serve any crops. It would make for a device that can be readily adapted to accommodate a range of uses, such as crop and livestock management and tracking, as well as retail sales to local retailers and customers. Such a method will be devoid of all spatial or ethnic constraints, and it will be able to support a wide range of IoT in farming.

(3) Protection: IoT device protection along with end-to-end information security may lead to being hot topics in science. In order to improve IoT devices that may reinforce newer encryption schemes, like the state-of-the-art signcryption approach, further research is needed. To avoid eavesdropping and unwanted modification of classified information, signcryption blends digital signature along with cryptography. Security measures to protect IoT devices from physical attackers and intruders must be scrutinized, and newer approaches must be designed.

(4) Energy Competency: To meet the LPWA specifications, various approaches like narrowband channels along with spread spectrum are utilized. Newer technology that may accommodate speedier data, lengthy distance provision, enormous track-loss connection costs, along with increased battery viability are expected as more LPWA compliant solutions are deployed. Currently, the most cellular NB-IoT structures accept frequency bands that run in frequency division duplex mode. In bands that use time division duplex modes, further work is required. Other testing problems, such as pilot pollution, will arise as a result of this.

    Although LPWA focuses for a 10-year battery life, IoT devices also need energy-efficient mechanisms because performance is mainly based on the use of node. Various approaches for energy efficiency in WSNs have been developed, including classification along with inter-network processing approaches. Various power-saving IoT systems, capacity in forecasting the sleep duration of IoT appliances depending on the residual battery level, historical use experience, and the quality of knowledge needed by a specific application, may be investigated additionally. The use of excellent wireless energy transmission allowed IoT transceiver frameworks, parallel wireless records and energy transmission in IoT, and power collecting IoT appliances is anticipated to pique attentiveness in the research community.

(5) QoS: Research on IoT QoS indicates that QoS is expected at any level of the framework. A need to certify that a computer that wants to transmit vital information will do it by utilizing IoT and various networking technologies is also a research field in progress. In contrast to LoRa, the usage of NB-IoT transmission technique guarantees a higher quality of service. Major work is to be maintained to develop mechanisms, which ensure quality of service across the various IoT network levels.

(6) Artificial Intelligence and Data Analytics: Various researches into the usage of AI to prototype crop growing along with illness organization depending on agricultural information and weather knowledge are required. The utilization of ML for illness identification through pictures sent via mobile phones is an example. It is anticipated that DA algorithms can be built, which can exercise vast amounts of information at a much greater speed than IoT contact time.

(7) Privacy Preservation: To address the problem of IoT data privacy breaches, terminal-to-terminal secured-preservation approaches that facilitate the extrication of information from information while protecting the security of one-self is suggested. Examples of the proposed strategies for maintaining a minimum degree of security when optimizing the usefulness of information are categorized depending on the information life-cycle period where privacy is assured. Further study into the implementation of the proposed privacy protection approaches and how they can increase IoT adoption in the agriculture field is possible.

(8) Data Compression: While more IoT devices become connected, advanced compression and multiplexing techniques would be needed for data sharing from hundreds to lakhs of wireless sensors to a centralized position. When using NB-IoT cellular connectivity, this will be especially important for transmitting images and video data. Multiplexing would also aid in the consolidation of information from various farmlands into a unit position, allowing for support, monitoring, along with maintenance from a lone location.

(9) Spontaneous-Time Tracking: Since thousands of various categories of sensors will be installed for the area in spontaneous-time tracking, a basic internetwork management protocol will be needed in allowing connectivity amidst entities along with the server containing the least amount of overhead. Present protocols are depicted primarily for internetwork equipment and which results in increased data traffic and network latency and also increased energy demands for IoT appliances.

5.11.2 Scenarios for Implementation

Software frameworks and IoT applications are currently being developed, and research on connectivity technology that may provide lower-price IoT arrangements is continuing. The majority of the current work is focused on small-scale prototyping and research. To assess the accessibility and utility in IoT frameworks in farming, large-scale pilots are needed. More larger-scale pilots in the whole supply chain along with agricultural-food implementations will be conducted in near future, not just in developed countries but also in emerging nations in Asia along with Africa.

5.11.3 Marketability Along with Business

(1) Expenditure curtailing: The cost for IoT solutions for agriculture is projected to decrease as the power demand of IoT devices is minimized, physical size is reduced, and mass production is increased. Future studies will include the invention of less expensive sensors, research into the use of a combination of authorized and unauthorized transmission techniques in reducing setup along with operational costs, and exploration of the usage of mixed authorized and unauthorized transmission technique in reducing layout and utilization costs.

(2) Strategies and Rules: Much effort is needed to be done on policy compliance and similarity in the usage of IoT in farming. When designing policies and regulations for IoT in agriculture, government participation or involvement from the agriculture department must be assured, as described in Section VI-C. It may help IoT acquisition in farming to get off to a good start.

5.12 Conclusion

In this article, an outline of Internet of Things and Data Analytics in farming is given. Several aspects of IoT application in agriculture have been thoroughly explored. According to a review of the literature, there is a lot of work being done to evolve IoT technologies that can be used to improve plant and livestock operating production and productivity. This paper explains and addresses the advantages of IoT and DA, as well as transparent problems. The agricultural industry is supposed to benefit from the Internet of Things in a number of ways. However, a variety of problems must be tackled in order for small- and medium-scale farmers to manage them. Security and cost are the most critical factors. As the agriculture market becomes more competitive and more favorable policies are adopted, the adoption rate of IoT in agriculture is projected to rise. The application of LPWA connectivity technologies for agricultural purposes is one big field that is expected to receive a lot of research interest. Among the LPWA innovations, the NB-Internet of Things is anticipated to stand out. This is due to telco operators' implementation of the 3GPP open standard.

References

1. Aba EN, Olugboji OA, Nasir A et al (2021) Petroleum pipeline monitoring using an internet of things (IoT) platform. SN Appl Sci 3:180. https://doi.org/10.1007/s42452-021-04225-z
2. Amoran AE, Oluwole AS, Fagorola EO, Diarah RS (2021) Home automated system using Bluetooth and an android application. Sci Afr **11**
3. Afreen H, Bajwa IS (2021) An IoT based real-time intelligent monitoring and notification system of cold storage. IEEE Access Digit Object Identif. https://doi.org/10.1109/ACCESS.2021.3056672
4. Ahmad I (2021) Discover internet of things editorial, inaugural issue. Discov Internet Things 1:1. https://doi.org/10.1007/s43926-021-00007-6
5. Alilou M, Tousi B, Shayeghi H (2021) Multi-objective energy management of smart homes considering uncertainty in wind power forecasting. Electr Eng. https://doi.org/10.1007/s00202-020-01165-6
6. Villa-Henriksen A, Edwards GTC, Pesonen LA, Green O, Sørensen CAG (2020)
7. Barth M (2021) A case study on data portability. Datenschutz Datensich 45:190–197. https://doi.org/10.1007/s11623-021-1416-3
8. Bozorgi SM, Hajiabadi MR, Hosseinabadi AAR et al (2021) Clustering based on whale optimization algorithm for IoT over wireless nodes. Soft Comput 25:5663–5682. https://doi.org/10.1007/s00500-020-05563-7
9. Chehri A, Chaibi H, Saadane R, Hakem N, Wahbi M (2020) A framework of optimizing the deployment of IoT for precision agriculture industry. Procedia Comput Sci 176:2414–2422
10. Wu CH, Cheng TY, Liu HC (2014) A multi-to-one short-range wireless communication system for the smart ICU physiology telemetry system. In: IEEE International conference on consumer electronics, Taiwan, Taipei, Taiwan, pp 25–26. https://doi.org/10.1109/ICCE-TW.2014.6904083
11. Cvitić I, Peraković D, Periša M et al (2021) Ensemble machine learning approach for classification of IoT devices in smart home. Int J Mach Learn Cyber. https://doi.org/10.1007/s13042-020-01241-0
12. Divyapriya S, Amudha A, Vijayakumar R (2021) Design of solar smart street light powered plug-in electric vehicle charging station by using internet of things. J Inst Eng India Ser B. https://doi.org/10.1007/s40031-021-00548-y
13. Duraimurugan S, Avudaiammal R, Vincent PMDR (2021) Enhanced QoS through optimized architecture for video streaming applications in heterogeneous networks. Wirel Pers Commun. https://doi.org/10.1007/s11277-021-08109-8
14. Feng D, Lai L, Luo J et al (2021) Ultra-reliable and low-latency communications: applications, opportunities and challenges. Sci China Inf Sci 64:120301. https://doi.org/10.1007/s11432-020-2852-1
15. Fizza K, Banerjee A, Mitra K et al (2021) QoE in IoT: a vision, survey and future directions. Discov Internet Things 1:4. https://doi.org/10.1007/s43926-021-00006-7
16. Gautam AK, Kumar R (2021) A comprehensive study on key management, authentication and trust management techniques in wireless sensor networks. SN Appl Sci 3:50. https://doi.org/10.1007/s42452-020-04089-9
17. Goel SS, Goel A, Kumar M et al (2021) A review of Internet of Things: qualifying technologies and boundless horizon. J Reliab Intell Environ 7:23–33. https://doi.org/10.1007/s40860-020-00127-w
18. Huo C, Liu L, Bai HF (2021) Physical impairments awareness based virtual network mapping strategy of elastic optical networks. Optoelectron Lett 17:36–39. https://doi.org/10.1007/s11801-021-0029-2
19. Hu Q, Jiang C, Du L et al (2021) Control system design and implementation at flexible, distributed offshore sensor test sites in the Yangtze Estuary area. J Ocean Univ China 20:285–295. https://doi.org/10.1007/s11802-021-4469-x

20. Samanta D, Sanyal G (2012) A novel approach of SAR image classification using color space clustering and watersheds. In: 2012 Fourth international conference on computational intelligence and communication networks, Mathura, India, pp 237–240. https://doi.org/10.1109/CICN.2012.27.
21. Khamparia A, Singh PK, Rani P, Samanta D, Khanna A, Bhushan B (2020) An internet of health things-driven deep learning framework for detection and classification of skin cancer using transfer learning. Trans Emerg Tel Tech e3963. https://doi.org/10.1002/ett.3963
22. Hossain MA, Samanta D, Sanyal G (2012) Statistical approach for extraction of panic expression. In: 2012 Fourth international conference on computational intelligence and communication networks, Mathura, India, pp 420–424. https://doi.org/10.1109/CICN.2012.189
23. Althar RR, Samanta D (2021) The realist approach for evaluation of computational intelligence in software engineering. Innov Syst Softw Eng. https://doi.org/10.1007/s11334-020-00383-2
24. Singh RK, Begum T, Borah L, Samanta D (2017) Text encryption: character jumbling. In: 2017 International conference on inventive systems and control (ICISC), Coimbatore, India, pp 1–3. https://doi.org/10.1109/ICISC.2017.8068691.
25. Guha A, Samanta D (2021) Hybrid approach to document anomaly detection: an application to facilitate RPA in title insurance. Int J Autom Comput 18:55–72. https://doi.org/10.1007/s11633-020-1247-y
26. Agarwal M, Sarkhel D, Samanta D (2018) Architecture of 'loop' without 'for' & 'while'. In: 2018 2nd International conference on inventive systems and control (ICISC), Coimbatore, India, pp 491–494. https://doi.org/10.1109/ICISC.2018.8399121.
27. Samanta D, Sivaram M, Rashed A, Boopathi CS, Sadegh Amiri I, Yupapin P (2020) Distributed feedback laser (DFB) for signal power amplitude level improvement in long spectral band. J Opt Commun. https://doi.org/10.1515/joc-2019-0252
28. Chakrabarti S, Samanta D (2015) Notice of removal: a novel approach to digital image steganography of key-based encrypted text. In: 2015 International conference on electrical, electronics, signals, communication and optimization (EESCO), Visakhapatnam, India, pp 1–6. https://doi.org/10.1109/EESCO.2015.7254009.
29. Pramanik S, Samanta D, Bandyopadhyay S, Ghosh R. A new combinational technique in image steganography. Int J Inf Secur Privacy (IJISP) 15(3). ISSN: 1930-1650|EISSN: 1930-1669
30. Ibrahim M, Abdullah MT, Abdullah A et al (2021) The impact of memory-efficient bots on iot-wsn botnet propagation. Wirel Pers Commun. https://doi.org/10.1007/s11277-021-08320-7
31. Jan MA, He X, Song H et al (2021) Machine learning and big data analytics for IoT-enabled smart cities. Mob Netw Appl. https://doi.org/10.1007/s11036-020-01702-4
32. Jo S, Lee J, Han J et al (2020) P2P computing for intelligence of things. Peer-to-Peer Netw Appl 13:575–578. https://doi.org/10.1007/s12083-020-00887-5
33. Jurcut A, Niculcea T, Ranaweera P et al (2020) Security considerations for internet of things: a survey. SN Comput Sci 1:193. https://doi.org/10.1007/s42979-020-00201-3
34. Khanna A, Kaur S (2020) Internet of Things (IoT), applications and challenges: a comprehensive review. Wirel Pers Commun 114:1687–1762. https://doi.org/10.1007/s11277-020-07446-4
35. Kilian A, Obi E, Mansiangi P et al (2021) Variation of physical durability between LLIN products and net use environments: summary of findings from four African countries. Malar J 20:26. https://doi.org/10.1186/s12936-020-03549-2
36. Koutras D, Stergiopoulos G, Dasaklis T, Kotzanikolaou P, Glynos D, Douligeris C (2020) Security in IoMT communications: a survey. Sensors 20(17):4828. https://doi.org/10.3390/s20174828
37. Kuzlu M, Fair C, Guler O (2021) Role of artificial intelligence in the internet of things (IoT) cybersecurity. Discov Internet Things 1:7. https://doi.org/10.1007/s43926-020-00001-4
38. Leduc G (2000) Verification of two versions of the challenge handshake authentication protocol (chap). Ann Télécommun 55:20–30. https://doi.org/10.1007/BF02997769
39. Lee B, Lee JH (2017) Blockchain-based secure firmware update for embedded devices in an Internet of Things environment. J Supercomput 73:1152–1167. https://doi.org/10.1007/s11227-016-1870-0

40. Li W, Chai Y, Khan F et al (2021) A comprehensive survey on machine learning-based big data analytics for IoT-enabled smart healthcare system. Mob Netw Appl. https://doi.org/10.1007/s11036-020-01700-6
41. Liu D, Xu X, Liu M et al (2021) Dynamic traffic classification algorithm and simulation of energy Internet of things based on machine learning. Neural Comput Appl. https://doi.org/10.1007/s00521-020-05457-7
42. Liu Q, Mkongwa KG, Zhang C (2021) Performance issues in wireless body area networks for the healthcare application: a survey and future prospects. SN Appl Sci 3:155. https://doi.org/10.1007/s42452-020-04058-2
43. Mahbub M (2020) NB-IoT: applications and future prospects in perspective of Bangladesh. Int J Inf Tecnol 12:1183–1193. https://doi.org/10.1007/s41870-020-00469-x
44. Mouton S (2021) Generalized spectral perturbation and the boundary spectrum. Czech Math J. https://doi.org/10.21136/CMJ.2021.0046-20
45. Nadian-Ghomsheh A, Farahani B, Kavian M (2021) A hierarchical privacy-preserving IoT architecture for vision-based hand rehabilitation assessment. Multimed Tools Appl. https://doi.org/10.1007/s11042-021-10563-2
46. Navarro E, Costa N, Pereira A (2020) A systematic review of IoT solutions for smart farming. Sensors 20(15):4231. https://doi.org/10.3390/s20154231
47. Nazarov LE, Zudilin AS, Kaevitser VI et al (2021) Algorithms for the encoding and reception of OFDM signals based on manipulation with minimum frequency shift. J Commun Technol Electron 66:56–61. https://doi.org/10.1134/S106422692101006X
48. Olsson M (2020) Error handling. In: PHP 8 quick scripting reference. Apress, Berkeley, CA. https://doi.org/10.1007/978-1-4842-6619-9_29
49. Orsini F (2020) Innovation and sustainability in urban agriculture: the path forward. J Consum Prot Food Saf 15:203–204. https://doi.org/10.1007/s00003-020-01293-y
50. Panahi P, Bayılmış C, Çavuşoğlu U et al (2020) Performance evaluation of lightweight encryption algorithms for IoT-based applications. Arab J Sci Eng 46:4015–4037. https://doi.org/10.1007/s13369-021-05358-4
51. Podder SK, Samanta D (2019) Impact of climate changes on rural livelihoods and re-orienting the situation through human resources towards a sustainable society. In: Proceedings of international conference on sustainable computing in science, technology and management (SUSCOM), Amity University Rajasthan, Jaipur-India, February 26–28, 2019. Available at SSRN: https://ssrn.com/abstract=3355347 or https://doi.org/10.2139/ssrn.3355347
52. Pradhan KN, Siddappa M, Kavitha S, Samanta D (2019) Analysis & improvement of wireless network security based on biometrics. In: Proceedings of international conference on sustainable computing in science, technology and management (SUSCOM), Amity University Rajasthan, Jaipur, India, February 26–28, 2019. Available at SSRN: https://ssrn.com/abstract=3356360 or https://doi.org/10.2139/ssrn.3356360
53. Karthikeyan MP, Samanta D, Banerjee A, Roy A, Inokawa H (2021) Design and development of terahertz medical screening devices. In: Chakraborty M, Jha RK, Balas VE, Sur SN, Kandar D (eds) Trends in wireless communication and information security. Lecture notes in electrical engineering, vol 740. Springer, Singapore. https://doi.org/10.1007/978-981-33-6393-9_40
54. Althar RR, Samanta D (2021) Building intelligent integrated development environment for IoT in the context of statistical modeling for software source code. In: Kumar R, Sharma R, Pattnaik PK (eds) Multimedia technologies in the internet of things environment. Studies in Big Data, vol 79. Springer, Singapore. https://doi.org/10.1007/978-981-15-7965-3_7
55. Podder SK, Samanta D, Gurunath R (2020) Impact of business analytics for smart education system and management functions. In: Sharma H, Govindan K, Poonia R, Kumar S, El-Medany W (eds) Advances in computing and intelligent systems. Algorithms for intelligent systems. Springer, Singapore. https://doi.org/10.1007/978-981-15-0222-4_45
56. Sarkhel D, Deka D, Samanta D, Kumudavalli M, Le DN (2020) GUI-based percentage analysis for curing breast cancer survivors. In: Satapathy S, Bhateja V, Nguyen B, Nguyen N, Le DN (eds) Frontiers in intelligent computing: theory and applications. Advances in intelligent systems and computing, vol 1013. Springer, Singapore. https://doi.org/10.1007/978-981-32-9186-7_33

57. Praveen B, Samanta D, Prasad G, Ranjith Kumar C, Prasad MLM (2020) Protecting medical research data using next gen steganography approach. In: Jain L, Peng SL, Alhadidi B, Pal S (eds) Intelligent computing paradigm and cutting-edge technologies. ICICCT 2019. Learning and analytics in intelligent systems, vol 9. Springer, Cham. https://doi.org/10.1007/978-3-030-38501-9_34
58. Guha A, Samanta D (2020) Real-time application of document classification based on machine learning. In: Jain L, Peng SL, Alhadidi B, Pal S (eds) Intelligent computing paradigm and cutting-edge technologies. ICICCT 2019. Learning and analytics in intelligent systems, vol 9. Springer, Cham. https://doi.org/10.1007/978-3-030-38501-9_37
59. Chakrabarti S, Samanta D (2016) Image steganography using priority-based neural network and pyramid. In: Shetty N, Prasad N, Nalini N (eds) Emerging research in computing, information, communication and applications. Springer, Singapore. https://doi.org/10.1007/978-981-10-0287-8_15
60. Samanta D, Sanyal G (2012) Novel Shannon's entropy based segmentation technique for SAR images. In: Venugopal KR, Patnaik LM (eds) wireless networks and computational intelligence. ICIP 2012. Communications in computer and information science, vol 292. Springer, Berlin, Heidelberg. https://doi.org/10.1007/978-3-642-31686-9_22
61. Hossain MA, Samanta D, Sanyal G (2012) Extraction of panic expression from human face based on histogram approach. In: Venugopal KR, Patnaik LM (eds) Wireless networks and computational intelligence. ICIP 2012. Communications in computer and information science, vol 292. Springer, Berlin, Heidelberg. https://doi.org/10.1007/978-3-642-31686-9_48
62. Samanta D, Sanyal G (2011) Development of edge detection technique for images using adaptive thresholding. In: Venugopal KR, Patnaik LM (eds) Computer networks and intelligent computing. ICIP 2011. Communications in computer and information science, vol 157. Springer, Berlin, Heidelberg. https://doi.org/10.1007/978-3-642-22786-8_85
63. Park DS (2018) Future computing with IoT and cloud computing. J Supercomput 74:6401–6407. https://doi.org/10.1007/s11227-018-2652-7
64. Pham HX, Shamseldin AY, Melville BW (2021) Projection of future extreme precipitation: a robust assessment of downscaled daily precipitation. Nat Hazards. https://doi.org/10.1007/s11069-021-04584-1
65. Qin J, Li Z, Wang R et al (2020) Industrial internet of learning (IIoL): IIoT based pervasive knowledge network for LPWAN—concept, framework and case studies. CCF Trans Pervasive Comp Interact 3:25–39. https://doi.org/10.1007/s42486-020-00050-2
66. Qiu S, Allan R, Nilavalan R et al (2021) Performance analysis of a fail-safe wireless communication architecture for IoT based fire alarm control panels. SN Appl Sci 3:379. https://doi.org/10.1007/s42452-021-04400-2
67. Rachit BS, Ragiri PR (2021) Security trends in internet of things: a survey. SN Appl Sci 3:121. https://doi.org/10.1007/s42452-021-04156-9
68. Raghavendra YM, Mahadevaswamy UB (2021) Energy efficient intra cluster gateway optimal placement in wireless sensor network. Wirel Pers Commun. https://doi.org/10.1007/s11277-021-08247-z
69. Rajasekar SJS (2021) An enhanced IoT based tracing and tracking model for COVID-19 Cases. SN Comput Sci 2:42. https://doi.org/10.1007/s42979-020-00400-y
70. Rehman Au, Syed AR, Khan IU et al (2020) IoT-enabled smart socket. Wirel Pers Commun 116:1151–1169. https://doi.org/10.1007/s11277-020-07043-5
71. Saini J, Dutta M, Marques G (2021) Sensors for indoor air quality monitoring and assessment through Internet of Things: a systematic review. Environ Monit Assess 193:66. https://doi.org/10.1007/s10661-020-08781-6
72. Sandoval MM, Flores LAR, Cumplido R, Hernandez JJG, Feregrino C, Algredo I (2021) A compact FPGA based accelerator for curve based cryptography in wireless sensor networks. J Sens. https://doi.org/10.1155/2021/8860413
73. Savaglio C, Fortini G (2021) A simulation driven methodology for IoT data mining based on edge computing. ACM Trans Internet Technol. https://doi.org/10.1145/3402444

74. Schmickl S, Faseth T, Pretl H (2021) Microwatt power management: challenges of on-chip energy harvesting. Elektrotech Inftech 138:31–36. https://doi.org/10.1007/s00502-020-00859-w
75. Shafique K, Khawaja BA, Sabir F, Qazi S, Mustaqim M (2020) Internet of things for next-generation smart systems: a review of current challenges, future trends and prospects for emerging 5G-IoT scenarios. IEEE Access. https://doi.org/10.1109/ACCESS.2020.2970118
76. Singh M, Baranwal G, Tripathi AK (2020) QoS-aware selection of IoT-based service. Arab J Sci Eng 45:10033–10050. https://doi.org/10.1007/s13369-020-04601-8
77. Singh KK, Elngar AA, Izonin (2021) Reliability and usability of machine learning and IoT for urban intelligence. J Reliab Intell Environ 7:1–2. https://doi.org/10.1007/s40860-021-00135-4
78. Spanaki K, Sivarajah U, Fakhimi M et al (2021) Disruptive technologies in agricultural operations: a systematic review of AI-driven AgriTech research. Ann Oper Res. https://doi.org/10.1007/s10479-020-03922-z
79. Rao KR, Samanta D, Somashekara MT, Gurunath R, Paul A (2019) Automatic segmentation based graphical interface for recognition of tomography image analysis of damage cell. In: 2019 Third international conference on inventive systems and control (ICISC), Coimbatore, India, pp 52–55. https://doi.org/10.1109/ICISC44355.2019.9036343
80. Gurunath R, Agarwal M, Nandi A, Samanta D (2018) An overview: security issue in IoT network. In: 2018 2nd International conference on I-SMAC (IoT in social, mobile, analytics and cloud), Palladam, India, pp 104–107. https://doi.org/10.1109/I-SMAC.2018.8653728
81. Ghosh G, Samanta D, Paul M (2016) Approach of message communication based on twisty "Zig-Zag". In: 2016 International conference on emerging technological trends (ICETT), Kollam, pp 1–5. https://doi.org/10.1109/ICETT.2016.7873676
82. Dhanush V, Mahendra AR, Kumudavalli MV, Samanta D (2017) Application of deep learning technique for automatic data exchange with air-gapped systems and its security concerns. In: 2017 International conference on computing methodologies and communication (ICCMC), Erode, India, pp 324–328. https://doi.org/10.1109/ICCMC.2017.8282701.
83. Hossain MA, Samanta D, Sanyal G (2012) Extraction of panic expression depending on lip detection. In: 2012 International conference on computing sciences, Phagwara, India, pp 137–141. https://doi.org/10.1109/ICCS.2012.35
84. Hossain MA, Samanta D, Sanyal G (2012) A novel approach for panic-face extraction based on mutation. In: 2012 IEEE International conference on advanced communication control and computing technologies (ICACCCT), Ramanathapuram, India, pp 473–477. https://doi.org/10.1109/ICACCCT.2012.6320825.
85. Wang J, Zhang Y (2021) Using cloud computing platform of 6G IoT in e-commerce personalized recommendation. Int J Syst Assur Eng Manag. https://doi.org/10.1007/s13198-021-01059-1
86. Wang H, Zhang Z, Taleb T (2018) Special issue on security and privacy of IoT. World Wide Web 21:1–6. https://doi.org/10.1007/s11280-017-0490-9
87. Recent trends in computational intelligence enabled research, 1st ed. https://www.elsevier.com/books/recent-trends-in-computational-intelligence-enabled-research/bhattacharyya/978-0-12-822844-9. Accessed 22 Apr 2021
88. Amazon.In. https://www.amazon.in/Fundamentals-Data-Structures-Students-Samanta/dp/9351109283. Accessed 22 Apr 2021
89. Samanta D, Sanyal G (2011) A novel statistical approach for segmentation of images. J Glob Res Comput Sci (JGRCS) 2(10):9–13. ISSN: 2229-371X

Chapter 6
Transformation of Intelligent IoT in the Energy Sector

Abstract Consolidation in renewable power and power efficiency are critical designers of clean energy transformations and weather switch mitigation. New technology, like the IoT, can be used in a range of ways in the power field, having power supply, communication along with supply, and requirement. The Internet of Things may be utilized to improve power usage, increase the use of renewable power, along with reduction of the ambient consequences of power use. This manuscript concentrates on the contemporary survey on the usage of IoT in power systems, as well as smart grids in particular. We also go through some of the IoT's supporting technologies, such as cloud computing and various data analysis platforms. We also look at some of the confrontations of implementing IoT in the power quarters, like security and privacy, as well as few strategies, like blockchain technology. This manuscript gives power lawmakers, financial experts, along with proprietors an outline of the role in IoT in power system optimization.

Keywords Smart power frameworks · Intelligent grid · Power repository · IoT · Power proficiency · Power in constructions

6.1 Introduction

6.1.1 Concepts

A technical uprising progresses through four phases. New forms of power were found to power the nodes during the first revolution. Coal pile mining and the invention of steam energy organizations were also important growth times during this time span. The second industrial revolt [1], also known as abundance manufacturing and power generation [2], was marked by massive-quantity iron and steel development. Several large-scale businesses with assembly lines were established during this time span, resulting in the rise of new professions. During the third industrial revolution, the node and the first generation of transmission infrastructures, such as telephony networks [3], were put in place, allowing supply chains [4] to be automated.

D. Samanta and A. Banerjee, *Computationally Intensive Statistics for Intelligent IoT*,
Studies in Autonomic, Data-driven and Industrial Computing,
https://doi.org/10.1007/978-981-16-5936-2_6

The fourth transition is expected to be driven by a wide range of newer frameworks, including transmission networks (such as 5G) [5], automated robots [6], and the Internet of Things [7]. Through allowing appliances, individuals, records, and exercises to communicate in real time, the Internet of Things links them. As a result, by accumulating along with refining vast volumes of records, IoT will assist in rendering multiple processes more quantifiable and observable. The Internet of Things has the power to change people's lives in a number of ways, including patient care, smart cities [8], the building sector, manufacturing [9], resource resources, and the energy business. It is made possible by increasing the use of real-time automated decision-making [10] and promoting the use of devices that assist with such decision-making.

6.1.2 Motivation

In 2020, global power demand is expected to grow by 2.5% compared to 2017, the largest increase since 2012. As a result, CO2 emissions from the power industry surpassed peak amounts in 2018. Global warming is estimated to exceed 1.5 °C by the middle of the twenty-first century. Climate warming [11] will surpass the 3 °C target if existing rates persist, posing a significant danger to the planet's inhabitants. Climate warming, regional air pollution, water scarcity for high temperature energy production, along with the finiteness of fossil fuel reserves are all examples of the increasing need for better efficiency electricity usage and the usage of sustainable energy sources (RESs) [12]. Several research, whether at the country level, regionally, or internationally, have indicated that a non-fossil power grid is virtually impractical to achieve bereft of successful power usage and/or demand reduction, as well as a high degree of RES incorporation.

According to the United Nations Sustainable Development Goals plan, electricity production is an important driver in economic growth. Furthermore, power generation has long-term economic advantages by lowering the costs of fuel import/supply, electricity storage [13], and pollution associated with power generation. For the electricity generation and optimizing power storage in the energy supply chain, efficient real-time data analysis is critical. From resource output to practical delivery to end consumers, the power supply chain is divided into three parts: I power supply, which includes upstream processing; (ii) power transition processes, which includes utility provider communication and dispersal; and (iii) power demand, which includes power usage in households, conveyance [14], and organizations. Figure 6.1 depicts all three components, as well as the pieces that go with them. This essay examines the role of the Internet of Things for every facet in the power supply chain. The goal of this presentation is in demonstrating how the Internet of Things will assist in energy conservation, demand reduction, and enhanced renewable energy use.

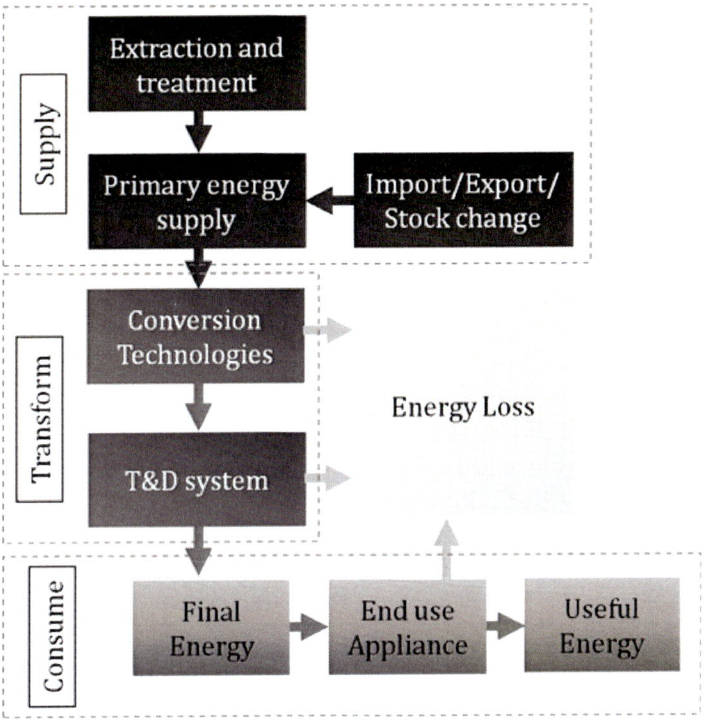

Fig. 6.1 Supply chain of energy

In the Internet of Things, sensors and networking systems are used to detect and relay real-time data, allowing for quicker computations and better decision-making. Additionally, the Internet of Things would help in the shift from a centralized to a mobile, smart, and integrated control structure in the power sector. It is a critical demand for implementing regional, dispensed renewable energy sources like breeze and sunlight, along with interchanging various smaller-number power terminal utilizing into prosumers by accumulating the production along with maximizing the request where it is necessary to the IoT-based networks that make use of sensors [15] and networking technologies [16] to streamline, incorporate, and track activities. Wide information gathering and the utilization of smart algorithms in instant-time data analysis will facilitate with the identification and tracking of different users' and devices' power consumption patterns over time scales.

6.1.3 Methodologies for Testing

The usage of IoT in various quarters along with organizations is extensively studied and assessed in the literature. Additionally, the risks along with the benefits of deploying one or more IoT devices, such as sensors or 5G networks, have been carefully assessed. The bulk of survey study in the power sector has concentrated on a particular subsector, such as buildings or the power sector's technical capabilities for a given IoT technology. For example [17], look at IoT intelligent home apps including how they can be adapted into an environment powered by IoT. The methods, latest innovations, and implementation of 5G are only discussed from the viewpoint of power demand in a paper by researchers [18]. The role of the Internet of Things in maximizing the power proficiency of homes along with public transit was addressed in [19] looking at the main issues concerning the appropriateness of IoT record sharing along with networking protocols for using in intelligent grids.

Contrary to the majority of the literature discussed, which focuses on either a particular subsector of the power quarter or specific IoT techniques, this manuscript discusses IoT's use in the power quarters starting from creation to communication along with dispersal and request management. Thus, the primary handout of the manuscript is to contribute to the current level of expertise by offering a detailed analysis of the possibilities and disputes of registering IoT through the entire electricity quarters to power regulators, analysts, power experts, and managers. In this section, we offer a brief summary of the Internet of Things architecture and supporting infrastructure to pave the basis for addressing the IoT architecture along with its enabling mechanizations in the power sector.

In order to regulate this study, a methodical search was conducted to gather along with examining current literature of the importance of IoT in the power field. Firstly, we looked for the denominations "Internet of Things" along with "Power" in the titles, abstracts, along with buzzwords of publishing in the various reputed databases. Technology, economics, and management were used to narrow down the search results wherever possible. After that, publications written before 2012, as well as several conference papers that lacked facts regarding the peer-review phase, were withdrawn. After that, the papers were divided into three categories: power generation [20] (energy manufacturing units, additional assistances, along with advanced green energy [21]), transmission and distribution systems (electricity, coal, along with district steaming internetworks, as well as intelligent grids), along with demand management (inclusive of power usage in homes, conveyance, along with the industry quarters). Rather than discussing particular cases and their drawbacks, we emphasize on IoT implementations [22] which are popular in most power systems. For instance, we talk about the functions of IoT in intelligent homes except going into detail regarding home categorization, materials, occupant power consumption habits, home appliance form and quantity, and so on.

The remainder of the chapter will be formatted in this manner. The IoT and relevant technologies, such as sensors and networking, cloud computing, and computer processing units, are addressed in Sects. 6.2 and 6.3. Section 6.4 discusses the IoT position in the energy sector. Section 6.5 considers the advantages along with disadvantages of IoT deployment, and Sect. 6.6 discusses subsequent upgrades. The essay comes to a close with Sect. 6.7.

6.2 Internet of Things

The IoT is an internetwork which connects computers and other electronic devices. The IoT is a digital internetwork which connects physical devices (or "things") through the Internet. Physical instruments include things like household items and heavy equipment. If these instruments were equipped with the requisite sensors and communication networks, they would be able to provide data. Individuals with access to a wealth of information and resources intelligently monitoring the usage of building electricity, for example, will help reduce energy costs. Manufacturing and architecture are only a couple of the sectors that might profit from the Internet of Things. IoT applications include environmental surveillance [23], hospital networks and services, effective energy use in homes, and drone-dependent devices. Figure 6.2 shows the IoT platform constituents.

While developing IoT applications, that are the beginning phase in implementing IoT frameworks, the choosing of IoT structures like sensor modules, transmission protocols, data repositories, along with computation must be suitable for the considered use. An IoT GUI [24], for example, will use applicable environmental sensors and acceptable networking technology to detect warming, chilling, along with air cooling in a home. Various components of an IoT platform are illustrated in Fig. 6.2.

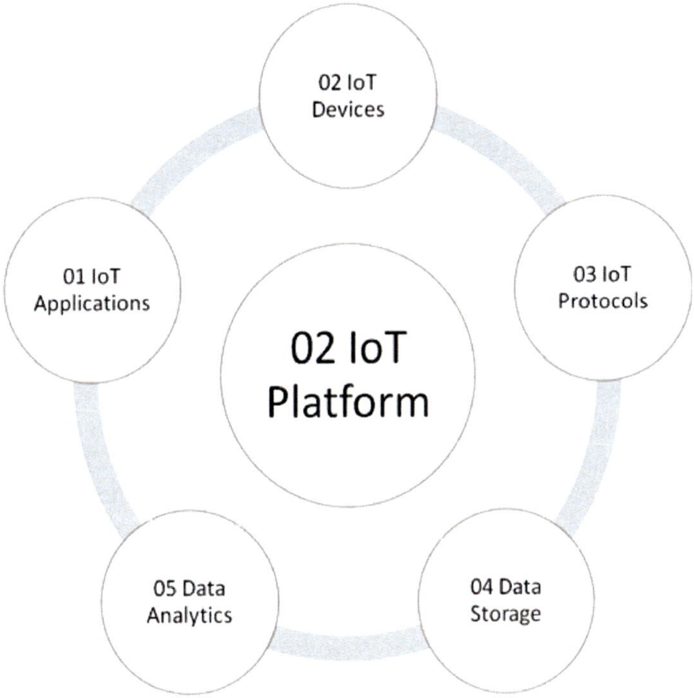

Fig. 6.2 IoT platform constituents

IoT networks, that are the second aspect of IoT systems, are made up of actuators, IoT gateways and sensors, and any other unit which participates in the loop of information acquisition, storage, along with transmission. Viz. an IoT gateway [25] computer facilitates information to be routed via an IoT infrastructure and bidirectional connections to be formed between the gateway, cloud and the device.

Transmission protocols, which allow various appliances to connect along with sharing information with controllers or conclusion-making centers, are the third feature of the IoT network. IoT architectures offer you the option of selecting the networking architecture (each with its own set of features) that best meets your requirements. These systems consist of Zigbee, Bluetooth [26], and Wi-Fi [27] along with wireless networking innovations like 5G along with LTE-4G [28] internetworks. Information storing is the fourth constituent in the IoT architecture, and it allows for the management of sensor data.

In principle, the total amount of data collected by the instruments is enormous. As a consequence, a strategy for data storage in cloud centers or at the network's edge is needed. Processed info that is utilized in computational purposes is the fifth feature in IoT platforms. Once the records have been analyzed, data analytics may be done either offline or in real time, and the findings are used to make device operational choices. Depending on the situation, data analytics may be done both offline and in real time. Off-line analytics modeling methods are used to recover the processed data, which is then visualized on-premises. With cloud or edge storage, real-time analytics visualization, such as stream analytics, is possible.

6.3 The Breakthroughs that Would Make It Possible

The IoT is a term that mentions the usage of sensors, actuators, and processors to enable artifacts and computer components to communicate and provide useful services to one another. Sensors in IoT networks identify and capture data, which is then routed via gateways to benchmark centers or the cloud for future storing, analysis, along with conclusion-making. When the conclusion is taken, a counterpart request is directed back to the actuator stationed on the device, along with the sensed information. Since there are various sensor and actuator systems, transmission mechanizations, along with information processing approaches, we discuss new technologies that empower IoT in this segment. Then, with the aid of the literature, we illustrate how these advancements contribute to power generation.

6.3.1 Instruments That Are Pleasant to Listen to

In the Internet of Things, sensors play a crucial function. They're used to store and exchange data in real time. Sensors increase the IoT's accuracy and durability, and they're essential to its performance. Sensors are available in a wide range of sizes and shapes, and they can be utilized in various domains of implementations. Among the uses are drainage, water monitoring, hospital networks and services, and public protection. The electricity sector, which includes power transmission and production as well as power storage, processing, and distribution, employs several of these sensors [29]. In the power quarter, sensors are utilized to save money and energy. Intelligent power administration systems benefit from sensors because they allow real-time power use and the development of new control load management strategies. The aim of the sensor system research and future trends is to improve sensor technologies that will increase load creation and consumer recognition, as well as advanced facilities that will promote sustainable energy performance. Finally, as part of the Internet of Things, utilizing sensor sensors in the power sector increases diagnostics, decision-making, analytics, optimization processes, and automated output assessments [30]. We'll go through a few instances of commonly used sensor instruments in power generation and use since there are too many sensors used in the power industry.

Warmth sensors are utilized in tracking changes in the warming and freezing of a framework. Warmth is a significant environmental parameter that is widely used. In the power field, the fundamental proposition of energy production is the technique of transforming mechanical power into electrical power. The method of converting mechanical energy into electrical energy is the fundamental principle of power generation in the power quarters. The fundamental mechanism of power production in the power industry is the technique of converting mechanical energy into electrical energy [31]. The method of translating mechanical power into electrical power is the fundamental theory of power generation in the power sector. Mechanical power is provided by heat power, such as thermal energy firms, breeze, water movement, along with solar power firms, and it is the technique of converting mechanical power into electrical power which denotes the fundamental principle of power generation in the power sector. These power transformations are carried out using thermal, or temperature, transitions. Temperature controls are used to improve a system's reliability as the temperature changes during normal operations while still saving energy. Temperature controls, for example, can decide whether heating and cooling systems should be switched on or off in a household setting, making for more efficient power use and energy saving.

Humidity meters are used to measure the difference between relative humidity and the amount of moisture in the air. The ratio of wetness in the atmosphere to the optimum quantity of wetness at a given atmospheric temperature is what relative humidity is shown in [32]. In the electricity sector, humidity sensors are used in a number of applications. For instance, they're often used in the production of wind energy. Humidity sensors are becoming particularly necessary with the construction of offshore wind turbines (because of the increased level of wetness in the atmosphere). To provide continuous moisture control, humidity checking sensors could be installed at the top and beneath the wind turbines. This enables operators to adapt rapidly to adjustments in turbine operating circumstances, resulting in more effective operations, improved performance, and lower power costs. The luminance (amount of light in the environment) or intensity of a light is determined using light sensors.

Light sensors are used in a number of manufacturing and consumer applications because of their low power consumption. Lighting is an important cause of energy usage in homes, accounting for about 15% of total electricity use. Light is responsible for about 20% of all energy use on a global scale. As a result, light sensors may be used to sense lighting conditions both inside and outside, switch lights on and off or dimming them in response to ambient light shifts. As a result, the amount of energy used for lighting in indoor environments may be decreased [33].

PIR (passive infrared) cameras, also referred to as motion sensors, monitor infrared light produced by objects in their surroundings. In order to conserve electricity, these sensors are mounted in houses. Human presence may be detected in enclosed spaces using PIR sensors, for example. The light control unit turns off the lights when there is no activity in the building, which is known as smart lighting control. As a result, the need for electricity in buildings is lowered. Air conditioning systems are no exception, accounting for about 40% of overall building energy demand.

Proximity sensors are used to track the position of near targets without the need for explicit contact. A good example is the use of proximity sensors in wind energy generation. These sensors have long-term performance as well as precise location sensing in wind turbines. Proximity sensors are used in wind turbines to monitor rotor speed and sense brake wear, as well as adjust blade pitch, yaw angle, and rotor and yaw brake location [34].

6.3.2 Actuators Are Automated Systems That Keep Track of the Movement of Information

Actuators are mechanical machines which converts one configuration of energy into another. All keep track of machines and appliances by converting electrical feedback from control devices to motion and then tracking it with Internet of Things systems. Actuators may produce a broad spectrum of motion patterns, including linear, oscillatory, and revolving motions. Based on their power origins, actuators are classified into the following groups. Pneumatic actuators are operated by compressed air. The motive force of pneumatic actuators is produced by a piston or a diaphragm. These actuators are used to track processes that involve fast and reliable responses without using a lot of motive power. Water is used to power hydraulic actuators. Hydraulic actuators consist of a cylinder or a fluid motor which uses hydraulic power to conduct mechanical activities. As an output, the mechanical system produces a semi-linear, spinning, or wavering movement. These actuators are utilized for high-speed and high-force industrial process control applications [35].

Thermal actuators operate by using a heat source to produce actual motion. Thermal actuators translate thermal energy into kinetic energy, which can then be used to drive objects. A diaphragm acts as a temperature-sensing substance that presses against a socket to drive a piston in thermostatic actuators. As the warmth-detecting medium, you may use any fluid/wax-alike solid, or other substance which transposes dimensions in response to heating. With the assistance of external power sources including batteries, electric actuators are able to travel. Electrical actuators are mechanized tools competent in transforming electrical energy to kinetic energy in a lone linear or rotary motion. The frameworks of the actuators are dependent on the devices' expected operations.

In the power sector, such as in power stations, pneumatic actuators have long been used to control valves. To attain power output, electric control-valve actuator technology is employed. They're also regarded as the ultimate command and control center for power plant activities. Furthermore, actuators designed specifically for the power sector, such as the LINAK electrical actuator, can help reduce energy loss in wind turbines by opening hatches and locking brakes, as well as creating motion in solar monitoring panels. A variety of articles have been reported in the literature to illustrate how actuators are used in IoT applications. The researchers [36] propose a wireless sensor network for an IoT-dependent autonomous smart computer. The proposed design reduces overall power consumption by optimizing the activity of IoT sensors and computers over time.

6.3.3 Technology That Allows for Communication

The Internet of Things is propelled by wireless networking networks. Sensor devices are linked to IoT gateways through wireless networks, allowing for terminal-to-terminal record connectivity between the IoT modules. WSNs are designed utilizing a number of wireless protocols, and the one that is used banks on the needs of the device, like transmission range, bandwidth, along with energy utilization. Renewable energy origins like breeze along with sunlight power projects are widespread in rural areas. As a result, maintaining secure IoT links in distant locations is challenging. The deployment of IoT frameworks on the websites necessitates the choosing of appropriate communications framework which may maintain a secure communication link along with allowing spontaneous-time information transmission while using fewer resources. We'll spend a lot of time in this chapter talking about communication technologies because it's so important in the IoT. We will have few examples of how they can be used in the field of control.

Wireless fidelity (Wi-Fi) and other short-range wireless networks have been thoroughly investigated for IoT implementations in the electricity quarter. Wi-Fi is mostly used for electricity metering and building resource use in the utility industry. Wi-Fi, on the other hand, is not a good option for the service industry because of its high power requirements. In terms of power use, narrowband IoT (NB-IoT), Bluetooth low power, and modern LPWAN gadgets like LoRa, and LTE-M handling in an illegal band are safer options. These new LPWAN technologies are ideal for smart power management solutions since they require the deployment of an effective, lower-expenditure, lower-speed, longer-range, mechanization. As a consequence, the focus of this article will be on short-range and recent LPWAN developments, as well as certain power-related applications. We regularly address the value of satellite networks in bringing global IoT access to remote industrial sectors. The different characteristics of these technologies are mentioned in Table 1.

Bluetooth is a wireless technology that permits one to link to different gadgets. BLE (Bluetooth Low Power) [37] is a short-range wireless networking device for the Internet of Things that allows data to be exchanged over short radio wavelengths. BLE is less costly to install and allows for the creation of an immediate personal area network [38] since it has a standard range of 0–30 m. BLE was developed for Internet of Things (IoT) applications that need relatively little power to transmit very limited volumes of data. Businesses in the power sector can use IoT technologies to create various types of node-to-node and node-to-human transmission with well-designed IoT software. BLE is widely used in the power industry to track energy use in residential and industrial buildings. The researchers describe a smart workplace power management device that utilizes Bluetooth Low Energy to reduce the amount of power used by computers, displays, and lamps. Another research [39] suggests a smart home power control system that uses Bluetooth Low Power (BLE) for connectivity between home appliances to reduce power consumption. Similarly, with the aim of optimizing the home power control system, [40] proposes a fuzzy-based technique for intelligent power management in a building automation environment. Zigbee is a networking application that helps you to build a small-scale personal area network. Zigbee is a lower-expenditure, lower-data-rate, along with high efficient lower-energy network that is easy to set up. A mesh network specification is often used in Zigbee, which links computers by several interconnections. When mesh networking is used, the real communication range of Zigbee is significantly expanded, going up to 100 m. In the power market, Zigbee IoT technologies provide lighting frameworks (homes along with roadway lights), intelligent grids [41] (e.g. automatic energy meters), and building monitoring units, along with factory automation. The demonstrations are designed in illustrating how to more easily employ authority. In the literature [42], the effectiveness of a home power management framework is studied by developing a Zigbee-based wireless sensor network with the aim of lowering consumer power costs. The authors of [43] further provide intelligent home interfaces, which permit exchangeability between Zigbee networks, electric appliances, along with intelligent meters, resulting in more effective power consumption. The outline is a Zigbee-based control scheme for reducing energy use by controlling and switching the power of household appliances at outlets and lamps. Another research addresses field studies utilizing ZigbeeZigbee technology to monitor photovoltaic and wind power systems. Zigbee sensors, according to the study's results, may be used in dispersed renewable production along with intelligent metering applications [44].

Plan for the long run LoRa is a wireless network technology for the Internet of Things. LoRA is a lower-expenditure networking framework that will enable Internet of Things (IoT) computers last longer on their batteries. Longer-length communications having lower-energy utilization (greater than 10 km in countryside locations) can also be accomplished with LoRa. This technology's characteristics make it an excellent communication technology for use in power sector, especially in intelligent cities with intelligent grids along with home automation frameworks such as intelligent metering [45].

The research in [46] aims to minimize energy demand by deploying a LoRa-based building power management system, according to the literature. The research presents a forum for maximizing building capability by integrating a variety of technologies such as air conditioning, ventilation, and power management. The platform's growth resulted in a 20% drop in electricity usage. The researchers [47] describe the development of a LoRa-powered smart controller for a commercial building's HVAC system that is focused on machine learning. When the smart controller notices that a room is empty, it switches off the HVAC device, saving up to 19.8% on energy consumption. Another study [48] integrates LoRa technologies into an interconnected system for evaluating the energy efficiency of public buildings. When the platform was put to the test, it was discovered that it saved 40% of the energy that an illuminating framework needed.

Sigfox is a WAN infrastructure that utilizes ultra-narrow bands. Sigfox enables low-power appliances to transmit with one another, allowing for the creation of IoT implementations. Sigfox, according to [49], is the most successful lower-power applicants in intelligent metering in order to deliver real-time power services to households. Additionally, [50] compares and contrasts a range of lower-power WAN technologies before deciding that Sigfox is a feasible elucidation for smart building electric plug sensors. The Narrowband Internet of Things (NB-IoT) is a lower-power broad-area network (LPWAN) networking infrastructure that enables a wide range of IoT devices and networks to connect at high data rates with low latency. The Narrowband Internet of Things (NB-IoT) standard is a lower-cost, high-coverage, longer-battery-life option. NB-IoT is a possible option for smart power transmission networks, according to the makers of [51], because of its low-cost communications for smart meters. The researchers [52] also discuss the use of NB-IoT technologies in smart metering. The thesis in [53], which contrasts NB-IoT to other transmission networks in terminology of data transmission rate, latency, along with network spectrum as a likely alternative in intelligent grid transmissions, is another use of NB-IoT in the power sector.

3GPP (third-generation cooperation project) produced LTE-M as a machine-type communication (MTC) norm with the aim of reducing system sophistication. LTE-M provides for reliable networking, a wide spectrum of coverage, and a versatile platform. LTE-M provides reduced latency and better throughput services as compared to NB-IoT. This device also helps low-power networks receive energy-efficient electricity, making it an excellent fit for intelligent meters along with intelligent grid transmissions [54].

Weightless is a free wireless protocol which enables a vast range of Internet of Things devices along with computers to communicate with one another. Weightless is a smart metering system with future uses in the energy market. According to a paper published in [55], weightless is a realistic wireless system that may be utilized in intelligent house IoT networks in intelligent metering and intelligent grid transmissions.

Satellite is another networking choice, with a wide range of coverage and the ability to reinforce lower-data-transmission-rate implementations in a host-to-host manner. IoT instruments and computers in remote areas may benefit from satellite technologies. The researchers define a node-to-node satellite transmission device which is based on the Internet of Things and can be used in smart grid applications, especially in the communication and dispersal industry. A related survey illustrates the significance of utilizing satellite-dependent IoT transmissions in the power sector, like sunlight and breeze power ventures [56].

6.3.4 Data and Computation in the Internet of Things

For more in-depth analysis, more dependable software responses, and more accurate machine power usage decisions, IoT data can be computed and analyzed. Manipulation of IoT results, on the other hand, is a demanding undertaking. IoT data is often referred to as "Big data" because it relates to vast amounts of organized and non-structured information produced by a variety of IoT device elements, like sensors, software programs, intelligent computers, and transmission internetworks. Big data must be quickly comprehended and analyzed due to its characteristics, such as length, velocity, and range. Traditional big data processing techniques, like storing it on regional hard discs, collecting it, and then analyzing it, are ineffective. Advanced computational and mathematical approaches are required to deal with big data. In the parts that follow, we'll look at cloud computing and fog analysis, two methods for storing and processing big data that are widely utilized [57].

6.3.5 The Term "Cloud Computing" Indicates a Form of Computation That Makes Use of the Internet

Cloud computing denotes a form of information refining which links internet-connected IoT computers to the internet and offers software, applications, storage, and computation. The phrase "cloud" denotes the "Web", and "computing" denotes the functionality of the method to calculate and collect data. Both Internet-based infrastructure frameworks and data center-based hardware models are used in cloud computing. Cloud computing necessitates the processing of vast amounts of data while still enabling sophisticated calculations to be performed. The researchers benefit by the primary advantages of utilizing cloud-based systems like (i) reducing hardware costs; (ii) growing computation power along with repository capability; and (iii) utilizing multi-core frameworks to make information handling easier [58]. Cloud infrastructure refers to a protected network that enables people to access resources, computing space, and storage from anywhere in the world. The characteristics of cloud storage allow easy analyzing, handling, and sorting of vast amounts of data produced by IoT applications. When utilizing cloud computing, the costs of purchasing machines and applications, as well as the costs of running IoT data processing algorithms, are also minimized, resulting in a substantial decrease in the amount of power available for local data computation [59].

As discussed in the Fog of Computing, cloud computing, while being one of the most powerful, is also one of the most costly technical paradigms for IoT data processing. Because of the delays and bandwidth constraints of centralized data processing services, more reliable solutions are needed. Fog computing refers to a dispersed computing platform along with cloud augmentation that brings computing and analytics closer to the network's edge. Fog computing is a form of cloud computing that allows users to maximize the size of their workloads. Any device that can measure, store data, and communicate with the internet is referred to as a fog node in fog computing. These networks provide home computers, factory controllers, switches, routers, and embedded servers, to name a few examples. Instead of sending IoT data to the cloud, fog saves and stores it locally on IoT computers in this computational model. This solution has a number of advantages, including improved secure services, which are needed by various IoT applications, along with decreased inter-network congestion along with latency. As a consequence, unlike cloud storage, fog offers quicker and more effective data and processing services. This allows for the making of choices and the taking of acts [60].

6.4 The Energy Sector and the Internet of Things

Currently, the energy market is largely subjected on fossil fuels, which account for about 85% of global concluding power output. Uncontrolled usage of fossil fuels has detrimental implications for the atmosphere, public health, and the economy, including increased air pollution and climate change. Energy efficiency, or using less oil to produce the same amount of energy, along with the usage of renewable energy sources are two important options for reducing the negative effects of fossil fuel usage [61].

The segment explores the part of IoT for the power industry, from fuel extrication to power generation property operation and maintenance (O&M), as well as power end-usage. The Internet of Things has the potential to reduce energy waste and CO2 pollution significantly. An IoT-based power management system can monitor real-time power usage and raise consciousness about power accomplishment at a point in the supply chain. In the section, the usage of IoT in the power production steps is addressed initially. Then we will look at smart cities, which are an overarching word for a number of IoT-dependent sub-systems like intelligent grids, intelligent houses, intelligent factories, and smart conveyance. Following that, we will go through individual components discussed above one by one.

6.4.1 Power Production Along with the Internet of Things

Industrial process control, supervisory oversight, and data processing technologies were both introduced in the power sector throughout the 1990s. In the early stages of the Internet of Things, the power sector was able to reduce the possibility of a supply loss or outage by monitoring and controlling devices and processes. Reliability, performance, environmental impacts, and maintenance problems are all major concerns with older power plants. Because of the age of the power sector's facilities, as well as maintenance problems, severe power shortages and unreliability may occur. Any of the structures that are older than 40 years are very valuable, and cannot be replaced. Many of these problems with power plant technologies would be resolved by the Internet of Things. IoT sensors may sense any service malfunction or unwanted decrease in power usage, alerting connected devices to the need for maintenance. This improves system stability and efficiency while also lowering repair costs. In accordance with [62], a newer IoT-dependent energy plant would deposit 240 million dollars over its life span, versus 50 million dollars for a current plant with the same size.

Many countries are embracing green energies as a means of decreasing fossil fuel usage along with reducing dependence on regional power sources. Wind and solar power, which are weather-dependent or intermittent renewable energy (VRE) sources, pose new threats to the power grid, which have been dubbed the "intermittency crisis". Due to supply and demand differences, matching energy output with demand in a power grid with a significant share of VRE is challenging, resulting in time scale mismatch. IoT systems allow for more versatility in matching generation to demand, which simplifies VRE integration and leads to higher renewable energy integration shares and lower GHG emissions [63]. Furthermore, utilizing machine learning algorithms to assess the optimal combination of supply and demand technologies, IoT may be used to achieve more productive power use. For example, artificial intelligence algorithms can combine a thermal power plant's power output with in-house power generation sources such as aggregating multiple smaller-scale cosmic PV panels.

6.4.2 Intelligent Cities

Rapid urbanization coupled with overpopulation has resulted in a slew of global problems, including air and water pollution, energy shortages, and environmental challenges. Supplying cities with clean, stable, and affordable power sources is one of the most pressing issues in this sector. Recent technical advances have fueled the creation of intelligent, IoT-dependent elucidations for the current intelligent city concerns. Intelligent plants, intelligent houses, energy firms, along with farms could all be connected in one location, with data on their power use obtained at different times during the day. When one section of the grid, such as suburban areas, requires the most electricity in the afternoon, power to other sections of the grid, such as warehouses, is immediately restricted to maintain the system stable at the lowest possible cost and chance of congestion or failure [64].

Knowledge communication and networking, smart recognition, position resolution, tracking, routing, contamination reduction, and identification protection would all benefit from IoT technology in a smart city. The Internet of Things (IoT) will allow for the identification of people in specific locations. Households, towns, transportation, power grids, and infrastructure will all benefit from the usage of sensors. These links may support a power-efficiency intelligent city by constantly tracking information collected through sensors. For example, IoT may be used to monitor cars and regulate street lighting, allowing for the most productive use of electricity. Officials would have access to the results, which will enable them to make better judgments about alternative forms of transportation and energy demand [65].

6.4.3 The Smart Grid is an Interactive System That Enables You to Keep Track of Your Energy Use

Intelligent grids are specialized grids that utilize the best efficient and reliable ICT framework to map and optimize power sources, T&D grids, along with end usage. By integrating multiple intelligent meters, an intelligent grid offers a numerous-directional drift in data that may be utilized for infrastructure maintenance and reliable electricity supply. Smart grid networks may either concentrate on particular elements of the power system, such as power production, homes, or conveyance, or they may take a more holistic approach [66].

In regular grids, adapters with power cables and an AC/DC inverter are used to reconnect batteries. These batteries may be charged wirelessly in an intelligent grid due to inductive charging framework. Data from an IoT app is often used in smart grids to monitor end-user energy usage patterns, such as the amount of time spent charging mobile phones or electric vehicles. After that, the computer or car will be charged at the closest wireless battery charging station, where it will be assigned a time slot. Another benefit of the Internet of Things is that it will enhance battery-driven vehicle servicing and monitoring, resulting in better power supply and ensuring that they are still powered up. As a result, there will be a substantial decline in the consumption of non-sustainable fuels [67].

The Internet of Things (IoT) may also be used in isolated and micro-grids for one-of-a-kind islands or organizations, particularly when constant power is required, such as in databases. In such networks, grid-connected assets and non-grid-connected assets will communicate. The power demand of each commodity is often shown. Power management may be precisely regulated anywhere and wherever it is required as a consequence of this relationship. This depicts how various parts of an intelligent city fitted with IoT-dependent intelligent grids may be linked together in terminologies of the cooperative effect of intelligent grids.

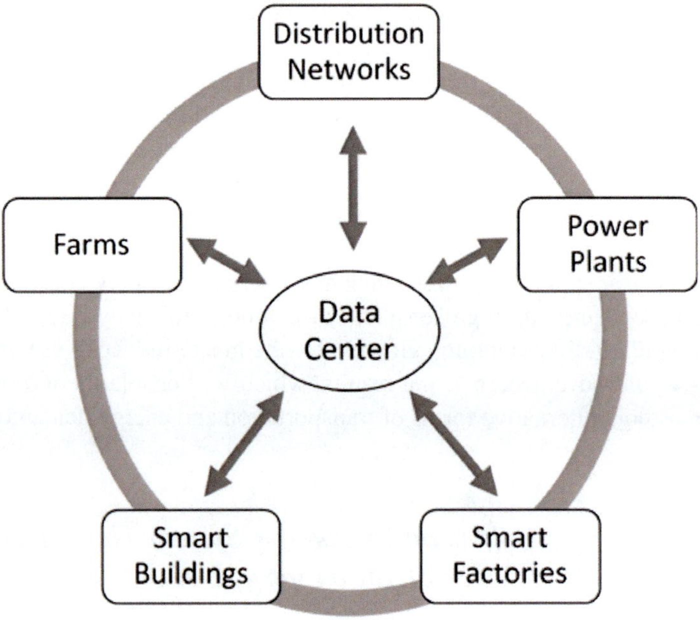

Fig. 6.3 A smart city definition of unified data access

The smart grid will warn mechanics through intelligent devices before a serious difficulty arises as a result of mutual contact between various industries. Continuous monitoring, for instance, will detect when energy demand reaches the grid's capability. Authorities which utilize a number of methods as a product of real-time forecasts, and power usage may be rescheduled to a time when performance is predicted to be smaller. Smart (or dynamic) pricing tariffs for flexible power rates have been considered under some situations. At a period when electricity demand is predicted to rise, real-time pricing (RTP) contracts and the energy price would be higher. Using data gathered from smart grid systems, far-sighted approaches will perfectly optimize and monitor power consumption and generation. Two other IoT implementations are active voltage management to minimize transmission losses in T&D networks and a network of smart meters to reduce non-technical losses [68]. Figure 6.3 express smart city definition of unified data access.

6.4.4 Intelligent Building

A smart city model of centralized data networking is depicted in Fig. 6.3. Residential (domestic); industrial (services), which involves supermarkets, offices, and schools; and transportation are the three different categories of power usage in communities. Household power use in the domestic quarter comprises illumination, facilities, household warm water, boiling, refrigeration, ventilating systems, cooling, along with air conditioning (Fig. 6.4). HVAC energy narrates most of the electricity usage in most households. Controlling the HVAC function, as a consequence, is important for reducing energy usage. Figure 6.4 shows residential energy consumption as a percentage. As technology advances, IoT devices can become more critical in reducing energy losses in HVAC systems. Finding wireless thermostats that are occupancy-dependent, for example, may be used to fill empty spaces. Any power-saving steps may be implemented prior to the formation of an unoccupied space. For example, HVAC systems can turn off appliances in unoccupied areas, saving and wasting a significant amount of electricity.

A smart city model of centralized data networking is depicted in Fig. 6.3. Residential (domestic); industrial (services), which involves supermarkets, offices, and schools; and transportation are the three different categories of power usage in communities. Household power use in the domestic quarter comprises illumination, facilities, household warm water, boiling, refrigeration, ventilating systems, cooling,

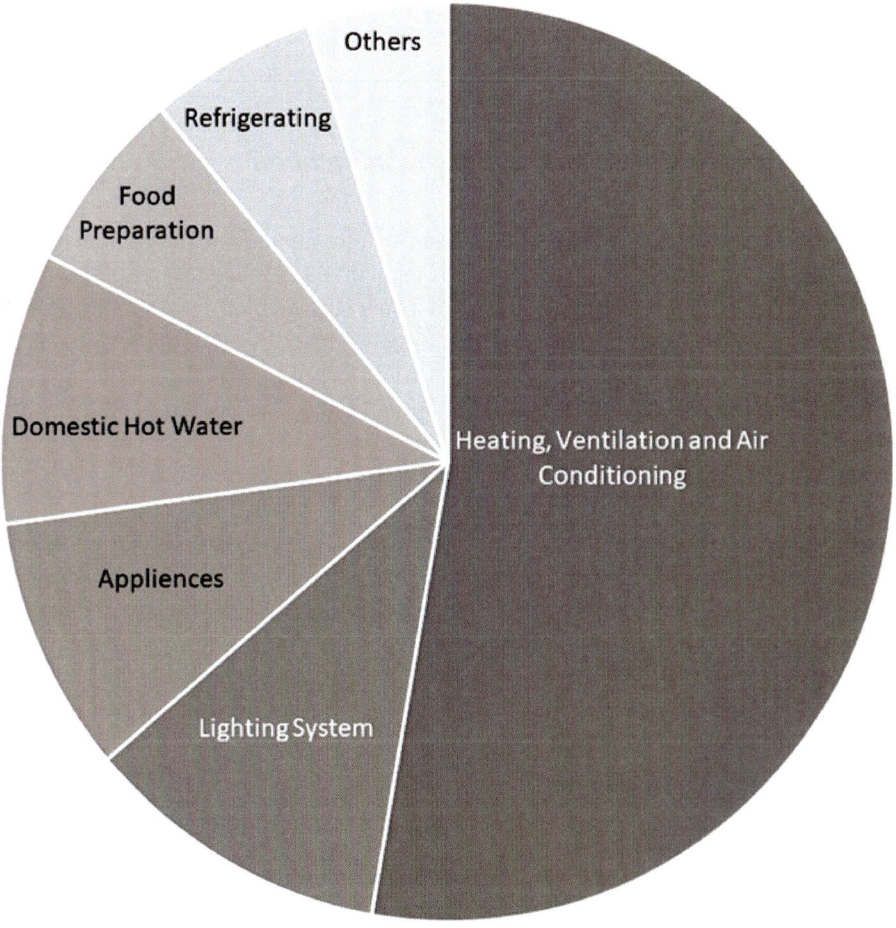

Fig. 6.4 Residential energy consumption as a percentage

along with air conditioning (Fig. 6.4). HVAC energy narrates most of the electricity usage in most households. Controlling the HVAC function, as a consequence, is important for reducing energy usage. Figure 6.4 shows residential energy consumption as a percentage. As technology advances, IoT devices can become more critical in reducing energy losses in HVAC systems. Finding wireless thermostats that are occupancy-dependent, for example, may be used to fill empty spaces. Any power-saving steps may be implemented prior to the formation of an unoccupied space. For example, HVAC systems can turn off appliances in unoccupied areas, saving and wasting a significant amount of electricity.

It's also possible to use the Internet of Things to track power shortages in lighting systems. IoT-based lighting systems, for example, could warn consumers when their energy consumption exceeds the usual limit. Furthermore, due to a reliable study of spontaneous-time information, load from high-peak levels may be transferred to low-peak levels. It makes a major offering to the effective usage of electrical power along with the elimination of greenhouse gas discharges. As a result of the Internet of Things, market reaction will be mostly flexible and elastic, along with tracking and demand side management would be more capable.

6.4.5 Industrial Intelligent Power Application

The Internet of Things (IoT) will be used in the automotive industry to create a completely integrated and distributed system that saves money while increasing performance. Oil is used extensively in conventional plants to manufacture the finished product and calculate demand. Keeping track of all activities also necessitates the usage of human resources. Instead of recording products at the end of the production line, smart factories employ an agile and flexible approach that allows for simultaneous fault detection. As a consequence, immediate action is expected to minimize excess demand and the surplus energy produced as a result.

Industrial process management depends strongly on the Internet of Things (IoT) and its supporting technology. Portal systems, IoT pivotal internetworks, database repositories, along with cloud vendors are all part of the monitoring system, and they can all be accessed through intelligent mobile devices (like smart-phones or PCs). Wireless networking, like Bluetooth and Wi-Fi, as well as wired networks, like a LAN, will link all pieces of equipment. Furthermore, sensors installed in a manufacturing location can detect constituents which use more power than they can handle, allowing IoT to be used more efficiently. As a result, each subsystem can be maintained effectively, computer faults can be overcome, and power consumption for each part can be managed. As a result, it is expected that smart factory power losses can be minimized [69].

Data analysis is a critical component of a smart factory's overall operation since it enables data from the cloud network (which acts like a brain) to be analyzed in real time, enabling managers to make smarter judgments. When it comes to repairing and rebuilding plant machinery, system and mechanical unit degradation is a major concern for factories. To decrease wear and tear along with related maintenance expenditures, the right device size may be selected using an appropriate IoT platform and equipment. Because of IoT-dependent contingent regulation, the mechanical appliance never gets to its threshold restriction. Clearly stated, this prolongs the existence of the machine and decreases the amount of errors. Errors that occur in a lack of power must be corrected on a daily basis [70].

Client, seller, and business coordination will be made simpler with IoT-based agile programs. As a result, in response to a specific request from a client, a new product may be created. As a result, the volume of labor needed to manufacture modern components, as well as the amount of capital lost in factories to purchase replacement parts, will be drastically decreased. The ability to manufacture and handle a small range of various types of materials allows for greater resource efficiency and output consistency.

6.4.6 Transportation That Is Intelligent

One of the important sources of atmospheric contamination and electricity disasters in major cities is the too much use of personal conveyances rather than general conveyance. In comparison to a traditional conveyance system, where every system runs separately, using IoT technology in conveyance, also known as "digital transportation", has a global management network. Furthermore, real-time statistics processing is needed for traffic management. Many facets of the transportation system could be linked together, and data from each could be merged. Smart mobility solutions that include traffic control and smart parking services provide interactive maps. Consumers who use smart transportation will choose the cheapest route with the shortest distance and quickest lane, saving time and passion. People would schedule ahead of time and guess the time it would take them to arrive at. Figure 6.5 represents IoT in an intelligent Energy Framework. As a result, mass transit will be more efficient, and electricity use will be decreased dramatically. This has the potential to dramatically decrease CO2 pollution and other toxins released into the air as a result of conveyance [71].

This section depicts the IoT technologies in the power quarter, which range from intelligent power grids to power usage. Digitalization allows for the transformation of a power source dependent on the Internet of Things from a unidirectional to an integrated power infrastructure, i.e. from production to power grids to buyers. The different components of an embedded smart power grid are depicted in Fig. 6.5.

6.5 Confrontations in Soliciting IoT

Aside from the various benefits of IoT in terms of energy quality, introducing IoT in the power sector presents a variety of concerns that must be tackled. In this

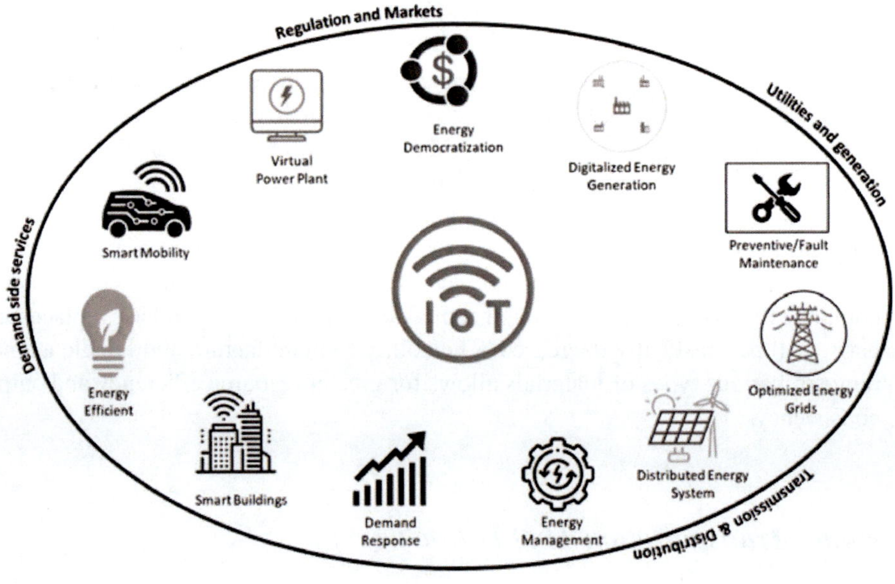

Fig. 6.5 IoT in an intelligent energy framework

segment, the problems and current solutions for integrating IoT-based power systems are addressed.

6.5.1 Consumption of Electricity

Power grids use a lot of energy, and IoT platforms are working hard to reduce the consumption. A large number of IoT devices relay data in order to enable IoT contact in power systems. Operating the Internet of Things networks and relaying the large quantities of data provided by IoT devices needs a considerable amount of resources. As a result, power consumption in IoT systems appears to be a major concern. In the other side, different approaches to lowering IoT system power consumption have been sought. Put the sensors in sleep mode, for instance, and then use them when absolutely necessary. It's been extensively researched how to construct successful communication protocols that enable distributed computing procedures to facilitate resource-efficient communications. The use of a framework that incorporates radio optimization procedures like modulation optimization along with cooperative collaboration was settled upon. Once upon a time, cluster architectures along with multi-path routing schemes were considered to be the most energy-efficient routing methods [72].

6.5.2 Subsystems of the Internet of Things (IoT) Are Being Incorporated

It is challenging to incorporate an IoT computer into a power system's subsystems. Because of their special design, power sector subsystems use a mix of sensor and data transmission approaches. As a result, solutions for organizing data sharing among the subsystems of an IoT-enabled power system are required. Modeling an interconnected infrastructure for the power grid is a technique for solving the integration issue by taking into account a subsystem's IoT requirements. Another possibility is to develop control system co-simulation models that embed the system and reduce subsystem synchronization delay error.

6.5.3 Security of the Consumer

Owners of a person or collective possession have the right to keep personal details exchanged with a single person secret. As a consequence, reliable data on energy users, along with the number and range of goods that use electricity, is inaccessible. In fact, IoT data collection aids in power management, delivery, and utilization decisions. To prevent invading customers' privacy, energy suppliers may seek consent to utilize their data, which means that the data is not exchanged with various alliances. Implementing a protected privacy protection system that allows power users full control of their data and privacy is another alternative.

6.5.4 Apprehensions Concerning Protection

From output to storage and distribution to consumption, the usage of IoT and networking technology in power networks increases the [72] to cyber attacks on consumers' information and power infrastructure. The challenge to the electricity sector's stability is defined in these threads. Furthermore, in the power industry, IoT-based control systems are widely used to move energy around broad geographic regions. IoT devices are more susceptible to cyber attacks because of their widespread use. One solution, according to a study, is to encrypt power data to secure it from cyber attacks. Distributed control frameworks that allow control at various IoT device levels are also recommended to minimize the chance of cyber attack while also expanding machine reliability.

6.5.5 *The Internet of Things (IoT) Has Developed a Series of Principles*

By combining technologies and ideas, the Internet of Things (IoT) connects a unit computer to a huge quantity of others. A new problem is the lack of consistency between IoT devices that use different specifications. There are two types of guidelines in IoT-enabled networks: network protocols and networking protocols, data processing criteria, and valid data security and privacy standards. The implementation of specifications in the IoT is hampered by unstructured data storage criteria, data security and privacy concerns, and legal guidelines for data markets. One approach to the standardization problem of IoT-based power systems is to provide a community of networks with a common consensus that all members will connect to and use in the same manner. Transparent information specifications, models, and protocols may also be established by the cooperating parties. As a result, the general public's expectations will be clear and equitable.

6.5.6 *IoT Networks Connect an Increasing Number of Smart Integrated Devices and Sensors*

IoT networks connect a growing number of smart integrated devices and sensors using a variety of technologies. The aim of the Internet of Things (IoT) is to provide self-contained, ad hoc contact with all relevant providers at any time and from any place. This indicates that, depending on the use, IoT systems are framed with complicated, decentralized, and ambulatory features. Because of the particular features and parameters of each IoT implementation, recommended framework may not be a one-size-fits-all solution. As a result, IoT framework demand heterogeneous reference architectures that is both transparent and consistent with industry requirements. Thanks to architectures, consumers are no longer limited to preset and end-to-end IoT experiences.

6.5.7 *Transmission System Primary Variable Sensing and Actuation*

Since the 1965 Northeast Blackout, the transmission grid had to mount tracking and sensing systems. Modern sensing instruments have become more relevant as the North American power grid has progressed, allowing for a greater view of its electricity network overall. The transmission grid, as seen in this section, uses a series of devices in power lines and power stations to control "traditional" parameters including power systems, procedures, and unit limitations. When it comes to preserving system integrity and performance, power, voltage, switching frequency, power flow, and voltage magnitude are all critical considerations. Detectors which track impedance, identify defects, and perform preventive modeling perform line monitoring in the transmission system.

Transmission controls can also be used to track the physical condition of power plants and determine where employees can be sent for maintenance or failure protection. Such detectors will be useful in power stations, aerial cables, and submerged lines used in submarine cable networks. Sensors in the transmission device can also send data to already-running databases, which can aid decision-making and keep the system safe. The reader is guided to [73] for a more in-depth look at current events.

The requirement for impulse control prompted the creation of sensing devices. Sensor networks, as described in this section, are really a series of device attached to a standardized interaction system that enables physical devices to external decision-making points. These sensed data are spatially dispersed throughout the electricity network to create an integrated control and information layer. The very first or even well of these sensor nodes is the SCADA function seen in this part. SCADA is a voltage, frequency, along with electricity flow tracking system that sends data to centralized operations control centers in substations and distribution feeders. PLCs can submit external triggers to modify generation speeds, pass electrical systems, and control devices in SCADA systems. As part of a broader emphasis on connectivity networks, this part delves further into SCADA systems along with other sensor networks. The SCADA architecture is used to describe many of the embedded sensors in this section.

Despite the transmission system's complex SCADA-based sensing network, many issues must be resolved before eIoT can be successfully implemented. For starters, the communication infrastructure is dispersed across a large geographic area, constantly making collection of data complicated. Since communication equipment is typically located in remote locations, the cost of mobilizing personnel for scheduled repair tests is high. Several of the detectors are mounted on distribution networks, which range in number from 60 to 125 per substation. The distance between two carrier ranges between 500 and 900 m. A standard infrastructure of 25,000 km of 68 kV transmission lines and millions of transmission lines, connectors, and circuit breaker is projected to also have 1 million separate detectors distributed across a 60–20,000 km region.

Outside threats include climate (like hurricanes or excessive heat), age, physical damage, as well as other environmental conditions. Because of the large global number and variety of sensors connected, manual measurements are less accurate than gathering signals from automated sensors. EPRI also recommends condition-based data sharing and transmission mechanism automation over time-based data sharing and automation. To escape faults and correct sub-optimal situations, probabilistic (rather than deterministic) methods can be used to assess transmission system susceptibility. Real-time data is necessary in all circumstances to track transmission system conditions protection and reliability.

Second, in intermittent and minimal transmission stabilization designs, the latest SCADA approach fails to detect complex phenomena. Estimating complex condition over even a large region is challenging because SCADA's sampling rate is only 2–4 s. Rather, SCADA information is frequently used in manual decision-making strategies that use static system identification equations. The lack of organized time stamp calculations in SCADA makes complicated state estimation much more difficult.

To resolve these concerns, SCADA system has to be able to display temporal variations with higher resolution and consistency. Such parameters point to improved SCADA terminal synchronization and usability. Wide-area computing advances are aimed at improving regulatory responses to system-wide disturbances. Data processing, delivery, and interpretation can all be improved with modern electric grid sensors. Since sensor power is scarce, sensor network integration is impractical. The majority of sensors use microprocessors, cellular terminals, circuit boards, power supplies, along with other energy-intensive equipment. Figure 6.6 shows fiber optic lines and power stations for wearable sensors.

Memory storage systems are also available. This dilemma, however, can be solved by using batteries or other environmentally sustainable power sources. When developing devices with offshore correspondence, renewable energy use and affordability are important factors. In an effort to reduce cost of maintenance, devices should be designed in such a manner whereby they optimize hardware and system power usage by using energy storage capacity.

Manufacturers must maximize the usage of passive elements like capacitors, along with electrodes, as well as other energy-saving methods, to limit switching losses and shifting thresholds [74]. Decrease the energy dependency of detectors mostly on electricity grid to avoid rippling faults here between actual electricity network and the advanced machine learning communication module. The combined reliability of the two networks is improved by decoupling the energy national grid sensors with individual power flows.

The use of phasor measurement units (PMUs) in the transmission system was motivated by sensing problems (that is, synchrophasors). Because of their higher sampling rates, phasor measurements can record complex system activity and provide a dynamic viewpoint on grid operations. PMUs will measure volts, variables, amplitude, and transition angles 130 times each electricity circuit. It's even possible to verify the voltage and current. The diagram of a PMU is seen in Fig. 6.7. The whole PMU information gains computational complexity error detection, system identification for reliability and accuracy solution consistency, and trialability right away. PMUs, according to simulations and field experience, will have a huge effect on how the electric grid is managed and regulated. The deployment of PMUs including the management systems, on the other hand, will be difficult due to budget reasons. A fully measurable interface requires a lot of PMUs, which appliances typically introduce in stages [75].

Recent research examined algorithms for optimum PMU placement in order to reduce the amount of PMUs needed to capture enough data. The global positioning system (GPS) is used to synchronize PMU measurements in PMU-based wide-area control systems (WAMS). Throughout the proper research of grid faults, these coordinated calculations cause two components to also be contrasted. PMUs improved power system performance by allowing for wide-area control and synchronization, which had previously been hampered by SCADA's sluggish state adjustments. Synchrophasors have also allowed for precise time stamping of voltage and

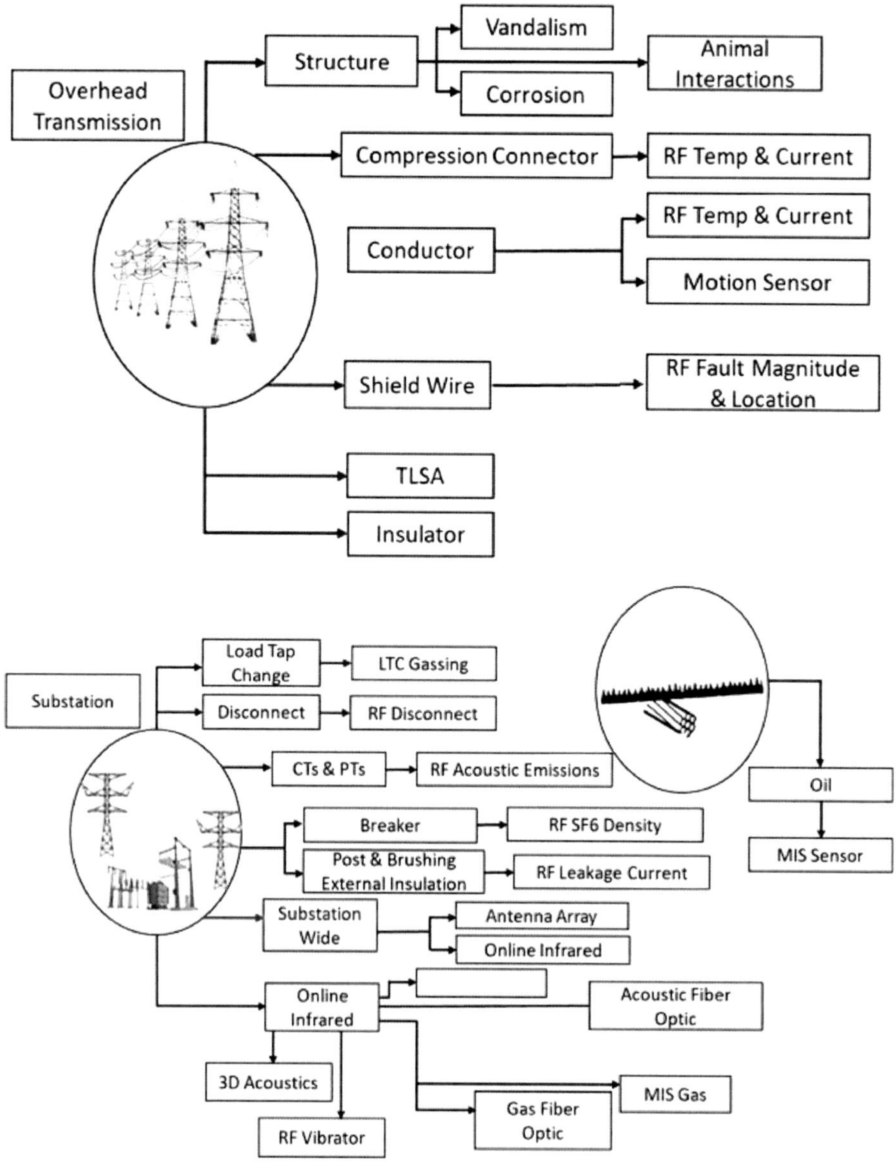

Fig. 6.6 Fiber optic lines and power stations for wearable sensors

current data from various locations, allowing for real-time device state measurements. Synchrophasors are also used in defensive systems, but owing to the rigorous criteria for safety systems, their complete incorporation into line security is still debatable. Wide-area surveillance, protection, and control mechanisms, as well as post-disturbance experiments and model validation, are increasingly using synchrophasors.

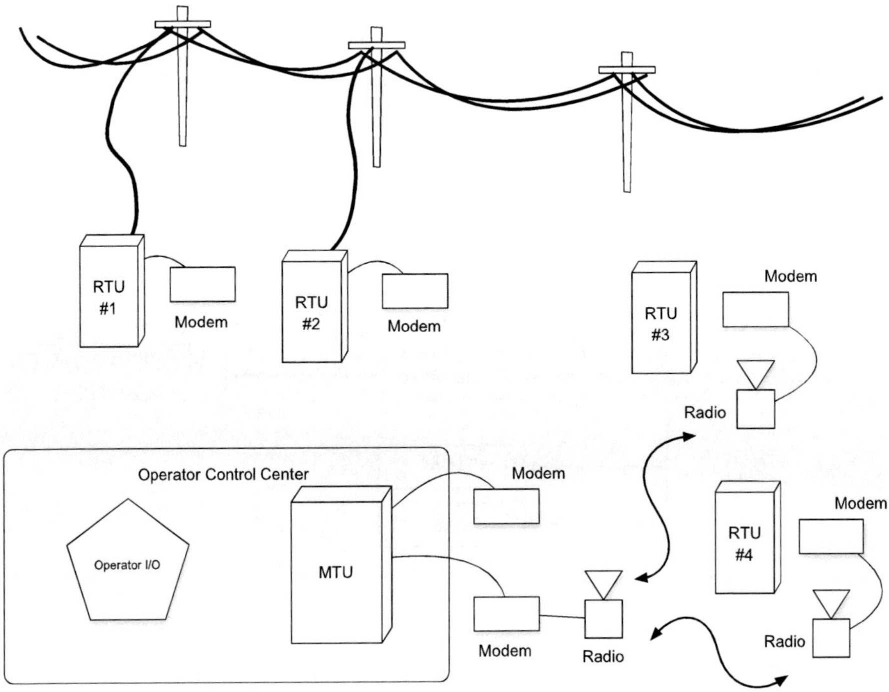

Fig. 6.7 SCADA is defined as an internetwork of various sensors connected by modems and radios to a central processing unit through naturally available energy sources like thermal, solar, seismic, and hydraulic energy. Few detectors will toggle between such a static "asleep" mode as well as a variable "awake" state as required

Although introducing PMUs into another power system will boost depth perception in the power system, it will not be adequate for the entire grid. Second, PMUs are built for transmission and are unreliable in the delivery system to a large degree. They're still useless when it comes to analyzing consumers' energy use patterns. In this respect, the application of new meters has delivered an even service. PMUs, on the other hand, can only compute current and voltage phasors. As a consequence, they can have much-needed information on grid conditions, but they can't explain why they happen. Secondary assessments of these amounts are becoming more critical because as electricity system becomes focused on interrelated technology, environmental patterns, and customers' complex actions. In this case, secondary measurements can depend heavily on sensors from other industries.

6.6 Future Possibilities

As mentioned in previous posts, there are many advantages of using recent IoT frameworks to build power-capable advances in the power field. However, in order to improve IoT performance and address related problems, new strategies and trends are needed for IoT implementation in the power domain. In this section, we'll look into how Blockchain technology and Green IoT might help solve some of the problems.

6.6.1 The Internet of Things (IoT) and Blockchain

The majority of today's IoT installations are driven by cloud-based networks. The bulk of IoT installations necessitate the synchronization of thousands of IoT modules and machines, which can be complicated. Furthermore, since the Internet of Things is centralized and client–server, if one system is compromised or corrupted, all related artifacts can be easily accessed or manipulated, raising questions about user security and privacy. Fortunately, Blockchain will assist in the resolution of this issue.

The blockchain is a decentralized, open, and democratic framework that runs without the use of a third party. Any IoT node involved in the blockchain consensus network must demonstrate that it is operating towards the same end as the others. Checked transactions are often stored as a block that is attached to the previous one to guarantee that the evidence is never lost. Each node's inhabitants would be able to register and view transaction history. As a result, any modifications to each block are immediately available to all on the blockchain. Furthermore, thousands of IoT computers can be securely clustered thanks to blockchain's shared ledger. To create a reliable distributed ledger, blockchain consensus algorithms based on peer-to-peer networks can be used. As a result, blockchain will have a stable IoT that is intended to be decentralized and confidential.

The blockchain, in particular, allows app updates to be stored and exchanged can platforms. It's difficult to remove or change an update after it's been added to the blockchain as a legal block. There are nodes that affirm the authenticity of updated knowledge and defend it from attacks like a modern node. As a result, IoT-based networks will profit from the availability and safe side of blockchain.

The use of blockchain in the power sector would boost power stability and performance by creating a decentralized network for distributed power generation and storage systems. People would have convenient access to power data without needing the help of a third party, and real, high-quality data would be exchanged between machines in a relaxed manner. Only their immediate neighbors should be able to use their resources. People's trust will be improved, the costs of subscribing to centralized networks will be minimized, and political interference will be prevented. Another benefit of Blockchain is that it allows electricity production firms to monitor demand data and simplify power distribution to specific locations from a single place. In addition, smart grid technology would benefit from blockchain-based IoT networks for diagnosis and monitoring. The direct deployment of blockchain technologies in an IoT-dependent environment is currently out of question because of a shortage of processing power, bandwidth, and the requirement to conserve energy. Cloud and fog processing implementations, on the other hand, would extend the use of blockchain technologies in the IoT.

6.6.2 *IoT Power Use That Is Long-Term and Economically Friendly*

The usage of IoT power is a major issue, particularly when these systems become more commonly distributed in the near future. The millions and millions of computers which would be coupled to the World Wide Web would need a tremendous amount of energy. There will be a lot of electrical waste because of the large number of IoT devices. Low-carbon, high-efficiency transmission networks would be needed to solve these concerns. These requirements, luckily, culminated in the formation of the green IoT. In the green IoT life cycle, which includes design, growth, deployment, and eventual disposal, power-efficient characteristics are significant.

The G-IoT loop may be incorporated into a variety of IoT deployments. For example, identifiers that use radio frequency identification (RFID). RFID tags are shrinking in size in order to reduce the volume of difficult-to-recycle content in each tag. Another example is green M2M communications, which uses algorithmic and distributed computing techniques to allow low-power transmission and more powerful communication protocols. Sensor nodes in wireless sensor networks can also go to sleep and only wake up when they are required. To reduce the nodes' power consumption, radio optimization strategies like modulation optimization and co-operative collaboration may be used. Cluster frameworks or multi-path routing are two power-saving routing approaches that can be useful. Finally, the methods and explanations presented above will assist IoT systems in energy conservation.

6.7 Conclusion

The electric grid is on the verge of undergoing a significant transition. Due to the widespread usage of VRE in distributed power systems, as well as the need for further power, system-wide, structural approaches to mitigating power system socioeconomic and environmental impacts are needed. In this regard, emerging technology such as the Internet of Things (IoT) could aid the power quarter move from a bureaucratic, centralized supply chain to a decentralized, intelligent, and streamlined system. This article addresses the role of the Internet of Things in the power industry, as well as smart grids in particular.

From generation to power grids to end-user industries, we categorize different IoT consumption cases in every quarter of the power supply chain. The advantages of Internet-of-Things-based power management systems for increasing power generation and combining renewable energy sources are examined and the discovery is summarized. Temperature, humidity, illumination, rpm, passive infrared, and proximity sensors, as well as their uses in the power industry, are all addressed. Cloud computing and data processing systems, for example, may be used to capture and model data for a large variety of smart power applications, from homes to towns.

At various stages, like intelligent cities, intelligent grids, intelligent homes, and smart transportation, we investigate how the IoT is being utilized in the energy supply chain. Item identification, big data management, reliability issues and sophistication, subsystem synchronization, protection and privacy, IoT power specifications, standardization, and architectural design are only a couple of the difficulties that using IoT in the power sector presents. According to us, two potential research avenues for addressing these issues are blockchain and green IoT.

References

1. Aba EN, Olugboji OA, Nasir A et al (2021) Petroleum pipeline monitoring using an internet of things (IoT) platform. SN Appl Sci 3:180. https://doi.org/10.1007/s42452-021-04225-z
2. Abel EE, Latiff MSA (2021) The utilization of algorithms for cloud internet of things application domains: a review. Front Comput Sci 15:153502. https://doi.org/10.1007/s11704-019-9056-6
3. Attaran M (2021) The impact of 5G on the evolution of intelligent automation and industry digitization. J Ambient Intell Human Comput. https://doi.org/10.1007/s12652-020-02521-x
4. Bansal S, Kumar D (2020). IoT ecosystem: a survey on devices, gateways, operating systems, middleware and communication. Int J Wirel Inf Netw 27:340–364. https://doi.org/10.1007/s10776-020-00483-7
5. Bilandi N, Verma HK, Dhir R (2021) An intelligent and energy-efficient wireless body area network to control coronavirus outbreak. Arab J Sci Eng. https://doi.org/10.1007/s13369-021-05411-2
6. Bertino E, Jahanshahi MR, Singla A et al (2021) Intelligent IoT systems for civil infrastructure health monitoring: a research roadmap. Discov Internet Things 1:3. https://doi.org/10.1007/s43926-021-00009-4
7. Bhushan S, Kumar M, Kumar P et al (2021) FAJIT: a fuzzy-based data aggregation technique for energy efficiency in wireless sensor network. Complex Intell Syst. https://doi.org/10.1007/s40747-020-00258-w
8. Brambilla M, Umuhoza E, Acerbis R (2017) 2017 Model-driven development of user interfaces for IoT systems via domain-specific components and patterns. J Internet Serv Appl 8:14. https://doi.org/10.1186/s13174-017-0064-1
9. Bunruangses M, Arumona AE, Youplao P et al (2021) Realizing THz RFID using silicon chip space-time control circuit. Silicon. https://doi.org/10.1007/s12633-021-00960-5
10. Cheddadi Y, Cheddadi H, Cheddadi F et al (2020) Design and implementation of an intelligent low-cost IoT solution for energy monitoring of photovoltaic stations. SN Appl Sci 2:1165. https://doi.org/10.1007/s42452-020-2997-4
11. Cvitić I, Peraković D, Periša M et al (2021) Ensemble machine learning approach for classification of IoT devices in smart home. Int J Mach Learn Cyber. https://doi.org/10.1007/s13042-020-01241-0
12. Dash SP (2020) The impact of IoT in healthcare: global technological change & the roadmap to a networked architecture in India. J Indian Inst Sci 100:773–785. https://doi.org/10.1007/s41745-020-00208-y
13. Deng DJ, Benslimane A (2021) Editorial: innovation and application of internet of things for smart cities. Mobile Netw Appl. https://doi.org/10.1007/s11036-020-01715-z
14. Deng L, Li D, Cai Z et al (2020) Smart IoT information transmission and security optimization model based on chaotic neural computing. Neural Comput Appl 32:16491–16504. https://doi.org/10.1007/s00521-019-04162-4
15. Elhadi S, Marzak A, Sael N (2021) Operating models of network protocols IoT: long-range protocols. In: Ben Ahmed M, Rakıp Karaș İ, Santos D, Sergeyeva O, Boudhir AA (eds) Innovations in smart cities applications, vol 4. SCA. Lecture notes in networks and systems, vol 183. Springer, Cham. https://doi.org/10.1007/978-3-030-66840-2_81

16. Al-Turjman F, Abujubbeh M (2019) IoT-enabled smart grid via SM: an overview, future generation computer systems. 96:579–590. ISSN: 0167-739X. https://doi.org/10.1016/j.future.2019.02.012
17. Ferrara P, Mandal AK, Cortesi A et al (2021) Static analysis for discovering IoT vulnerabilities. Int J Softw Tools Technol Transf 23:71–88. https://doi.org/10.1007/s10009-020-00592-x
18. Gautam AK, Kumar R (2020). A comprehensive study on key management, authentication and trust management techniques in wireless sensor networks. SN Appl Sci 3:50. https://doi.org/10.1007/s42452-020-04089-9
19. Hassan MB, Alsharif S, Alhumyani H et al (2021) An enhanced cooperative communication scheme for physical uplink shared channel in NB-IoT. Wirel Pers Commun. https://doi.org/10.1007/s11277-021-08067-1
20. Qinxia H, Nazir S, Li M, Ullah Khan H, Lianlian W, Ahmad S (2021) AI-enabled sensing and decision-making for IoT systems. Complexity 2021:9. Article ID 6616279. https://doi.org/10.1155/2021/6616279
21. Park H, Lee D, Park G, Park S, Khan S, Kim J, Kim W (2019) Energy harvesting using thermoelectricity for IoT and E-skin sensors. J Phys Energy 1(4)
22. Iraji S, Mogensen P, Ratasuk R (2017) Recent advances in M2M communications and Internet of Things (IoT). Int J Wirel Inf Netw 24:240–242. https://doi.org/10.1007/s10776-017-0362-3
23. Jan MA, He X, Song H et al (2021) Editorial: machine learning and big data analytics for IoT-enabled smart cities. Mobile Netw Appl 26:156–158. https://doi.org/10.1007/s11036-020-01702-4
24. Jurcut A, Niculcea T, Ranaweera P et al (2020) Security considerations for Internet of Things: a survey. SN Comput Sci 1:193. https://doi.org/10.1007/s42979-020-00201-3
25. Kasrin N, Benabbas A, Elmamooz G et al (2021) Data-sharing markets for integrating IoT data processing functionalities. CCF Trans Pervasive Comput Interact 3:76–93. https://doi.org/10.1007/s42486-020-00054-y
26. Sadique KM, Rahmani R, Johannesson P (2018) Towards security on Internet of Things: applications and challenges in technology. Proc Comput Sci 141:199–206. ISSN: 1877-0509.https://doi.org/10.1016/j.procs.2018.10.168
27. Khan H, Kushwah KK, Singh S et al (2021) Smart technologies driven approaches to tackle COVID-19 pandemic: a review. 3 Biotech 11:50. https://doi.org/10.1007/s13205-020-02581-y
28. Khanna A, Kaur S (2020) Internet of things (IoT), applications and challenges: a comprehensive review. Wirel Pers Commun 114:1687–1762. https://doi.org/10.1007/s11277-020-07446-4
29. Khoie R, Bose A, Saltsman J (2021) A study of carbon emissions and energy consumption of wind power generation in the Panhandle of Texas. Clean Technol Environ Policy. https://doi.org/10.1007/s10098-020-01994-w
30. Kishorebabu V, Sravanthi R (2020) Real time monitoring of environmental parameters using IOT. Wirel Pers Commun 112:785–808. https://doi.org/10.1007/s11277-020-07074-y
31. Konur S, Lan Y, Thakker D et al (2021) Towards design and implementation of Industry 4.0 for food manufacturing. Neural Comput Appl. https://doi.org/10.1007/s00521-021-05726-z
32. Kumari A, Tanwar S (2021) A secure data analytics scheme for multimedia communication in a decentralized smart grid. Multimed Tools Appl. https://doi.org/10.1007/s11042-021-10512-z
33. Kuzlu M, Fair C, Guler O (2021) Role of artificial intelligence in the Internet of Things (IoT) cybersecurity. Discov Internet Things 1:7. https://doi.org/10.1007/s43926-020-00001-4
34. Kwon S, Park S, Cho H et al (2021) Towards 5G-based IoT security analysis against Vo5G eavesdropping. Computing 103:425–447. https://doi.org/10.1007/s00607-020-00855-0
35. Le DN, Parvathy VS, Gupta D et al (2021) IoT enabled depthwise separable convolution neural network with deep support vector machine for COVID-19 diagnosis and classification. Int J Mach Learn Cybern. https://doi.org/10.1007/s13042-020-01248-7
36. Guha A, Samanta D, Banerjee A, Agarwal D (2021) A deep learning model for information loss prevention from multi-page digital documents. IEEE Access 9:80451–80465. https://doi.org/10.1109/ACCESS.2021.3084841

37. Mekala MS, Patan R, Islam SKH, Samanta D, Mallah GA, Chaudhry SA (2021) DAWM: cost-aware asset claim analysis approach on big data analytic computation model for cloud data centre. Secur Commun Netw 2021: 16. Article ID 6688162. https://doi.org/10.1155/2021/6688162
38. Samanta D, Karthikeyan MP, Banerjee A, Inokawa H (2021) Tunable graphene nano-patch antenna design for on-chip integrated terahertz detector arrays with potential application in cancer imagining. Nanomedicine. ISSN:1743-5889. https://doi.org/10.2217/nnm-2020-0386
39. Biswal AK, Singh D, Pattanayak BK, Samanta D, Yang M-H (2021) IoT-based smart alert system for drowsy driver detection. Wirel Commun Mobile Comput 2021:13. Article ID 6627217. https://doi.org/10.1155/2021/6627217
40. Maheswari M, Geetha S, Selva Kumar S, Karuppiah M, Samanta D, Park Y PEVRM: probabilistic evolution based version recommendation model for mobile applications. IEEE Access. https://doi.org/10.1109/ACCESS.2021.3053583
41. Gomathy V, Padhy N, Samanta D et al (2020) Malicious node detection using heterogeneous cluster based secure routing protocol (HCBS) in wireless adhoc sensor networks. J Ambient Intell Human Comput 11:4995–5001. https://doi.org/10.1007/s12652-020-01797-3
42. Sivakumar P, Nagaraju R, Samanta D et al (2020) A novel free space communication system using nonlinear InGaAsP microsystem resonators for enabling power-control toward smart cities. Wirel Netw 26:2317–2328. https://doi.org/10.1007/s11276-019-02075-7
43. Khamparia A, Singh PK, Rani P, Samanta D, Khanna A, Bhushan B (2020) An internet of health things-driven deep learning framework for detection and classification of skin cancer using transfer learning. Trans Emerg Telecommun Technol e3963. https://doi.org/10.1002/ett.3963
44. Althar RR, Samanta D (2021) The realist approach for evaluation of computational intelligence in software engineering. Innov Syst Softw Eng. https://doi.org/10.1007/s11334-020-00383-2
45. Guha A, Samanta D (2021) Hybrid approach to document anomaly detection: an application to facilitate RPA in title insurance. Int J Autom Comput 18:55–72. https://doi.org/10.1007/s11633-020-1247-y
46. Samanta D, Sivaram M, Rashed A, Boopathi CS, Sadegh Amiri I, Yupapin P (2020) Distributed Feedback Laser (DFB) for signal power amplitude level improvement in long spectral band. J Opt Commun.https://doi.org/10.1515/joc-2019-0252
47. Pramanik S, Samanta S, Bandyopadhyay S, Ghosh R A new combinational technique in image steganography. Int J Inf Secur Priv (IJISP) 15(3). Article 4, ISSN: 1930-1650|EISSN: 1930-1669. https://doi.org/10.4018/IJISP.2021070104.
48. Biswas J, Kayal P, Samanta D (2021) Reducing approximation error with rapid convergence rate for non-negative matrix factorization (NMF). Math Stat 9(3):285–289. https://doi.org/10.13189/ms.2021.090309
49. Lee H, Gu B, Cha SW et al. (2021) Model based automated calibration for shift control of automatic transmission. Int J Autom Technol. https://doi.org/10.1007/s12239-021-0026-2
50. Li L, Aphale SS, Zhu L (2021) High-bandwidth nanopositioning via active control of system resonance. Front Mech Eng. https://doi.org/10.1007/s11465-020-0619-x
51. Li W, Chai Y, Khan F et al (2021) A comprehensive survey on machine learning-based big data analytics for IoT-enabled smart healthcare system. Mobile Netw Appl 26:234–252. https://doi.org/10.1007/s11036-020-01700-6
52. Mahbub M (2020) NB-IoT: applications and future prospects in perspective of Bangladesh. Int J Inf Technol 12:1183–1193. https://doi.org/10.1007/s41870-020-00469-x
53. Manuel MP, Daimi K (2021) Implementing cryptography in LoRa based communication devices for unmanned ground vehicle applications. SN Appl Sci 3:397. https://doi.org/10.1007/s42452-021-04377-y
54. Maroli AA, Narwane VS, Raut RD et al (2021) Framework for the implementation of an Internet of Things (IoT)-based water distribution and management system. Clean Technol Environ Policy 23:271–283. https://doi.org/10.1007/s10098-020-01975-z
55. Mishra M, Choudhury P, Pati B (2021) Modified ride-NN optimizer for the IoT based plant disease detection. J Ambient Intell Human Comput 12:691–703. https://doi.org/10.1007/s12652-020-02051-6

56. Możaryn J, Petryszyn J, Ozana S (2021) PLC based fractional-order PID temperature control in pipeline: design procedure and experimental evaluation. Meccanica 56:855–871. https://doi.org/10.1007/s11012-020-01215-0
57. Mylonas G, Paganelli F, Cuffaro G et al (2021) Using gamification and IoT-based educational tools towards energy savings—some experiences from two schools in Italy and Greece. J Ambient Intell Human Comput. https://doi.org/10.1007/s12652-020-02838-7
58. Nasajpour M, Pouriyeh S, Parizi RM et al (2020) Internet of Things for current COVID-19 and future pandemics: an exploratory study. J Healthc Inf Res 4:325–364.https://doi.org/10.1007/s41666-020-00080-6
59. Nguyen VD, Duong TQ, Vien QT (2020) Editorial: emerging techniques and applications for 5G networks and beyond. Mobile Netw Appl 25:1984–1986. https://doi.org/10.1007/s11036-020-01547-x
60. Otero P, Chowdhry BS, Zeng H et al (2021). Special issue: underwater communications and sensors technologies. Wirel Pers Commun 116:955–961. https://doi.org/10.1007/s11277-020-08031-5
61. Pahlavan K, Krishnamurthy P (2021) Evolution and impact of Wi-Fi technology and applications: a historical perspective. Int J Wirel Inf Netw 28:3–19. https://doi.org/10.1007/s10776-020-00501-8
62. Park DS (2018) Future computing with IoT and cloud computing. J Supercomput 74:6401–6407. https://doi.org/10.1007/s11227-018-2652-7
63. Qin J, Li Z, Wang R et al (2021) Industrial Internet of Learning (IIoL): IIoT based pervasive knowledge network for LPWAN—concept, framework and case studies. CCF Trans Pervasive Comput Interact 3:25–39. https://doi.org/10.1007/s42486-020-00050-2
64. Rachit, Bhatt S, Ragiri PR (2021). Security trends in Internet of Things: a survey. SN Appl Sci 3:121. https://doi.org/10.1007/s42452-021-04156-9
65. Rajab H, Cinkler T, Bouguera T (2020) IoT scheduling for higher throughput and lower transmission power. Wirel Netw. https://doi.org/10.1007/s11276-020-02307-1
66. Saha R, Biswas S, Sarmah S et al (2021) A Working prototype using DS18B20 temperature sensor and Arduino for health monitoring. SN Comput Sci 2:33. https://doi.org/10.1007/s42979-020-00434-2
67. Richa E (2021) IoT: security issues and challenges. In: Senjyu T, Mahalle PN, Perumal T, Joshi A (eds) Information and communication technology for intelligent systems. ICTIS 2020. Smart innovation, systems and technologies, vol 196. Springer, Singapore. https://doi.org/10.1007/978-981-15-7062-9_9
68. Sequeiros H, Oliveira T, Thomas MA (2021) The Impact of IoT smart home services on psychological well-being. Inf Syst Front. https://doi.org/10.1007/s10796-021-10118-8
69. Seiger R, Kühn R, Korzetz M et al (2021) HoloFlows: modelling of processes for the Internet of Things in mixed reality. Softw Syst Model. https://doi.org/10.1007/s10270-020-00859-6
70. Simeone A, Zeng Y, Caggiano A (2021) Intelligent decision-making support system for manufacturing solution recommendation in a cloud framework. Int J Adv Manuf Technol 112:1035–1050. https://doi.org/10.1007/s00170-020-06389-1
71. Sodhro AH, Pirbhulal S, Muzammal M et al (2020) Towards blockchain-enabled security technique for industrial internet of things based decentralized applications. J Grid Comput 18:615–628. https://doi.org/10.1007/s10723-020-09527-x
72. Yadav S, Luthra S, Garg D (2021) Modelling Internet of things (IoT)-driven global sustainability in multi-tier agri-food supply chain under natural epidemic outbreaks. Environ Sci Pollut Res 28:16633–16654. https://doi.org/10.1007/s11356-020-11676-1
73. Yang F, Gu S (2021) Industry 4.0, a revolution that requires technology and national strategies. Complex Intell Syst. https://doi.org/10.1007/s40747-020-00267-9
74. You X, Wang CX, Huang J et al (2021) Towards 6G wireless communication networks: vision, enabling technologies, and new paradigm shifts. Sci China Inf Sci 64:110301. https://doi.org/10.1007/s11432-020-2955-6
75. Zhu XN, Peko G, Sundaram D et al (2021) Blockchain-based agile supply chain framework with IoT. Inf Syst Front. https://doi.org/10.1007/s10796-021-10114-y

Chapter 7
Abnormality Diagnosis from Ambient Data: IoT Data Sequences in Real Time

Abstract Modern sensor networks are being propelled by the Internet of Things (IoT) model to track a wide variety of phenomena, including environmental control, medical care, manufacturing operations, along with intelligent metropolis. These meshwork function as pivot facilitators to a Digital Earth Nervous System by offering a constant pulse of the almost limitless events taking place in physical space. Nonetheless, the accelerated transforming for these sensor information sequences resumes posing a problem for conventional data-handling strategies, necessitating the creation of new approaches. We suggest a generalized approach to this problem that could be used to help all aspects of dispensed instantaneous inspection. For working along with multiple types of record origins, this impartial technique utilizes a brokering approach and web-based specifications to ensure interoperability. We used the technique to identify peculiarities instantaneously and related it with the field of atmospheric management as a proof of concept. The built framework is capable of identifying irregularities, carrying out alerts, and showing the user the current situation.

Keywords IoT · Artificial neural network · Sensor data · Big data

7.1 Introduction

Thousands of wireless sensor networks (WSNs) track nearly any normal and man-made phenomenon. Any of these networks can be used in our everyday lives for various monitoring purposes, such as environmental monitoring (meteorological, air quality, traffic, and so on), smart cities (smart parking, smart lighting, and so on), medical-care tracking, industrial tracking, or online media monitoring. Every sensor in the internetwork creates a data stream, and subject to the reviving time, each sensor will produce a large number of measurements, which will be compared to those from different sensors within the internetwork. The IoT paradigm authorized the WSNs in connecting to Internet through the TCP/IP, along with their connectivity becoming more accessible. In addition, IoT facilitates large-scale observation retrieval and provides a direct link to WSN.

D. Samanta and A. Banerjee, *Computationally Intensive Statistics for Intelligent IoT*, Studies in Autonomic, Data-driven and Industrial Computing,
https://doi.org/10.1007/978-981-16-5936-2_7

With these capacities, we are moving closer to the Artificial Neural Network [1] and others expected in 2020. However, when the raw values are collected, it becomes impossible to evaluate any of these observations. The researcher infers that efforts in enhancing the transforming capacities are ongoing; we also lack the capacity to facilitate regarding such a neural network. We lack an approach to incorporate the Modern Earth vision which solves the IoT's diverseness and need norms, enabling all in reaching and managing newer diverse information sources from the denationalized and government sectors simultaneously.

Here, the authors propose a framework for evaluating the burgeoning overflow of tracking information. We define a method along with devising architecture for analyzing scrutiny from various sensor internetworks when they are created. The proposed solution's potentials are demonstrated and tested in a utilization which senses abnormalities in surrounding sensor internetworks spontaneously. The generating method is built on cutting-edge approaches for rapidly processing vast volumes of streamed information, meaning that each and every information are properly analyzed and that every algorithm can be applied to the data stream. We expand and generalize our preceding job so that the ultimate approach may be extended to some form of Web-based sensor internetwork. Newer offerings comprise of (1) various appliances for communicating accompanied by sensor information origins regardless of data category; (2) the capability in interpreting vast volumes of sensor records in spontaneous-time; (3) a method in translating non-quality sensor records to quality templates; (4) the capability in communicating with various agreements using an organizing result; and (5) a framing solution.

The IoT is an interdisciplinary paradigm where a large number of devices in our world are interconnected and linked to the Web in delivering different demand and enhance efficiency. The Internet of Things was made possible by wireless networking, lower-power computers, integrated sensors and actuators, Radio Frequency Identification, cellular telephones, along with cloud technology. Despite the fact that not one of these innovations is needed for any IoT system, these still contribute to the growth of IoT by offering a sufficient precondition. While RFID warrants lower-expenditure object recognition along with very-lower-power system-on-chips authorize battery-mechanized embedded computers, cloud computation along with fog computation may be utilized to offload calculations along with utilities to regional or worldwide servers, freeing up resources for handling vast volumes of data or performing increasingly complicated procedures. The networking of embedded IoT systems sets them apart from traditional embedded systems. In a wider sense and perception, the IoT is a public network of diverse, compute cluster embedded internetworks and entities. Thanks to communication capabilities, especially Internet networking, systems and mobile objects can interact and communicate with certain technologies and systems, WSN [3], Mobile Computing, Cyber Physical Systems, machine-to-machine communication, RFID, and other application domains. Many research efforts on IoT have been made in the fields of networking, object detection, and data services (information security), but it has gained lesser coverage from both the viewpoint of embedded computation.

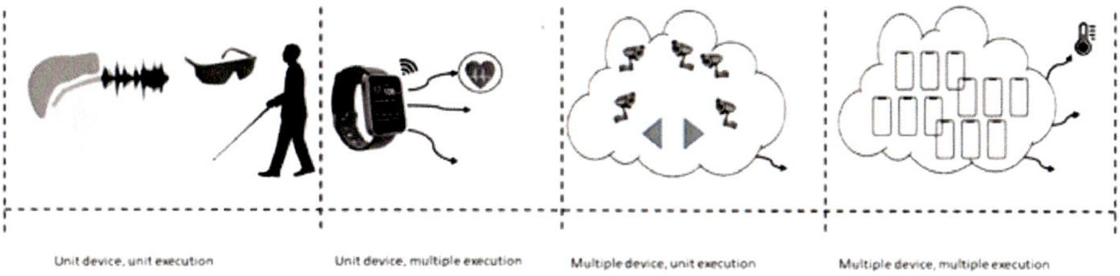

Fig. 7.1 Unit/multiple devices can be used by IoT applications to incorporate unit/multiple frameworks

It's impossible to present a succinct statement of IoT hardware and software requirements due to the vast variety of IoT applications and technologies. As a result, the IoT embedded designer is faced with tough questions, such as: Which wireless networking mechanization (1) spans the essential spectrum, (2) offers the requisite data rate, and (3) is though (ultra)-lower-power and encounters energy restraints. Figure 7.1 expresses Unit/multiple devices can be used by IoT applications to incorporate unit/multiple frameworks.

- What compromises can be made between (1) QoS [4] along with energy usage, (2) on-board production along with computing offloading, and so on?
- How do you cope with IoT systems' unpredictability and inconsistency (which is mostly attributable to transmission)?

This manuscript explores the Internet of Things along with its technological facilitators deriving out of the viewpoint. This paper not only examines essential IoT technology and emerging trends, but also provides defining IoT properties for the embedded domain, as well as a detailed IoT viewpoint for embedded systems, which is currently missing in existing surveys such as [5].

This chapter explores the Internet of Things and its technological enablers from this viewpoint. This paper not only examines essential IoT technology and emerging trends, but also provides defining IoT properties for the embedded domain, as well as a detailed IoT viewpoint for embedded systems, which is currently missing in existing surveys such as [6].

7.2 Properties of the Device and the Application

Domains of Application: The Internet of Things can have an impact on a multitude of application realms by allowing newer assistances or upgrading the functionality of prevailing ones amidst the attainable solicitations, we look at the main categories (which encompass a wider variety of various demands, mechanizations, and deployment challenges) as well as futuristic applications. These aren't the only types of IoT implementations that can be imagined; there's a lot more. In the other hand, their criteria, properties, and architecture issues are similar to those in our categories. The following pieces go into the main challenges and requirements.

In terms of allowing and improving healthcare services, the Internet of Things has shown a lot of potential. With IoT-dependent medicare services, continuing tracking of individual well-being position in spontaneous-time, everywhere, is possible. Electrocardiograms (ECGs) [7], electroencephalograms (EEGs) [8], electromyograms (EMGs) [9], body motion, and other vital bio-signals are collected. Spontaneous-time information may be preserved, analyzed, or sent to a distant machine (like a cloud server) for additional monitoring along with diagnosis. Problems such as ultra-lower power architecture and spontaneous-time limitations are encountered in these applications.

Assisted living is a term that refers to a type of care that aims to help i) the elderly, (ii) the mentally ill, and (iii) the disabled. A smart cane paired with a wearable IoT app, for example, can sense and avoid obstacles, gain access to houses, traverse indoor and outdoor spaces, and so on. Smart Buildings [10] and Homes using The Internet of Things (IoT) integrates embedded technologies, enabling apps that minimize costs, increase personal convenience, and enhance building and home security.

The word "smart city" refers to Smart cities using distributed IoT systems with a variety of sensors to improve transit and traffic safety [11], air grade tracking (e.g. noise, warmth, moisture) [12], intelligent parking [13], intelligent signage [14], and intelligent sprinkling gardens [15]. IoT-focused technologies for automation, supervision, and tracking in industrial realms like supply chain management, conveyance and logistics [16], and automation will boost organization by lessening operating and servicing costs along with improving service efficiency. One example is remote control of machines (for example, in farms, wind turbines, and so on) for predictive maintenance.

7.3 Implementations Versus Machines

The interaction for IoT implementations with the fundamental hardware or machine presents certain design confrontations which must be solved at the program or hardware level. There are four types of relationships among the quantity of appliances and the quantity of facilities along with apps offered:

- One-to-One: A single IoT unit is used for a single process. For example, a healthcare surveillance [17] device that collects real-time bio-signals [18] based on the Internet of Things.

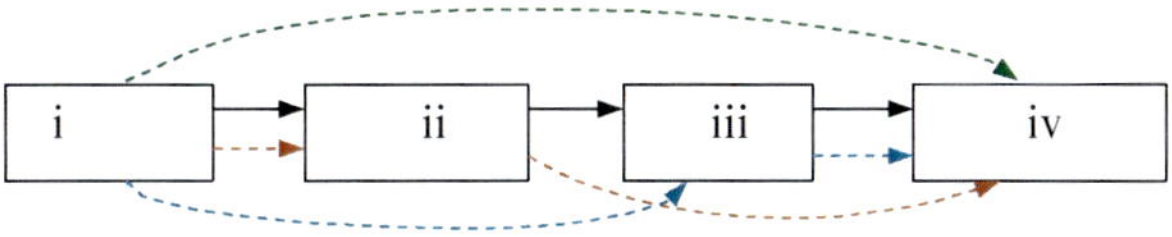

Fig. 7.2 Major levels in IoT execution

- One-to-many: A single Internet of Things device can execute several tasks. For example, a smart watch [19] is a fitness device with various sensors that can track a buyer's physique venture, heartbeat rate, and position. An intelligent meeting room [20], for example, utilizes an unit appliance to perform a variety of functions, including sensing the beginning/termination of a conference, inspecting the room's ambient factors (such as warmth and luminance), and manipulating auditory signals to monitor the meeting's activities, among others. In this category, the planner must make a decision on how to manage shared capital. The solutions range from conservative hardware selection (processor, memory, wireless ratio, etc.) to dynamically controlling and scheduling hardware consumption.
- Many-to-one: This type includes devices that are spatially distributed and have a single function. Distributed smart cameras, for example, are used for video monitoring [21]. When optimizing the method, this category normally has two properties that designers must consider: (1) There is a high level of computer access, and (2) there is a high level of repetition.
- Multiple-to-multiple communication: In certain IoT executions, many applications and utilities share a large number of computers. Smart Citizen [22] is a network of Internet of Things (IoT) embedded sensors [23] that gather data for executions which describe warmth, moisture, sound level, along with air quality.

WSNs that are shared are also included in this category. Figure 7.1 depicts these categories as well as few instances. Though shared IoT appliances minimize hardware and preservation costs, they also initiate newer problems such as linking, allotment, digital and execution time assets governance, and ensuring that applications that share a single machine adhere to scheduling restrictions, among others. Figure 7.2 expresses major levels in IoT execution.

7.4 Hardware and Software Framework for the IoT

The general operating levels for an IoT program are (1) data accession, (2) data analysis, (3) data repository, and (4) data transfer. The initial and ultimate phases, as well as the processing, are all included with any submission.

(i) Information acquiring
(ii) Information Processing
(iii) Information Repository
(iv) Information Communication.

Some programs may or may not have storage (see Figure 7.2).

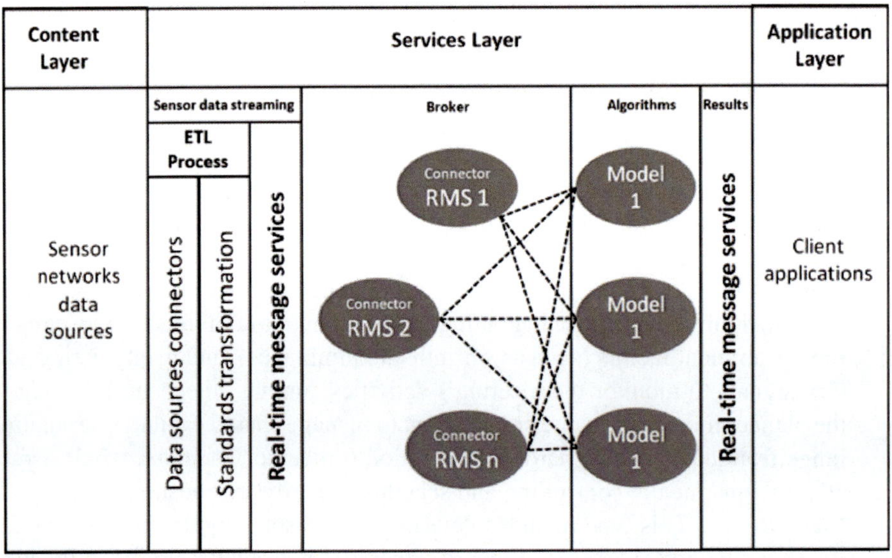

Fig. 7.3 Humanist description of the provided sensor streaming data analysis methodology

7.5 Efficiencies at Various Stages

7.5.1 Data Collection

At the hardware layer, lower-power amalgamated along with on-chip sensors based on Micro-Electro-Mechanical Systems automation may help minimize data acquisition energy consumption. Accelerometers, gyroscopes, microphones, and biosensors are examples of on-chip sensors.

At the system level, energy-efficient sensing schemes can take advantage of the spatial and temporal characteristics of the input data to collect fewer samples while maintaining the necessary signal quality. The energy required for transmission and storage is also affected by the diminished quantity of incoming data (depending on the quantity of specimens and resolution).

Compressed sensing (CS) [24] is an original approach that allows the signal to be repaired using fewer specimens than Nyquist theory, albeit at the expense of precision. Till the input data is sparse, a lesser quantity of specimens may arrest the necessary data, and CS may minimize the amount of data accumulated requiring losing remarkable data. The data sparsely property is present in many IoT applications, allowing them to take advantage of the CS paradigm. CS has been widely researched and analyzed in health tracking applications and wireless body sensor networks.

7.5.2 Information Processing

At the hardware level, (1) super lower-power cognitive models [25] and (2) effectively configured CPUs will lead to significant savings in a processor proposes and fabricates a diverse twin CPU [26] centered on the big.LITTLE model. Energy consumption for IoT systems is achieved by combining a super low power fairly close processor with a highly efficient processor and a task scheduling system.

7.5.3 Information Repository

At the system level, energy drain in storage has risen in popularity in the engineered systems engineering group, and there are many features unique to IoT systems which can be utilized to increase memory energy efficiency in IoT embedded systems even further. Many IoT applications, for example, are designed to withstand failure, data errors, that brings new opportunities with heterogeneous network structures made up of a mistake section (for better dependable data along with functioning) along with an erratum-prone portion (for lesser reliable data and operations) (for lesser significant records) proposing a unique memory centered on this property for low-power biomedical signal processors. Versatile–anti-volatile storage was already suggested for portable connected systems that require compact and curved types.

7.5.4 Transmission of Data

Data transmission can be enhanced at the hardware level by incorporating retrospectives onto SoCs, offering excellent micro radio processors, and so on. The most important current technologies, patterns, and challenges in communication and mobility. At the system level, modern compression algorithms techniques, specifically for data formats, are required to reduce the amount of data which is stored or transferred. This section depicts the overall structure of an IoT SoC platform's key components. Most, if not all of these components, can be found in an IoT embedded system, such as at least one RF component for communication.

7.5.5 Different Computing Layers

IoT devices can produce a large amount of information, namely, data streams, sound, and videos, which is referred to as big data. The challenges posed by evolving big data (e.g. large memory and stream processors demands, higher bandwidth, etc.) necessitate the transfer of computing along with processing to different underlying processing levels accessible in the IoT series. Figure 7.4 depicts various processing methods.

Through IoT embedded systems to Cloud [24] storage, there are several levels of computing. The data collected can be processed on either an IoT system or a computer or a portal, for example. As a result, for IoT applications that require data processing, deciding in which the processing must be performed (i.e. computing offloading) is a major challenge. Many factors influence the decision system goals (e.g. actual-time necessity, sustainable energy, etc.), and device requirements are examples of parameters and factors (e.g. energy exhaustion in information transmission and information communication on IoT appliance, transmission bandwidth, transmission delay, etc.). Different computing layers and platforms are shown in this section.

- Device-centric: An IoT device's microcontroller [25] may be used to conduct the processing. The main difficulties seem to be the scarce resources available on IoT connected systems (for example, on-chip storage and processor functionality) as well as meeting low-power requirements. To either conduct the calculation also on IoT embedded device [26] or unload it with other levels of computing is a vital task. When the response must be decided at running time (i.e. based on the process, reference results, source of energy status, as well as other transient variables), this decision-making becomes more difficult.
- Access (e.g. mobile phone): IoT gateway tools which are utilized to resolve heterogeneity between various networks and the Internet are typically gateway-centric having a higher computational capacity. As suggested in [27], gateway devices such as mobile phones could be utilized to conduct data analysis. Such framework was utilized in medical care and health-dependent based surveillance. The smartphone receives the captured ECG signal and processes it. The main challenge here is to ensure availability when adhering to the deadlines. Given the uncertainty of wireless technology and delay, this is difficult, particularly as the number of IoT devices grows.
- Fog-dependent: Fog computing [28] is an expansion of both the cloud computing model that may assist the IoT framework in containing the Big [29] issue. Fogs have more processing capacity and lower latency than IoT embedded along with gateway devices and the cloud servers (owing to the positioning and distribution). An ECG is a type of electrocardiogram which presents extraction of features for a medical tracking system, demonstrating the advantages of that same fog computing technology.
- Cloud-dependent: Cloud computation is a tool towards collecting and transporting large amounts of data. To have superior standards of service and to support strategic thinking, it necessitates a large amount of data storage and processing resources. Even so, because as number of IoT appliances grows, so does the amount of stream data, posing problems and challenges for cloud storage solutions such as scalability, high energy costs, latency, latency, and accessibility.
- Blended encounter: As each of the above options has its own set of benefits and drawbacks, micro and flexible delivery results are more powerful. As an instance, consider classification.

For patient health monitoring, methods such as SVM [30] devices are commonly used only for abnormality tracking and scene understanding. Software of a collection of SVMs is loaded into memory and will be utilized for classification at compilation time. Whenever the quantity of SVMs is high (i.e. the IoT system requires a lot of memory), it's more effective to retain most of them are on the interface (e.g. a mobile phone), rather than incrementing the repository capacity at design phase. If a function is far enough away again from SVMs installed onto the server, this approach is used. This must be transferred to a mobile and contrasted to certain other SVMs using an IoT system. By exploiting the benefits of every computational tier (e.g. greater storage, additional computer complexity, etc.), applications may improve their performance and meet their requirements. However, in a hybrid system, the key problem is to identify an accurate comparison among localized computation and computing unloading, as well as the ideal scheduling of offloading.

7.6 Exact Versus Approximate Computing

To achieve more performance, the new model of approximate computing takes advantage of applications' intrinsic durability and modifies the criterion of specific equality between description and execution. The majority of Internet of Things (IoT) systems communicate with the real universe using noisy incoming record. As a result, they are still concerned along with estimation. For example, in the Analog-to-Digital conversion, the first stage of approximation occurs, resulting in a quantization error. Although these applications accept certain failures, the final performance or QoS [31] should fall within a definite scope.

The error tolerance [32] property can be used in a variety of applications to exchange output efficiency for calculation attempt (e.g. energy utilization, interpretation, etc.). In the field of approximate computation for IoT, there are a few unsolved problems. The tolerable inaccuracy may be received and manipulated in a variety of hardware and software components:

- Data acquisition: During data processing, resolution and sampling rate decide the accuracy of input data (or frame rate). ECG signal, for example, is captured at 360 samples per second with an 11-bit resolution. While an IoT program permits fallacy, one way to take advantage of it is to lower the quality of input data. This will minimize energy utilization or latency.
- Information processing: Estimation can also be achieved in the fundamental hardware by constructing precise hardware units for complex arithmetic operations. Moreover, it may be accomplished at the program level using techniques such as stage skipping.
- Data storage: At the memory facility, the bearable fallacy should be used to minimize the magnitude of essential repository, the amount of memory accesses, or the computer's energy consumption. The researchers provide an instance of approximation in repository. Hybrid schemes, in which several steps take advantage of

approximation, are also feasible. The key problem here is deciding (1) at which point to apply approximation and (2) the quantity of approximation to apply for reduced computational work during satisfying QoS requirements.

7.7 Electronic Design Automation (EDA) Tools for the IoT

EDA tools would solve two facets of IoT design: (1) the rising need for embedded system design, and (2) the growing complication of IoT SoCs.

The growth of the IoT industry has resulted in the development of small design firms with more specific and creative products operating on a smaller scale, resulting in the exposure of IoT firms with a device design (rather than chip design) perspective. Reduced construction time and risks would be their primary considerations. Because of these issues, as well as a lack of chip design experience, IP cores seem to be a potential approach for managing design complexity and integration risk. Build IP cores (various hardware blocks which have previously been pre-established and evaluated) that are expected to drive IoT production, with IP companies experiencing exponential growth [33].

The IoT has two distinct characteristics: (1) physical interaction (via sensors and actuators) and (2) communication capability (intra and inter appliances). Mixed signal and analog are also involved in both of these properties. The most basic requirements of IoT platforms seem to be wireless radio, sensor Analog-to-Digital Converters, analog filters, and amplifiers. This complicates the design flow, mostly the identification and error correction of varied-signal SoCs. To meet the above IoT demands, there are two complementary patterns in EDA [34].

1. Design appliances to promote the development of IoT appliances (i.e. modular, inexpensive, quick designs): The tools provide standard EDA aids at a cheaper expenditure, with greater scalability and a short plotting time. IBM and SiCAD [35], for example, are collaborating on a cloud service that combines IBM EDA software with high-performance cloud services to make illustration, affirmation, and implementations quicker and much effective. Moreover, Silicon Cloud International targets IoT device developers with cloud-based “workflow as a service” for ASIC architecture.
2. IoT-dependent core design tools: It contains small and energy-dependent IP cores for wireless networking and analog front ends in IoT SoCs.

As the market for IP grows, newer cloud-dependent challenges must emerge. For example, before buying the IP core, the customer would be able to test it online (without installing it) by running simulations and testing its performance and power.

7.8 A Foundation for Implementing Sensor Information Sequences

For real-time approach, the suggested method exercises big data generated by sensors. The approach may be evaluated in a versatile manner and consistent as it (1) operates with a variety of sensor information origins with a variety of schemes and attachment functionalities; (2) permits for the real-time processing of large volumes of sensor observations; (3) permits in the implementation of any type of analysis; thus the specified method may be explained as quality-amenable; and (4) facilitates the findings utilizing a variety of methods.

7.8.1 *Layer Called Content*

The technique has been developed to operate on sensor data. It may be used in the model of atmosphere (humidity, air pressure, air temperature, and so on), atmospheric worthiness (carbon dioxide, carbon monoxide, and so on), fitness (pulse, blood pressure, and so on), and smart city phenomena (intelligent parking, intelligent light, etc.). Figure 7.3 expresses humanist description of the provided sensor streaming data analysis methodology.

Additional information sequences are interpreted by the system like a set of examinations generated by acknowledging nodes. Every acknowledging node has various revived tariff for producing newer findings, as well as the ability to use multiple sensors to quantify a number of occurrences. Every sensor creates a sequence of data that may be contextual or calculable in its category. This section demonstrates how various sensor information sequences come together to create a sensing node. A WSN is generated by a set of sensing nodes. One or both of these WSNs can be used in the content layer.

7.8.2 *Layer of Resources*

The service level creates interfaces in the sensor information origins, investigates the measurements, along with generating the information. To achieve an information sequence for every sensor, the authors open independent channels to each one. Real-time message system is a separate component that confines a series of transmission protocols that allows spontaneous information admittance. Next section explains how to link to various types of sensors and how to migrate to a regular data model when appropriate. For real-time data handling, different sensors can support different communication protocols and interfaces. Different protocols are harmonized in a corresponding brokering phase, allowing structured data to be handled through a common communication method. We produce the output as a complex information sequence by reutilizing the RMS after adding the individual generating techniques.

7.8.3 *Message Provider in Real Time*

The suggested algorithm functions in real-time, which ensures that newer quantities can be refined when they enhance accessibility over the Web. Internet-dependent services are typically obtained by sending HTTP requests to a web server [36], which subsequently returns the solicited resource (the request–response transmission). The protocol must be followed at each instance the customer demands entry to the facility. Figure 7.4 shows the sensing points and WSNs are made up of various sensor sequences.

While operating with information origins with fast reviving speeds, like market values or ambient sensor records, the web server must be queried continuously to remain updated. To resolve such problems, more successful and productive methods have been developed. They are dependent on electing approaches, in which the customer makes newer requisitions to the web server on a regular basis. If there is no new data on the server, it requests a suitable signal and shuts the interconnection. The customer then defers to the following submission to be received.

To pass sensor observations within the RMS, we use this method. For the sensor information sequencing framework, RMS is utilized in various sections of the assistance layer to plan sensor sequences. It will be used again to deliver the outcomes of the study. RMS may be deployed using Messaging-Oriented Middleware [37] (MOM), like the Java Messaging Services (which can provide a range of Message Brokers, including Apache ActiveMQ). Utilization of this series of software improves the versatility for accepted protocols (i.e. the ability in sharing data with a wide range of data origins and consumers) and sent messages (i.e. the ability in comprehending

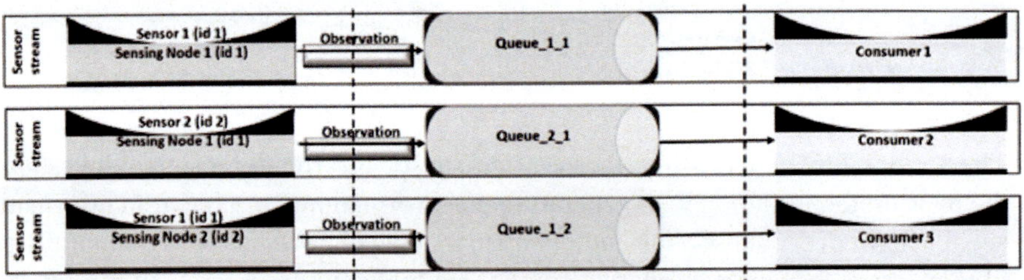

Fig. 7.4 The sensing points and WSNs are made up of various sensor sequences

the constituent of a wide range of statistical origins and be interpreted by several customers/clients).

The researcher's job employs two Message-Oriented Middleware theoretical concepts:

The messages are routed to a person in the point-to-point methodology to a customer who keeps track of incoming messages in a queue. Produce/advocate methodology: the technique enables notifications to be submitted to a specific Messaging Subject. Readers will show an attention in accepting Updates for a given information Subject by filling out a questionnaire. This work also makes use of the following JMS concepts:

Provider: a Message-Oriented Middleware execution for the JMS functionality.

Client: a program which sends and/or obtains communication.

A Customer who produces and transmits information is known as Producer/Publisher.

A Customer who accepts Messages is referred to as a Consumer/Subscriber.

Any data which requires to be conveyed utilizing JMS is referred to as a message.

Information which have been received and are continuing to be read are placed in a queue (by 1 client). A Queue means that all information is only processed once.

Topic: a system in disseminating information to numerous followers.

7.8.4 Streaming Sensor Data

The SDS part has two distinct functions. To begin, the SDS establishes connections with numerous sensors in order to collect data. As most openly accessible WSNs must not have quality entry to the record they create, Extract, Transform, and Load (ETL) [38] techniques turn non-quality data schemes into common ones. We consider three types of WSNs based on the data formats they help to make the job simpler and in reusing enduring tools like the organized WSNs, semi-organized WSNs, and non-organized WSNs.

The ETL method has two stages, as seen in Fig. 7.6. Data sources connectors, the first step, is in charge of collecting sensor information through various data origins. As previously stated, multiple types of sensor records are examined, along with the SDS functions as an agent in this regard since both organized and semi-organized sensor information must be interpreted, the SDS must be able to link to data origins which utilize a range of formats and agreements. To put it another way, it includes special linkers for every information origin. A single connector for quality WSNs may be reused for multiple WSNs that use the same solution. To obtain the unique observations that each sensor data source makes, a particular linker is facilitated for every origin. This phase necessitates a variety of metrics which are specified to information origin. It incorporates specifics related to the sensor information origin's relation, and the sensor refreshing tariff needed in acquiring newer monitoring when they are visible. Normal transformations are implemented in the second stage to acquire interoperable sensor data. Of observation made by a non-quality origin is converted into a proper configuration by a procedure.

Moreover, the RMS portion is used by the SDS to build the multiple data streams. An information agent with the P2P [39] methodology is utilized for this method, which guarantees full Message distribution to the User. As a consequence of this step, each sensor and sensing node has its own stream (Queue).

7.8.5 Brokering Policy

We use an organizing mechanism at the service level to admit data from various origins which utilize various communication agreements and information encodings. Figure 7.3 portrays the mechanism how a broker enables customers to link to information origins through a range of protocols. The system's stability, scalability, and interoperability are all improved by the ability to communicate with various sources. In order to communicate with the RMS, our suggested approach employs brokering. As a consequence, it is possible to use several RMS examples, each of which can use a different protocol.

As a User role, the technique provides link systems for various RMS protocols that are referred to as Linker RMS. Thus, every system offers a customer which can connect to plenty of protocols that are provided. Since the SDS is intended to operate with a single format, the existing version for the agent barely allows connections having various protocols; it doesn't accept several information schemes. Every Connector RMS provides a link between various sensor sequences facilitated by various RMSs. The findings are obtained in this manner as they are gained. Finally, the retrieved observations are forwarded to the algorithms in the next processing phase by these nodes [40].

7.8.6 Algorithm Implementation

Any algorithm can be extended to the observation sequence using the methods presented. To allow parallel computation, these algorithms are codified as separate nodes. Each node's outputs may be passed to subsequent nodes, allowing interconnection between algorithms, or distributed as a device output. Until conducting the necessary analysis, the algorithms must conform to the essence for the information presented by the information origin. Use of sensor stream standards simplifies data processing for review. The algorithm can generate various outputs facilitating on the category of survey.

It's vital to note how insights are exchanged between algorithms within the system's workflow. When relating with information sources, the location of every inspection in comparison to various stream components is important. Controlled by the method for inspection, the node will require in keeping every inspections in

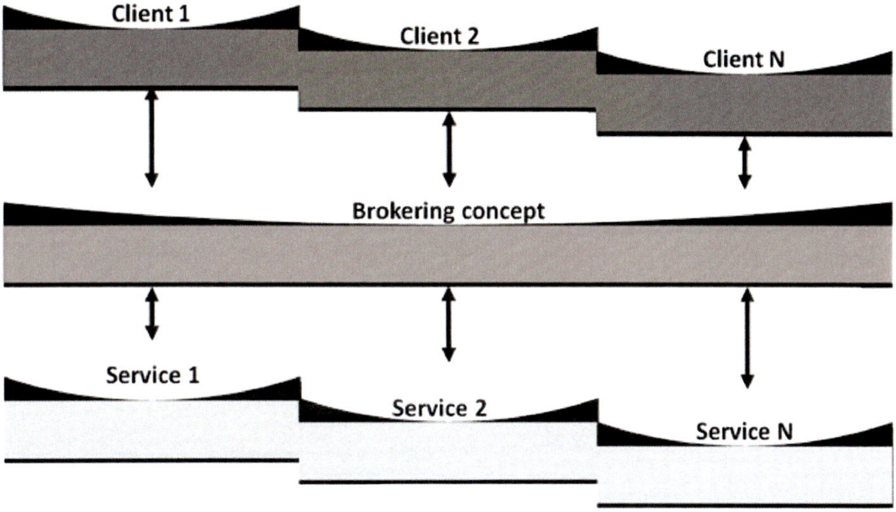

Fig. 7.5 Theoretical Organizing Method

the identical information sequence in the same order. Our technique means that all observations from each stream are evaluated, and it also helps you to preserve the sequence by which every individual item is prepared. Figure 7.5 shows theoretical Organizing Method.

7.9 Performance Distribution

The techniques can, for instance, extricate anomaly information from big data insertions and facilitate information that can be easily visualized [41]. These out comings may be coded utilizing the best suitable quality based on their form. The RMS is used to enhance interoperability by including a range of common communication protocols. The RMS is used in this case for a produce/support method that permits multiple subscribers in connecting to a single yield source along with an alert if necessary. This section illustrates an instance of an RMS with results for every sensor along with sensing node.

7.10 Application Layer

The service layer includes a range of transmission protocols along with some common schemes for building reusable clients. These features allow the development of clients that can be used in a number of circumstances. The server layer communicates with the RMS, which is the final component of the operation layer.

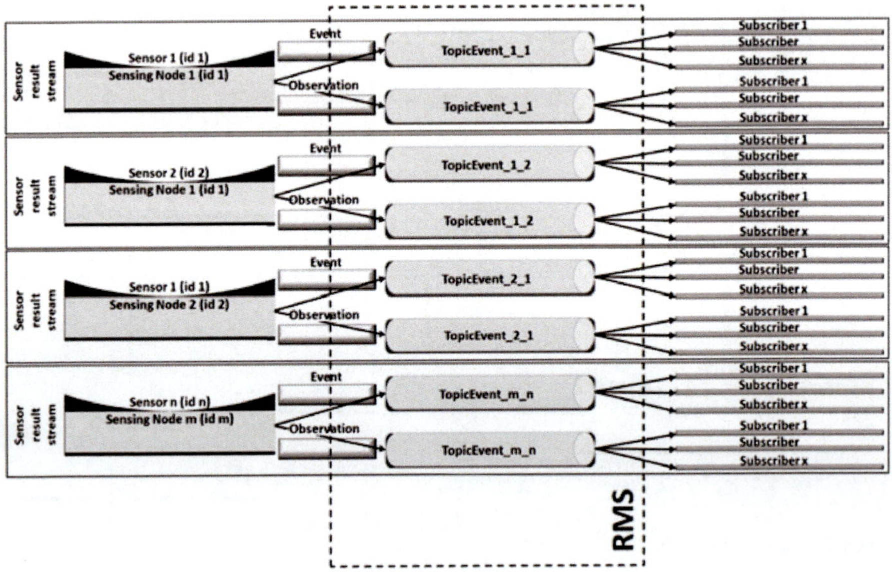

Fig. 7.6 Issued Method

7.10.1 *The CUSUM Algorithm is Used to Track Real-Time Events*

We used a technique in detecting an anomaly over real sensor information to validate the technique mentioned in the previous section. A warning must (1) initiate a conclusion-producing procedure and (2) notify regarding the abnormality which triggered the incident, as well as surrounding background information, as soon as an anomaly is identified. Since decision-making is time-sensitive, this support must also be given in (near) real-time. Figure 7.6 demonstrates Issued Method.

Due to the noticing of irregularities in information sequences from ambient surveillance, we chose the CUmulative SUM (CUSUM) technique. This algorithm can be used on any set of numbers. Anomalies are observed in spontaneous time. It contrasts two separate examples for the similar differential probability function regarding a data series in nature.

7.10.2 *Prior Implementations in the CUSUM Approach*

The CUSUM [42] technique was generated with the intention of regulating industrial processes. It has been successfully used in other fields in recent years. The algorithm is used by researchers [43] to identify potential disease outbreaks. The researchers [44] looked at 40-day mortality rate in heart surgery sufferers. In addition, CUSUM is used in WSNs to enhance contact. Two CUSUM modification-point identification techniques for information internetwork tracking implementations were developed by [45]. In addition to pattern recognition, CUSUM has been used in neural networks. The researcher's analysis suggests an ANN-dependent technique with many back propagation models, which includes a sample of these. The researchers equated the efficiency of the integrated Shewhart–CUSUM schemes with a substitute method in predicting operation supremacy based on ANN technique. CUSUM has since been used to address a variety in ambient issues. We chose to utilize CUSUM as section of the abnormality sensing method as a result of these successful examples. CUSUM is used to detect irregularities in air pollution in our execution instance. In the previously mentioned works, the accuracy of this algorithm was checked.

7.10.3 The CUSUM Algorithm is Defined

CUSUM takes into account a series of scrutiny (z_j), along with composed observations j = 1,…, m, where m is the quantity of information points. When a set has a mean and variance over a usual time and follows a normal distribution, the technique concludes that the scrutiny is in-command. When the method is under pressure, we can use the following expression to extract the total TOT (T_j) in an iterative manner:

$$T_j = T_{j-1} y_j, \tag{7.1}$$

where, $T^0 = 0$, y_j is the standard normal variable, $y_j = (z_j - z')/t$, x is the mean of the time series, and s is the SD value. Furthermore, by calculating the amounts as (Lucas 1982), the shift in terms of increasing or decreasing process mean may be observed.

$$T_{Hj} = \text{MAXIMUM}\left[0, \left(y_j - 1\right) + T_{Hj} - 1\right],$$

$$T_{Lj} = \text{MINIMUM}\left[0, \left(y_j + 1\right) + T_{Lj} - 1\right], \tag{7.2}$$

where, l denotes the relevant reference variable to choose. The term k governs the amount of "slack" allowed in the procedure and is normally adjusted to one-half of the mean to be observed. For the CUSUM control tables, the confidence limits (threshold) are h_x, where h = 6 and x is the SD value [45].

The algorithm detects irregularities as T_{Hj} or T_{Lj} surpass the threshold. If T_{Hj} crosses the threshold, the anomaly is due to a rise (up-event), while if T_{Hj} exceeds the threshold, the anomaly is due to a decline (down-event). The sensitivity of the findings is constrained by two features of CUSUM. To begin, the presumption that readings are statistically independent and follow a normal distribution is used to define an out-of-control operation. Second, observations of sensory phenomena may reveal seasonality and long-term patterns. This has the effect of allowing the threshold to be out of change [46].

7.11 A Device for Identifying Anomalies in the Atmosphere

By applying a framework to recognize abnormalities over environmental sensor records, we prove the computational architecture of our methodology. The technology used in each section of the device is summarized in Fig. 7.7. It suggests a technical approach for the sector-independent technique mentioned in chapter.

7.11.1 Layer of Material

The proposed framework, as described in next Section, assists the three categories of sensor records origins mentioned below, provided by the organizational attributes for the information form:

Organized WSN: there are two subcategories under this group. The sensor data sources in the first subcategory are supported in common sensor formats, such as using the Open Geospatial Consortium's Sensor Observation Server (SOS). The sensor data sources themselves, in the second subcategory, adopt a quality form coded with a hierarchical format, like very easy syndication. (The 28 South7 SOS implementation and Meteoclimatic8 to help RSS are used in our prototype). Semi-Structured WSN: a sensor information origin is stored in a semi-organized form, like the HTML here. To validate the suggested technique, we use an example of this kind, the Valencian Community government's air quality network8.

Sensor data sources in non-structured WSNs do not follow any structure. This form of WSN is exemplified by the SEnviro network. Lesser-price ambient sensors related to the Arduino platform are available from SEnviro. The sensor data is directly generated by the SEnviro nodes.

We selected a semi-organized airy standard sensor internetwork supported by the Spanish Community government in testing our methodology. As previously mentioned, the CUSUM technique requires two metrics (threshold and k) for each sensor that our machine examines. These parameters are procured from traditional evidence from information origin presented. This study was based on one year of past data. Fig. 7.7 shows a description of the technology used in the proof of concept for anomaly detection.

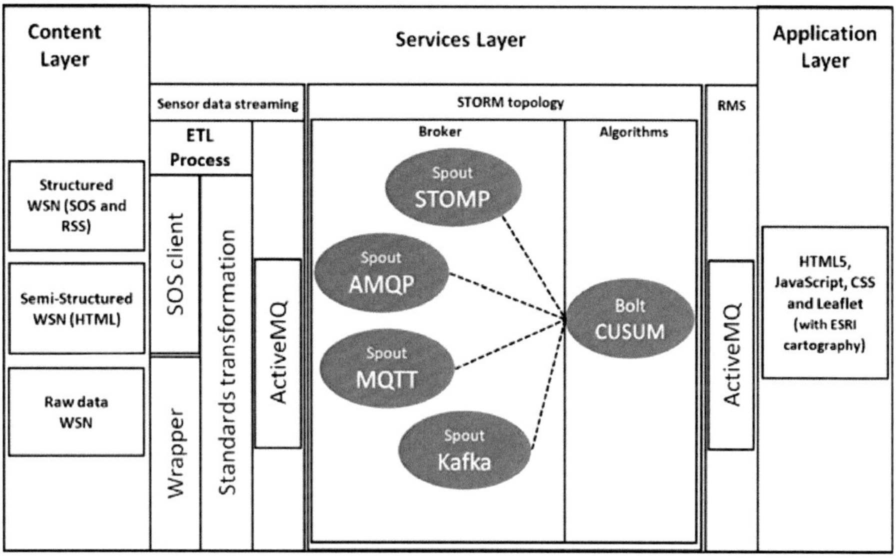

Fig. 7.7 A description of the technology used in the proof of concept for anomaly detection

7.11.2 Layer of Resources

An evidence of idea for the service layer was also applied. The mechanism utilized to construct an RMS example. The SDS is introduced in the following section. The mechanism utilized between the present obtainable results to interpret sensor information is defined in Section.

7.11.3 Message Provider in Real Time

We used ActiveMQ, a JMS system, for the RMS component. We provide a Client that connects to ActimeMQ through the Simple Text-Oriented Message Protocol; it may act as a promoter or receiver. The client permits two forms of connections: P2P along with produce/support. It was used to communicate with the RMS in the various comprehensive components.

7.11.4 Streaming Sensor Results

As previously mentioned, the SDS integrates and standardizes sensor data sources using an ETL procedure. The ETL method is divided into two stages as seen in Fig. 6. For the initial stage, we have two separate constituents, wrappers along with

SOS customer, and one of these two components establishes the relation based on the configuration of the data source. We created an SOS client for sources that already conform to the OGC's SOS specification, which implements the operation get observation by ID to retrieve each sensor's most recent observation. We'll need a special connector for all other sources. We build a special wrapper for each of these instances, based on preceding researches. This portion is in charge of linking and refining information for repository in this manner. This helps the device in scaling by allowing for the inclusion of additional data sources. This wrapper part collects observations from each sensor using site crawling techniques and is customized to each category of structured data. This module analyzes the information origins along with extraction of every monitoring with the help of some libraries. The frequency is modified by inclusion of the wrapper portion along with the SOS clients according to the number of publishing for every information origin. Moreover, the RMS adds the sensor measurements collected by the constituents from every individual sensor to the spontaneous-time interfaces [47].

As wrappers, SOS client must execute the relation using different parameters. We'll require enquiring the refreshing rate along with the URL for every individual sensor in order for this to happen. These parameters are stored in a custom XML format. It has one entry that specifies the sensor internetwork, as well as information related to every sensing connection, like an identifier, for example, name, state, or location. Each sensor which the sensing connection measures is represented by a separate element in the sensing node entry. Each of these components provides information about the phenomena being calculated, like an identifier, perceived property, scale of measurement, and refreshing time. This may provide the parameters for running the CUSUM approach (threshold and k). Moreover, every sensory activity involves a URL for connecting with the sensor information origin as well as a URL for connecting to the sensor data stream for connecting to the RMS. The SDS now provides a protocol for observation encoding and entry. When the machine makes a new observation, it undergoes a transition. Utilizing a DOM (Document Object Model) parser, every changed monitoring is coded in accordance to the OGC format for Observations and Measurements (O&M) [48].

The Client is utilized as a creator to associate to the RMS and facilitate a scrutiny data sequences for every sensor. The created monitoring is dispatched to the appropriate Queue, each for each sensor and observing node. This application in the RMS can be seen in this section. The researchers use the RMS P2P method in this case as it guarantees that the User receives every Message generated. A different XML folder is generated in describing the sensor stream link fixtures. When the stream is open, this folder contains the URLs along with protocol sort [49].

7.11.5 STORM Topology

Rain, S4, Samza, Borealis, MillWheel, and a variety of other spontaneous-time information processing tools are previously obtainable. We chose Storm for this analysis because it is one of the most common and has a large number of examples. It is used to execute the brokering and analysis phases as a single item. The Storm architecture, that disperses refined boundless sequences of information in spontaneous-time, is at the core of this aspect of our work [50].

We can evaluate several data sequences (having varying protocols) along with addition of committed abnormality perception techniques to them using the narrative implementation for Storm system in the IoT. Scalability is guaranteed as this technology is selected. Storm can send up to one million 100-byte data per second per node, along with it can test huge clusters of up to 3500 nodes [51].

The RMS connectors provide the brokering features. For each approved Message Broker protocol, these are executed utilizing separate Storm Spouts. Through supporting several protocols and permitting separate RMS examples for using, the system's interoperability improves. We designed four different Spouts for our broker, each assisting a disparate Message Broker protocol. The researchers picked the four most commonly used protocols: Kafka, MQTT, Stomp, and AMQP. Every Storm Spout is designed as a Customer for linking them to diverse RMS obtainable in collecting sensor observations from various data sequences [52].

Storm ensures a minimum of one implementing, but do not take into account the sequence by which information streams are emanated. When tuples are sorted, they must be in a separate manner. The order of the tuples must be preserved in order to meet the set targets. Trident13 is used to ensure this. Storm's Trident architecture is an upper-level abstraction structure for calculation. Trident uses Spouts as a root of data sources, much like the main Storm application programming interface (API). It consists of a clear, entirely a single semantics, making Trident Topologies use simple to think about. Various functioning, like filters, and collections from sequences of tuples, are already available [53].

Storm Bolts are used to execute the analysis phase. We can use some analysis algorithm within each Bolt. With the CUSUM algorithm, we generated a Bolt. This Bolt is accountable for adding CUSUM for the sequence of tuples given by the numerous Spouts. We use unique sensor identifiers to distinguish the tuples that come from the sensor networks for running the CUSUM technique for every occurrence-dependent estimation source. The Events Bolt utilizes the Message Broker Client for transmitting alerts to RMS as a contributor when CUSUM senses an anomaly. For every sensor and sensing connection, a Queue is generated once more [54].

The Publish/Subscribe paradigm is used once more.

The events are now available in a regular format encoded with the Traditional Alerting Protocol. A sensor identifier (forwarder field) and identifier for the specific monitoring which triggered the identifier field are also used with each event. CAP is a notification format that is used to carry out public notifications. It utilizes XML as a data-encoding form which was regulated by Association in the growth of Formal Information Standardization in 2010. The msgType field describes the detected occurrence, which may be an up-event or a down-event, based on whether the observed value is above or below thresholds [55].

A sensor identifier (sender field) along with the identifier for the specific monitoring which triggered the identifier field is also used with each event. The msgType field describes the detected occurrence, which may be an up-event or a down-event, based on whether the observed value is above or less than the thresholds. A second bolt allows you authorize the Spouts' most recent findings [56].

This Bolt is required in order for the tuples to be served equally and ingested by the concluding requests.

To link to RMS, the two Bolts utilize the Message Broker Client as a creator. Furthermore, all functionalities are introduced using the Publish/Subscribe paradigm, allowing multiple Users (final applications) in connecting to the similar Queue.

7.12 Case Management Dashboard

Data generated by service layer is visualized in an event dashboard. It illustrates the activated conclusion-deriving procedures by introducing details regarding observed irregularities for a spatiotemporal sense. This dashboard has a basic feature that we're using to validate our event prediction use case. More specialized dashboards may be produced based on the information and preferences of other users. This dashboard will provide pertinent details about the user's domain [57].

The client uses markers to represent every sensing system in an internetwork on a map. The number of episodes observed for this specific sensing node is shown within each marker. The marker turns red if this node causes an event; otherwise, it stays blue. Dashboard doesn't distinguish whether an incident is "up" (greater than the threshold) or "down" (lesser than the threshold) (falling below the threshold). Following the quantity of occurrences, a clustering technique was applied to the markers. The markers will be paired with the cumulative number of events found in the cluster while zooming out. If one of the cluster's sensing nodes activated an incident, the marker turns red. When a user clicks on a unit sensing node marker, a menu of newer markers appears as in this section. Every newer marker denotes a sensor connected with this specific sensing connection, and marker must turn red when a newer occurrence is registered. A newer window opens as a pop-up widget on the dashboard when we click on individual sensor markers, showing the most recent findings denoted by a graph. The service layer provides an insight inside the table. The graph is updated in real time with the most recent findings. The activities are defined by a red rhombus in the table. These incidents are also gathered from the operation layer. When a new discovery is taken, the map is changed. The user will view several graphs at the same time, like sensors through various sensing connections. By this process, the quantities of the similarly sensory event within the similar internetwork can be compared [58, 59].

We reused a mix of existing systems to provide a scalable, compatible, and standard-compliant approach. (1) Leaflet14 with ESRI15 basemap to find the creators. It is proven for being a simple and effective approach. Furthermore, it may be utilized in restricted settings, like smart-phones. (2) We have utilized Bootstrap as a library. 16 It has the potential to construct a flexible dashboard and it can react to the functionality of the unit. jQuery17 is also used to tackle pop-ups. (3)

Highchart Javascript [60] was another framework that was used. 18 It's an HTML5 [61] and JavaScript-based graphics library. In a web environment, the library offers a simple and immersive way to create graphs [62, 63].

7.13 The Proposed Approach is Discussed

Three views should be used to analyze the work discussed in this essay. The first paragraph describes how the presented work can be used to interpret data, especially data from environmental sensor networks [64, 65]. The following section looks at how the technique might be extended to additional sensor internetworks with various forms of sensor records, like social networks. The ultimate subsection delves into problems which are specifically relevant to the approach used along with the enabled information sources.

7.13.1 Sensor Internetworks as a Case Study

The suggested technique is intended to be used for data generated by wireless sensor networks (WSNs) (mobile sensing). Storm is being used for the first time in the IoT and environmental surveillance, as far as we know. It may be used to evaluate records from various other forms of WSNs in the IoT, like those used in the home, communities, electricity, health, agriculture, and so on. Both static and mobile sensing can be achieved with these WSNs [67].

In reality, depending on the format, our methodology took into consideration various categories of sensor internetworks. The advantage of combining multiple data sources is that it offers a common approach that can be extended to any situation with differing WSN characteristics. The technique allows for the relation of both normal and non-standard sensor data sources for this purpose. A client that meets the OGC SOS specification is provided for connecting to standard sources and may be explicitly reutilized in connecting to non-ambient sensor record origins. Ad hoc linkers must be required to receive observation sequences from non-standard sources. In this case, we consider using wrapping methods to make the relation. Extending the already existing brokering facilities to handle additional protocols will be all that is needed for adoption [68].

Another benefit of the proposed approach is the standardization of sensor data. Transformations must be extended to non-quality sensor information origins in this situation. The observation sequence can be managed directly by our solution once the ETL method from non-quality monitoring to O&M is established. We will enhance the development of applications by homogenizing the data format which the device uses internally along with moving it to the application layer by reinforcing O&M as a common form [69].

7.13.2 Expanding the Model to Other Contexts

The provided technique was used to evaluate data from environmental WSNs. The machine, on the other hand, is programmed to work with some collection of observations created by sensing systems, so it is unaffected by the existence of the observed phenomenon. The precise processing would be determined by the type of information given [70].

As a consequence, the technique can be extended to references given by mobile phones, laptops, wearable, and other gadgets. Sensors like the gyroscopes, accelerometers, GPS, sensors, and the remaining are gradually being built into such applications. Pervasive sensors can be utilized in delivering circumstances-receptive, adjustable, along with customized assistances which communicate directly alongside the environment. Pervasive sensors may also be utilized in inferring people's behaviors, resulting in a mechanism known as social sensing. People here create vast quantities of data and exchange it through Web 2.0 services (like Twitter or Instagram) [71]. The presented methodology could be used to evaluate the data generated by these services. The sensors in this situation are the people that have data sources. In reality, Twitter, Inc. created Storm specifically for this reason. (1) The researchers utilized Storm to remove trending hashtags from Twitter and sum-up circumstances of citations, and (2) The researchers utilized Storm to extract trending hashtags from Twitter and count occurrences of citations. (2) In [72], the authors use the Storm system to scrutinize records from magnetic sensor networks. (3) The researchers suggest a method for identifying water delivery network irregularities. (4) In [73], the writers use radio sensors to monitor the position of the players along with the ball in the course of a football game. They utilized Storm to do an instant-time scrutiny for this.

Each of these methods can be encapsulated by the solution provided in this article. Since all device modules have been developed to promote extensibility and reusability, it can be called a modular solution. To boost reusability, the modules are built in a modular manner. The RMS part, for example, is built on the idea of a Message Broker and can be used in a number of scenarios. The use of specifications and a number of protocols further enhances client communication. This causes the same client to be used in various situations [74].

Overall, we developed and approved an advanced along with flexible brokering platform which can combine several data sources at soaring refreshing costs and perform every kind of inspection. This technique is structured in communicating with societies with a range of outlets, such as metropolitan centers and intelligent Cities. The constituent is demonstrated to increase exchangeability for the processing of vast volumes of data from various sensor record origins.

7.13.3 Identification of Irregularities

We use the CUSUM technique to ascertain irregularities for air trait sensor information in the proof of concept implementation. We selected this technique as it is successfully demonstrated in similar functionalities that used the simple CUSUM technique to determine irregularities in a set of environmental data involving various sensory occurrences like carbon dioxide, and nitrogen oxide among others. However, when related to ambient evidence, the CUSUM technique has known limitations. The CUSUM algorithm senses sudden shifts in data sequences using a probability distribution function that is known. When a regular distribution is assumed, only a rapid change in the distribution's mean is taken into account; no alteration in the standard deviation value is predicted. It also lacks shifts in pattern or the recurrence of a given occurrence. The trait of each phenomenon can differ not only based on the season of the year, but also depending on the position of the sensor; for example, a measured phenomenon in a rural or commercial region may behave differently. Such specifics are not feasible to have in CUSUM [75].

This review does not address the modification of the study of each sensory phenomenon. The CUSUM technique is utilized to explain the technique along with furnishing an initial proof of idea. Our current work relies on a general approach that can extend any analysis over a sensor data source, while the CUSUM algorithm is only used to illustrate the procedure and provide a first proof of concept. Another anomaly detection technique may be used in the same way [76].

It would only be necessary to adapt its implementation to operate within the Storm system, which would be achieved in a similar fashion to the adaptation of the CUSUM algorithm. The most suitable algorithms must presumably be decided by the sensory phenomenon under examination.

7.14 Function that is Connected

There are several methods in the literature that are close to our idea. The works that follow both suggest a system for storing and processing data generated by IoT appliances.

The researchers describe a platform interface for sensor-dependent information collection for the circumstances of the Internet of Things. The framework assists big data analysis by allowing for the processing of huge data records collected through corporeal sensors. The design was authenticated using the SmartCampus scheme, but the job performed on information processing and repository was the key focus. In the future, the authors suggest using OGC specifications.

In [50], the authors define a cognitive-aligned IoT big data architecture. Through the IoT big data layering architecture function (COIB framework) for efficient data processing and information discovery in smart manufacturing systems, this architecture is used [77].

The researchers propose two separate methods for controlling discerning in their article storing services in the cloud and making them accessible as utility Sensor web enablement (SWE) specifications are used by Cloud4Sens, a cloud system. This system is used in two main applications: the first deals in risk control, and the second uses virtual sensors to identify potholes and track road surface conditions. The researchers propose a conglomerate framework for building a cloud computing infrastructure. Using the OGC's SWE standards, a solution is capable of storing vast volumes of miscellaneous data and provide them in a uniform fashion. The researchers suggest a new structure for working with data generated by IoT.

The authors define the design for a background smart framework in big data survey in organizational engineering along with other fields of study. The suggested use case employs audio frequency recognition technologies in detecting along with monitoring industrial processes, and the specified framework is used to control various aspects of these processes [78].

The researchers define a cloud network that can link diverse WSNs while retaining a high degree of protection diarizes them in compliance with the SWE specifications for processing; a business intelligence software layer is used. Finally, in order to communicate with the device, an implementation layer contains user interfaces. Danger identification in environmental and industrial processing is the use case for this study.

This section provides a contrast of the comprehensive works for comparing the previously examined jobs. It makes use of the following features: Big data: the study can be defined as high-level work that utilizes or does not utilize hardware constituents to build "smart stuff" Yes (which architecture)/No (which architecture).

GIS specifications: Indicates whether the framework supports GIS grading as an OGC format No/Yes on a scale of one to ten. The word "real-time" refers to whether or not a machine runs in real time. Analyze: Shows when the machine conducts an inspection Yes/No on a scale of one to ten.

User: If the device offers a customer to envision the sensors along with measurements, this value is set to true. Yes (what kind)/No on a scale of one to ten.

Intelligent factor: the intelligent factor that every estimate can solve. Intelligent world, intelligent people, intelligent economy, intelligent mobility, and so on are all examples of size. Analyze: Shows when the machine conducts an inspection Yes/No on a scale of one to ten.

User: If the device offers a client to visualize the sensors and measurements, this value is set to true. Yes (what kind)/No on a scale of one to ten. Smart factor: the smart factor that each project can solve. Smart world, smart people, smart economy, smart mobility, and so on is all examples of size.

The Storm system provides us with the only solution that ensures high scalability. Its goal is to be interoperable, and it is the only one that does so by using OGC standards like SWE. We also deliver spontaneous-time full-duplex transmission for providing sensor estimates as rapidly as viable. The key purpose is evaluating sensor record and has the ability to request various approaches to this type of record. Finally, the job discussed in this manuscript requires a Leaflet-based internet client. Our circumstances can be used in any "intelligent" case, but we've opted to use it in a smart world scenario.

7.15 Conclusion

In order to inspect data sequences from sensor internetworks in close by real-time, we developed a domain-independent methodology. Entry positions to numerous sensor information origins with numerous protocols are used in the technique. By using a brokering strategy, it enables a wide variety of devices to communicate with sensor information origins, nevertheless of the data categories it may include. This method also enables the device to connect to multiple real-time interfaces, allowing it to process vast volumes of sensor records in real time and obey the consequences in common forms.

The approach discussed here discusses two problems. The first challenge was to build a device that could process sensor data in real time. There are several sensor data sources that can be used. Our approach allows for a faultless review of each observation. Despite the poor refresh rates of the data source used, it could be scaled to higher refresh rates or several data sources could be applied to the same framework. The second task is to have a solution that is simultaneously flexible and interoperable. Our approach has a variety of characteristics that help to satisfy these criteria. The planned constituents may be reutilized in other cases having different traits for this reason. To have several connections with heterogeneous interfaces, a broker architecture pattern is often used. We introduce the execution of an evidence of notation which ascertains irregularities in information generated by ambient tracking terminals to validate and demonstrate this technique. While our verification instance concentrates on sector-dependent information, information from multiple domains (ambient, conveyance, healthcare, and so on) may be integrated in offering a hybrid-area approach in surveys investigating the effect of conveyance on the ambience, for instance.

New tools, like the stream processing system Storm and JMS, are included in this proof of concept. The CUSUM technique is shown to be efficient for identifying irregularities in a set of air attributes and meteorology measurements. CUSUM, on the other hand, has certain drawbacks that must be considered, like the assumption that every series obey a regular issuance and that a sequences of inspections may not have pattern shifts. Alternative algorithms, such as the one developed by the researchers, are still being researched. This can take into account approaches which may explain for occurrence-dependent probability dispersal in particular.

These implementations for a broader spectrum of occurrence, as well as the subsequent sensor internetworks, will permit us to conclude into a significant portion of our environment's senses. It will further help us to exercise the former information in spontaneous-time, making it an essential component for a Digital Earth Nervous System. The job may be specifically extended to expand the original application for various occurrences along with information points from a philosophical perspective.

It provides a platform for managing vast data streams in parallel from heterogeneous sources, addressing the IoT's lack of standards and helping us to acquire and exercise newer complicated information sequences from both the private and public sectors in actual time. Future work will concentrate on expanding the prototype to broader sensor networks and adding a broad range of data sources.

We suggest utilizing a newer initiation of information origins generated by mobile gadgets or wearables, like heartbeat rate sensors, accelerometers, gyroscopes, and henceforth, as a next phase. As well as over freely accessible records in Web 2.0, for ordering to conclude people's behaviors around the same time as anomalies arise. In a subsequent stage, the functions to exercise diverse-sensory amalgamation as proposed by the researchers will be created.

Another area we'd like to dig at is semantic interoperability in the sense of the Internet of Things. Because of the higher level of diverseness in occurrence of curiosity, perceived possessions, along with requested computation methods, the researchers discuss the SWE restrictions for the semantic field, particularly in the Internet of Things sense. As segment of the Semantic Web along with related information revolution, potential alternatives such as the World Wide Web Consortium's Semantic Sensor Network (SSN) Ontology have been constructed in recent years. According to Gomes and the researchers, new research into the implementation of semantic interoperability solutions is required to boost these problems.

References

1. Alenkar BM, Rios RA, Santana C, Prazeres C (2020) FoT-Stream: a fog platform for data stream analytics in IoT, vol 164, pp 77–87. https://doi.org/10.1016/j.comcom.2020.10.001
2. Alexandru A, Ianculescu M, Marinescu IA, Popescu TD (2019) Shaping the digital citizen into a smart citizen on the basis of IoT capabilities. In: 2019 22nd international conference on Control Systems and Computer Science (CSCS), Bucharest, Romania, 2019, pp 707–714. https://doi.org/10.1109/CSCS.2019.00126
3. Almeida A, Maciel DF, Sousa KF, Nascimento CTC, Koide S (2021) Vertical Electrical Sounding (VES) for estimation of hydraulic parameters in the porous aquifer, vol 13, issue 2. https://doi.org/10.3390/w13020170
4. Al-Omary A, AlSabbagh HM, Al-Rizzo H (2018) Cloud based IoT for smart garden watering system using Arduino Uno. In: Smart Cities Symposium 2018, Bahrain, 2018, pp 1–6. https://doi.org/10.1049/cp.2018.1401
5. Alvarado Moreno JD, Luis Garcia LC, Hernandez WC, Barrera Obando AM (2018) Embedded systems for Internet of Things (IoT) applications: a review study. In: 2018 Congreso Internacional de Innovación y Tendencias en Ingeniería (CONIITI) Bogota, Colombia, 2018, pp 1–6. https://doi.org/10.1109/CONIITI.2018.8587092
6. Amarlingam M, Mishra PK, Durga Prasad KVV, Rajalakshmi P (2016) Compressed sensing for different sensors: a real scenario for WSN and IoT. In: 2016 IEEE 3rd World Forum on Internet of Things (WF-IoT) Reston, VA, USA, vol 2016, pp 289–294. https://doi.org/10.1109/WF-IoT.2016.7845487
7. Babu SM, Lakshmi AJ, Rao BT (2015) A study on cloud based Internet of Things: CloudIoT. In: 2015 Global Conference on Communication Technologies (GCCT), Thuckalay, India, 2015, pp 60–65. https://doi.org/10.1109/GCCT.2015.7342624

8. Bajer M (2018) IoT for smart buildings—long awaited revolution or lean evolution. In: 2018 IEEE 6th International Conference on Future Internet of Things and Cloud (FiCloud), Barcelona, Spain, 2018, pp 149–154. https://doi.org/10.1109/FiCloud.2018.00029
9. Butpheng C, Yeh KH, Xiong H (2020) Security and privacy in IoT-cloud based e-health systems—a comprehensive review, symmetry, vol 12, issue 7. https://doi.org/10.3390/sym12071191
10. Caiza G, Saeteros M, Onate W, Garcia MV (2020) Fog computing at industrial level, architecture, latency, energy, and security: a review, vol. 6, issue 4. https://doi.org/10.1016/j.heliyon.2020.e03706
11. Chung CC, Huang CY, Guan CR, Jian JH (2019) Applying OGC sensor web establishment standards to develop a tdr multi-functional measurement model, sensors, vol 19, issue 19. https://doi.org/10.3390/s19194070
12. Ding K, Jiang P (2018) RFID-based production data analysis in an IoT-enabled smart job-shop. IEEE/CAA J Autom Sin 5(1). https://doi.org/10.1109/JAS.2017.7510418
13. Fersi G (2020) Study of middleware for internet of healthcare things and their applications. In: Jmaiel M, Mokhtari M, Abdulrazak B, Aloulou H, Kallel S (eds) The impact of digital technologies on public health in developed and developing countries. In: ICOST 2020. Lecture notes in computer science, vol 12157. Springer, Cham. https://doi.org/10.1007/978-3-030-51517-1_18
14. Gaddam A, Wilkin T, Angelova M, Gaddam J (2020) Detecting sensor faults, anomalies and outliers in the internet of things: a survey on the challenges and solutions. Electronics 9. https://doi.org/10.3390/electronics9030511
15. Galanopoulos A, Iosifidis G, Salonidis T (2018) Optimizing data analytics in energy constrained IoT networks. In: 2018 16th international symposium on modeling and optimization in mobile, ad hoc, and Wireless Networks (WiOpt) Shanghai, China, 2018, pp 1–8. https://doi.org/10.23919/WIOPT.2018.8362855
16. Gao C, Luo L, Zhang Y, Pearson B, Fu X (2019) Microcontroller based IoT system firmware security: case studies. In: 2019 IEEE International Conference on Industrial Internet (ICII), Orlando, FL, USA, 2019, pp 200–209. https://doi.org/10.1109/ICII.2019.00045
17. Gil D, Ferrandez A, Mora HM, Peral J (2016) Internet of things: a review of surveys based on context aware intelligent services. Sensors 16:1069. https://doi.org/10.3390/s16071069
18. Gomes P, Cavalcante E, Batista T et al (2019) A semantic-based discovery service for the Internet of Things. J Internet Serv Appl 10:10 (2019). https://doi.org/10.1186/s13174-019-0109-8
19. Hassan R, Qamar F, Hasan MK, Aman AHM, Ahmed AS (2020) Internet of things and its applications: a comprehensive survey. Symmetry 12:1674. https://doi.org/10.3390/sym12101674
20. Henrikson AV, Edwards GTC, Pesonen LA, Green O, Sorensen CAG (2020) Internet of things in Arable Farmimg. Biosys Eng 191:60–84. https://doi.org/10.1016/j.biosystemseng.2019.12.013
21. Hu Y, Li H, Yang H et al (2019) Detecting stealthy attacks against industrial control systems based on residual skewness analysis. J Wireless Com Netw 2019:74 (2019). https://doi.org/10.1186/s13638-019-1389-1
22. Idrees Z, Zou Z, Zheng L (2018) Edge computing based IoT architecture for low cost air pollution monitoring systems: a comprehensive system analysis, design, considerations and development. 18(9):3021. https://doi.org/10.3390/s18093021
23. Jiang X, Ding H, Shi H et al (2020) Novel QoS optimization paradigm for IoT systems with fuzzy logic and visual information mining integration. Neural Comput Applic 32:16427–16443 (2020). https://doi.org/10.1007/s00521-019-04020-3
24. Jo S, Lee J, Han J et al (2020) P2P computing for intelligence of things. Peer-to-Peer Netw Appl 13:575–578 (2020). https://doi.org/10.1007/s12083-020-00887-5
25. Jurcut A, Niculcea T, Ranaweera P et al (2020) Security considerations for Internet of Things: a survey. SN COomput Sci 1:193 (2020). https://doi.org/10.1007/s42979-020-00201-3
26. Krishnamurthi R, Kumar A, Gopinathan D, Nayyar A, Qureshi B (2020) An overview of IoT sensor data processing, fusion, and analysis techniques. Sensors 20:6076. https://doi.org/10.3390/s20216076

27. Laport F, Dapena A, Castro PM, Araujo FJV, Iglesia D (2020) A prototype of EEG system for IoT. Int J Neural Syst 30(7). https://doi.org/10.1142/S0129065720500185
28. Lee GM, Crespi N, Choi JK, Boussard M (2013) Internet of things. In: Bertin E, Crespi N, Magedanz T (eds) Evolution of telecommunication services. Lecture notes in computer science, vol 7768. Springer, Berlin, Heidelberg. https://doi.org/10.1007/978-3-642-41569-2_13
29. Biswal AK, Singh D, Pattanayak BK, Samanta D, Yang M-H (2021) IoT-based smart alert system for drowsy driver detection. Wirel Commun Mob Comput 2021, Article ID 6627217:13. https://doi.org/10.1155/2021/6627217
30. Pramanik S, Samanta D, Dutta S, Ghosh R, Ghonge M, Pandey D (2020) Steganography using Improved LSB approach and asymmetric cryptography. In: 2020 IEEE International Conference on Advent Trends in Multidisciplinary Research and Innovation (ICATMRI), Buldhana, India, 2020, pp 1–5. https://doi.org/10.1109/ICATMRI51801.2020.9398408
31. Maheswari M, Geetha S, Selva kumar S, Karuppiah M, Samanta D, Park Y (2021) PEVRM: Probabilistic Evolution based Version Recommendation Model for Mobile Applications. IEEE Access. https://doi.org/10.1109/ACCESS.2021.3053583
32. Kumar R, Kumar R, Samanta D, Paul M, Kumar (2017) A combining approach using DFT and FIR filter to enhance impulse response. In: 2017 International Conference on Computing Methodologies and Communication (ICCMC), Erode, India, 2017, pp 134–137. https://doi.org/10.1109/ICCMC.2017.8282660
33. Gomathy V, Padhy N, Samanta D et al (2020) Malicious node detection using heterogeneous cluster based secure routing protocol (HCBS) in wireless adhoc sensor networks. J Ambient Intell Human Comput 11:4995–5001. https://doi.org/10.1007/s12652-020-01797-3
34. Ghosh G, Samanta D, Paul M, Janghel NK (2017) Hiding based message communication techniques depends on divide and conquer approach. In: 2017 International Conference on Computing Methodologies and Communication (ICCMC), Erode, 2017, pp 123–128. https://doi.org/10.1109/ICCMC.2017.8282658
35. Sivakumar P, Nagaraju R, Samanta D et al (2020) A novel free space communication system using nonlinear InGaAsP microsystem resonators for enabling power-control toward smart cities. Wirel Netw 26:2317–2328. https://doi.org/10.1007/s11276-019-02075-7
36. Samanta D, Sanyal G (2012) A novel approach of SAR image classification using color space clustering and Watersheds. In: 2012 4th international conference on computational intelligence and communication networks, Mathura, India, 2012, pp 237–240. https://doi.org/10.1109/CICN.2012.27
37. Khamparia A, Singh PK, Rani P, Samanta D, Khanna A, Bhushan B (2020) An internet of health things-driven deep learning framework for detection and classification of skin cancer using transfer learning. Trans Emerg Tel Tech 2020:e3963. https://doi.org/10.1002/ett.3963
38. Hossain MA, Samanta D, Sanyal G (2012) Statistical approach for extraction of panic expression. In: 2012 4th international conference on computational intelligence and communication networks, Mathura, India, 2012, pp 420–424. https://doi.org/10.1109/CICN.2012.189
39. Althar RR, Samanta D (2021) The realist approach for evaluation of computational intelligence in software engineering. Innovat Syst Softw Eng. https://doi.org/10.1007/s11334-020-00383-2
40. Singh RK, Begum T, Borah L, Samanta D (2017) Text encryption: Character jumbling. In: 2017 International Conference on Inventive Systems and Control (ICISC), Coimbatore, India, 2017, pp 1–3. https://doi.org/10.1109/ICISC.2017.8068691
41. Guha A, Samanta D (2021) Hybrid approach to document anomaly detection: an application to facilitate RPA in title insurance. Int J Autom Comput 18:55–72. https://doi.org/10.1007/s11633-020-1247-y
42. Agarwal M, Sarkhel D, Samanta D (2018) Architecture of 'loop' without 'for' & 'while'. In: 2018 2nd International Conference on Inventive Systems and Control (ICISC), Coimbatore, India, 2018, pp 491–494. https://doi.org/10.1109/ICISC.2018.8399121
43. Samanta D, Sivaram M, Rashed A, Boopathi CS, Sadegh Amiri I, Yupapin P (2020) Distributed Feedback Laser (DFB) for signal power amplitude level improvement in long spectral band. J Opt Commun. https://doi.org/10.1515/joc-2019-0252

44. Chakrabarti S, Samanta D (2015) Notice of removal: a novel approach to Digital Image Steganography of key-based encrypted text. In: 2015 International Conference on Electrical, Electronics, Signals, Communication and Optimization (EESCO), Visakhapatnam, India, 2015, pp 1–6. https://doi.org/10.1109/EESCO.2015.7254009
45. S Pramanik, Debabrata Samanta, S Bandyopadhyay, R Ghosh, A New Combinational Technique in Image Steganography, International Journal of Information Security and Privacy (IJISP), ISSN: 1930–1650|EISSN: 1930–1669, vol 15, issue 3
46. Rao KR, Samanta D, Somashekara MT, Gurunath R, Paul A (2019) Automatic segmentation based graphical interface for recognition of tomography image analysis of damage cell. In: 2019 Third International Conference on Inventive Systems and Control (ICISC), Coimbatore, India, 2019, pp 52–55. https://doi.org/10.1109/ICISC44355.2019.9036343
47. Gurunath R, Agarwal M, Nandi A, Samanta D (2018) An overview: security issue in IoT network. In: 2018 2nd international conference on I-SMAC (IoT in Social, Mobile, Analytics and Cloud) (I-SMAC)I-SMAC (IoT in Social, Mobile, Analytics and Cloud) (I-SMAC), 2018 2nd international conference on, Palladam, India, 2018, pp 104–107. https://doi.org/10.1109/I-SMAC.2018.8653728
48. Ghosh G, Samanta D, Paul M (2016) Approach of message communication based on twisty "Zig-Zag". In: 2016 International Conference on Emerging Technological Trends (ICETT), Kollam, 2016, pp 1–5. https://doi.org/10.1109/ICETT.2016.7873676.
49. Dhanush V, Mahendra AR, Kumudavalli MV, Samanta D (2017) Application of deep learning technique for automatic data exchange with air-gapped systems and its security concerns. In: 2017 International Conference on Computing Methodologies and Communication (ICCMC), Erode, India, 2017, pp 324–328. https://doi.org/10.1109/ICCMC.2017.8282701
50. Hossain MA, Samanta D, Sanyal G (2012) Extraction of panic expression depending on lip detection. In: 2012 international conference on computing sciences, Phagwara, India, 2012, pp 137–141. https://doi.org/10.1109/ICCS.2012.35
51. Hossain MA, Samanta D, Sanyal G (2012) A novel approach for panic-face extraction based on mutation. In: 2012 IEEE International Conference on Advanced Communication Control and Computing Technologies (ICACCCT), Ramanathapuram, India, 2012, pp 473–477. https://doi.org/10.1109/ICACCCT.2012.6320825
52. Lee JW, Kim YW (2018) A study on smart IoT hub for intelligent signage services using trust information. In: 2018 International Conference on Information Networking (ICOIN), Chiang Mai, Thailand, 2018, pp 76–79. https://doi.org/10.1109/ICOIN.2018.8343089
53. Liu S, Zhang G, Wang L (2018) IoT-enabled dynamic optimization for sustainable reverse logistics. Proc CIRP 69:662–667. https://doi.org/10.1016/j.procir.2017.11.088
54. Machaka P, McDonald A, Nelwamondo F, Bagula A (2016) Using the cumulative sum algorithm against distributed denial of service attacks in internet of things. In: Vinh P, Alagar V (eds) Context-Aware systems and applications. ICCASA 2015. Lecture notes of the institute for computer sciences, social informatics and telecommunications engineering, vol 165. Springer, Cham. https://doi.org/10.1007/978-3-319-29236-6_7
55. Mahdavinejad MS, Rezvan M, Barekatain M, Adibi P, Barnaghi P, Shehth AP (2018) Machine learning for IoT data analysis: a survey. Digit Commun Netw 4(3):161–175. https://doi.org/10.1016/j.dcan.2017.10.002
56. Marques G, Garcia N, Pombo N (2017) A survey on IoT: architectures, elements, applications, QoS, platforms and security concepts. In: Mavromoustakis C, Mastorakis G, Dobre C (eds) Advances in mobile cloud computing and big data in the 5G Era. Studies in Big Data, vol 22. Springer, Cham. https://doi.org/10.1007/978-3-319-45145-9_5
57. Marquis G, Pitarma R, Garcia NM, Pombo N (2019) Internet of things architectures, technologies, applications, challenges, and future directions for enhanced living environments and healthcare systems: a review. Electronics 8(10):1081. https://doi.org/10.3390/electronics8101081
58. Patra MK (2017) An architecture model for smart city using Cognitive Internet of Things(CIoT). In: 2017 Second International Conference on Electrical, Computer and Communication Technologies (ICECCT), Coimbatore, 2017, pp 1–6. https://doi.org/10.1109/ICECCT.2017.8117893

59. Plageras AP, Psannis KE, Ishibashi Y, Kim B (2016) IoT-based surveillance system for ubiquitous healthcare. In: IECON 2016–42nd annual conference of the IEEE industrial electronics society. Florence, Italy, pp 6226–6230. https://doi.org/10.1109/IECON.2016.7793281
60. Poongodi T, Krishnamurthi R, Indrakumari R, Suresh P, Balusamy B (2020) Wearable devices and IoT. In: Balas V, Solanki V, Kumar R, Ahad M (eds) A handbook of internet of things in biomedical and cyber physical system. Intelligent systems reference library, vol 165. Springer, Cham. https://doi.org/10.1007/978-3-030-23983-1_10
61. Raj G, Prakash NR, Randhawa JS (2017) IoT based EMG monitoring system. Int Res J Eng Technol 4(7):355–361
62. Ray PP (2018) A survey on internet of things architectures. J King Saud Univ-Comput Inf Sci 30(3):291–319. https://doi.org/10.1016/j.jksuci.2016.10.003
63. Rane S, Dubey A, Parida T (2017) Design of IoT based intelligent parking system using image processing algorithms. In: 2017 International Conference on Computing Methodologies and Communication (ICCMC), Erode, India, 2017, pp 1049–1053. https://doi.org/10.1109/ICCMC.2017.8282631
64. Razafimandimby C, Loscri V, Vegni AM (2016) A neural network and IoT based scheme for performance assessment in internet of robotic things. In: 2016 IEEE first international conference on Internet-of-Things Design and Implementation (IoTDI), Berlin, Germany, 2016, pp 241–246. https://doi.org/10.1109/IoTDI.2015.10
65. Saralegui U, Anton MA, Arbelaitz O, Muguerza J (2019) Smart meeting room usage information and prediction by modelling occupancy profiles. Sensors 19(2). https://doi.org/10.3390/s19020353
66. Sarker VK, Jiang M, Gia TN, Anzanpour A, Rahmani AM, Liljeberg P (2017) Portable multipurpose bio-signal acquisition and wireless streaming device for wearables. In: 2017 IEEE Sensors Applications Symposium (SAS). Glassboro, NJ, USA, 2017, pp 1–6. https://doi.org/10.1109/SAS.2017.7894053
67. Scholtz B, Kapeso M, Van Belle JP (2019) An Internet of Things (IoT) model for optimising downtime management: a smart lighting case study. In: Strous L, Cerf V (eds) Internet of things. Information processing in an increasingly connected wWorld. IFIPIoT 2018. IFIP advances in information and communication technology, vol 548. Springer, Cham. https://doi.org/10.1007/978-3-030-15651-0_9
68. Sharmila KD, Kumar P, Ashok A (2020) Introduction to multimedia big data computing for IoT. In: Tanwar S, Tyagi S, Kumar N (eds) Multimedia big data computing for IoT applications. Intelligent systems reference library, vol 163. Springer, Singapore. https://doi.org/10.1007/978-981-13-8759-3_1
69. Shaown T, Hasan I, Mim MMR, Hossain MS (2019) IoT-based portable ECG monitoring system for smart healthcare. In: 2019 1st International Conference on Advances in Science, Engineering and Robotics Technology (ICASERT), Dhaka, Bangladesh, 2019, pp 1–5, https://doi.org/10.1109/ICASERT.2019.8934622
70. Shi Y, Li G, Zhou X, Zhang X (2012) Sensor ontology building in semantic sensor web. In: Wang Y, Zhang X (eds) Internet of things. Communications in computer and information science, vol 312. Springer, Berlin, Heidelberg. https://doi.org/10.1007/978-3-642-32427-7_38
71. Sin D, Shin D (2016) Performance and resource analysis on the javascript runtime for IoT devices. In: Gervasi O et al (eds) Computational science and its applications—ICCSA 2016. ICCSA 2016. Lecture notes in computer science, vol 9786. Springer, Cham. https://doi.org/10.1007/978-3-319-42085-1_50
72. Siddiqui S, Nesbitt R, Shakir MZ, Khan AA, Khan AA, Khan KK, Ramzan N (2020) Artificial neural network enabled internet of things architecture for music therapy. Electronics 9(12). https://doi.org/10.3390/electronics9122019
73. Stergiou C, Psannis KE, Plageras AP, Kokkonis G, Ishibashi Y (2017) Architecture for security monitoring in IoT environments. In: 2017 IEEE 26th International Symposium on Industrial Electronics (ISIE), Edinburgh, 2017, 1382–1385. https://doi.org/10.1109/ISIE.2017.8001447
74. Takiddeen N, Zualkernan I (2019) Smartwatches as IoT edge devices: a framework and survey. In: 2019 4th international conference on Fog and Mobile Edge Computing (FMEC), Rome, Italy, 2019, pp 216–222. https://doi.org/10.1109/FMEC.2019.8795338

75. Tastan I, Karaca M, Yurdakul A (2020) Approximate CPU design for IoT end–devices with learning capabilities. 9(1). https://doi.org/10.3390/electronics9010125
76. Ullo SL, Sinha GR (2020) Advances in smart environment monitoring systems using IoT and sensors. Sensors 2(11). https://doi.org/10.3390/s20113113
77. Vishal D, Afaque HS, Bhardawaj H, Ramesh TK (2017) IoT-driven road safety system. In: 2017 International Conference on Electrical, Electronics, Communication, Computer, and Optimization Techniques (ICEECCOT), Mysuru, India, 2017, pp 1–5. https://doi.org/10.1109/ICEECCOT.2017.8284624
78. Wang L, Li K, Chen X (2018) Internet of things security analysis of smart campus. In: Sun X, Pan Z, Bertino E (eds) Cloud computing and security. ICCCS 2018. Lecture notes in computer science, vol 11067. Springer, Cham. https://doi.org/10.1007/978-3-030-00018-9_37

Chapter 8
Future of Intelligent IoT

8.1 Introduction

More detail about the proposed prediction algorithm, as well as the many components that comprise our design, is given here. A Moving Window Regression with Adaptive Weights is an example of a regression model (AMWR). A new adaptive prediction technique, Adaptive Moving Window Regression (AMWR), for changing Internet of Things data is suggested and further developed in this article, which is available online. As a result of the limitations imposed by the massive amount of time needed for training, prediction classifiers are often built on a large quantity of archival data, and after the model has been tutored, it is simply not upgraded. Models of this kind are not intended to operate effectively in the face of phenomena such as concept drift, and as a result, they perform poorly. A change in the system's environment may occur, resulting in a decrease in the performance of the prediction model. This is conceivable. If you find yourself in this scenario, we recommend that you use a prediction model that uses a window size of records for constructing the classifier; and when the newer record is received, the model estimates an inaccuracy and fine-tunes the model suitably. An approach for finding the ideal magnitude for a training window was created by utilizing frequency lines in time series records, which was produced by using the Lomb Scargle approach. With frequent model updates, our suggested technique is adaptive in that it identifies and checks errors from generating farther down the chain of events, as shown in the following example: It is also adaptive in terms of the forecast window or forecast horizon, with the length of the window or forecast horizon being adjusted by the execution of the model for ensuring a certain degree of predictability. Three main stages are encountered throughout the planning process for the AMWR, as described below in the processes listed below.

D. Samanta and A. Banerjee, *Computationally Intensive Statistics for Intelligent IoT*,
Studies in Autonomic, Data-driven and Industrial Computing,
https://doi.org/10.1007/978-981-16-5936-2_8

There are three steps involved in this process:

(1) Selecting a regression technique;
(2) Establishing the optimum training window size; and
(3) Calculating the duration of the reference signal.

Determination of the regression algorithm to be used:

This includes the following steps: When it comes to time series regression (prediction), there is a wide range of methods accessible, extending from statistical to purely machine learning approaches [1]. Auto-regressive moving averages (ARMAs) and auto-regressive integrated moving averages (ARIMAs) have historically been used in time series regression analysis. This continues to be true in this instance. More sophisticated machine learning models, like many variations of support vector regression (SVR) and artificial neural networks (ANN), are becoming more popular as a result of their robustness and potential to facilitate more correct responses [2]. The SVR was selected for use in the construction of our approach because of its potential to represent unpredictable data utilizing kernel functions, which we found to be very useful. An improvement on the SVM method that is extensively utilized in regression scrutiny applications, SVR is a revision of the algorithm [3]. While the fundamental concepts of SVM remain the same, the major difference is that it uses neural networks to translate the training higher dimensional space feature space and finds the optimal function that best matches the datasets using a hyperplane in a higher dimension instead of a hyperplane in a lower dimension [4]. In addition, statistically significant variance reduction (SVR) approaches provide more complicated estimates than their comparable regression procedures, albeit at the expense of greater computational complexity. For datasets of this size and complexity, however, the extra complexity is practically non-existent due to our proposal to use a small training window in our algorithm. After testing different SVR versions, we came to the conclusion that SVR with radial basis function (RBF) kernel would be the most effective underlying regression technique in this research. In the meanwhile, researchers are still trying to figure out what is the best size of the training window for machine learning models to use [5]. According to the findings of the study, the accuracy of a prediction model improves in proportion to the amount of training data used. This highlights the importance of using extensive historical data to train prediction models in order to cover all potential patterns across time periods, which is demonstrated by the research. As previously stated, despite the fact that this approach provides broad and accurate models for prediction in the majority of cases, it has one important drawback: it is time-consuming [6]. The trained model will not be able to keep up with changes in the underlying data's behavior or statistics, which will result in erroneous readings and an increase in the degree of inaccuracy in future predictions. According to the researchers, the sliding window technique for learning the ML model is an alternate way that provides the models with the most up-to-date data available at any given time [7]. A challenging issue for which there is no universal solution is the selection of the optimum window size. In some cases, using a greater window proportion may yield extra precise outcomes, but it also enhances the accuracy of the algorithm, forming it inappropriate for real-time approaches; on the other hand, the use of a miniature window magnitude may lead to greater inaccuracy, which can have a negative impact on the system's dependability. For this issue, we suggest the Lomb Scargle methodology (a fruitful and general time series analysis tool), and our results are validated utilizing real-world records to demonstrate that our technique is successful. In our method, we made advantage of the naturally existing periodicity seen in the overwhelming majority of real-world time series data, which we found to be very useful [8]. A straightforward instance of temperature information collected by a sensor was installed in Rio de Janeiro, Brazil. Despite the fact that the temperature data are set to a very irregular standard, it is possible to observe a recurring sequence in the temperature data after each and every 24 h. In particular, we make advantage of the certainty that when the learning window utilized is equivalent to the built-in-frequency of the records, it may acquire all of the outs and, as a consequence, will be able to predict with more accuracy [9]. To be clear, our technique doesn't make the assumption that the underlying data are periodic, but rather looks for data that has the largest percentage of periods. Time series data may be detected for periodicity using the Fast Fourier Transform (FFT) method, which signifies the most widely utilized technique for this purpose. It finds significant peaks in the period gram, which is generated by executing a Fourier, transform on the time series data, and uses this information to make decisions [10]. With most IoT data, this is not always possible due to the need for an even number of points in the time series that is not always the situation. When it comes to the Internet of Things, missing values are common, and the incapability of FFT to assign with them compels it inappropriate for use with our framework. It is possible to identify the largest repeated element in a time series record for such systems using a method known as least-squares spectral analysis (LSSA), also called Lomb Scargle [11].

A variable-size prediction window, also known as the prediction horizon, is proposed in our research in order to ascertain a definite degree of accuracy in the forecasts. The prediction window, which is more often known as the prediction horizon, is more widely known as the prediction horizon [12]. The concept behind this method is to enhance the capacity of the prediction window when model precision is high and reduces the size of the prediction window when accuracy model performance is poor. The quality of a classifier may be estimated by contrasting the expected records with the authentic statistics that are obtained.

Additionally, there are several other components. The sections that follow offer a high-level overview of the components that make up our architectural design.

(1) Node-RED: Node-RED is a network of nodes that communicate with one another. This frontend interface for our architecture is utilized to interact with the rest of the system, and it is provided by Node-RED. For the first time, scientists have been provided with a global viewpoint thanks to the Internet of Things, which has enabled them to get access to a really varied set of data sources. They may be web services, MQTT record feeds, or various exterior information sources that can be accessed via the HTTP transport protocol. In the Internet of Things, data formats are not limited to a single kind of file format or format family. Data transmission formats like XML and JSON are some of

the generally utilized technologies for transmitting data from the Internet of Things, and they are both heavily utilized for this purpose. Additionally, data streams from a variety of sources may include information that is redundant for a specific application and must be removed before the data can be utilized [13]. As a result of the combination of all of these capabilities with the ability to prototype rapidly, Node-Red enables developers to build wrappers for a wide range of data sources in a very short period of time. When it comes to connecting devices together in the Internet of Things (IoT), Node-RED is a visual tool that is open source and extensively utilized [14].

(2) Also included are APIs for associating various constituents, as well as the ability to clean datasets and alter the configuration of data with the help of Java code provided by the user. Its goal is to provide the activity of connecting various elements along with data origins in the Internet of Things (IoT) more simple and clear [15]. We were able to decrease the amount of time spent on development by using Apache Kafka as a communication channel for real-time generated events, thanks to this technique. Additionally, it is a free and open source program that allows users to publish messages and data in real time, as well as to subscribe to messages and data. Because of its scalable architecture, it makes it feasible to have high-capacity data streams with very low latency. Later in 2011, it was declared open source by LinkedIn and made accessible to the general public as a free download. The Kafka messaging system, like other publishing messaging systems, organizes messages into subjects by grouping them together in feeds. Products are stored in topics, and consumers may obtain data from topics [16]. Topics are utilized by both producers and consumers. Given that Kafka ensures a distributed framework, data are separated and duplicated over many nodes in order to guarantee that they are constantly accessible. For a particular topic, it is possible to find one or even many customers. Messaging may be used to store any object in any format since it is stored as a byte array. The most common formats used by developers are the String, JSON, and Avro formats. In our approach, all communications are published in the JSON format, which is widely used in the web development community. When compared with other systems, Kafka's persistent feature, which enables it to retain messages for an extended length of time, sets it apart from the competition. It is composed of a log (instructed class of contents).

(3) Esper Complex Event Processing:
It is a technique for processing complicated events. A method for processing complicated events is called Esper Complex Event Processing (Esper CEP). Despite the fact that there exist various CEP systems present in the market, Esper is our chosen option owing to its enhanced Java built-in architecture, that enables a robust CEP feature classification while maintaining higher throughput [17, 18]. The fact that Esper is accessible as open source software is another significant factor in determining whether or not it is an appropriate option for the suggested design. Consequently, Esper is particularly suited for latency-sensitive practices that need huge amounts of streaming information to operate correctly, like trading systems, forgery identification systems, and

commercial intelligence frameworks. As opposed to different large-scale data refining approaches, that accumulate data and then execute queries on it, Esper accumulates questions and then runs datasets through them, similar to a conventional query-driven approach. The queries are programmed in Event Processing Language (EPL) that enables sliding windows to be used to conduct actions such as filtering, aggregating, and joining over single matches or groups of events. A SQL-alike language including words like SELECT, FROM, WHERE, GROUP BY, HAVING, and ORDER BY; however, emerging datasets restores tables and events serve as the fundamental unit of datasets in EPL. EPL is written in Java. Unlike other event-based systems, Esper stores events as Plain Old Java Objects (POJOs), which conform to the JavaBeans standards for representation. Complex events are recognized by EPL declarations, and as a result, POJOs are returned as a result of these Complex Events [19, 20].

In CEP, each functional component is further split into three sub-components, with the event collector serving as the first of these sub-components. When collecting data streams from a number of origins like Kafka or MQTT or some RESTful web service, the event collector is capable of reading data streams in a variety of data formats [21]. We have specified in our design that we would read data from Apache Kafka in JSON format, since we think this will be the most efficient way to do so. Data are collected and transformed into a suitable format (for example, POJOs for Esper) by the event collector, which then passes it on to the CEP engine for processing. This component contains the CEP engine, which determines occurrences by comparing trends utilizing EPL declarations, and then forwards disclosed complex occurrences to the available techniques in the necessary database schema utilizing adapters in the event builder constituent, which is located in the event producer component. Contains the event producer component, which contains the CEP engine, which is included inside this component [22].

The outcomes of the forecast chunk are given to CEP in the arrangement of an occurrence tuple, where the CEP engine recognizes the complex event based on pre-defined criteria, which is accomplished via the usage of Kafka. As an example of an abstracted event tuple (e = I, where each element denotes an occurrence, s represents a set of basic concepts, and t represents the time stamp associated with the event), the following is stated as follows: As a result of our design, every expected event is associated with an associated posterior probability, and the CEP links these events according to a set of criteria that we established. Prediction error introduces uncertainty into complex events, which has a detrimental effect on the overall dependability of the system as a result of this [23]. As a result, we utilized a probabilistic occurrence-driven technique for generating occurrence tuples, which is similar to the one described to create event tuples, to account for prediction error. As e = hs = val, pdf(1, 1), ti, and pdf denotes the probability density function of the estimate fallacy, enclosing the estimate fallacy with attribute's estimates in occurrence tuple. Here, we will show how this mistake is spread across the system by using a number of CEP pattern-matching rules and examples.

(1) Filtering the information:

By far the most basic component, event filtering acts as the basis for other, more complex patterns to be built on top of it. Some events may not be of interest to all consumers, and a user may only be interested in a subset of the events available. Consider the case of a simple temperature sensor that takes a measurement once per second. It is possible to specify a temperature threshold in the filtering process if a client is only concerned with temperatures that are higher than a certain threshold value [24]. If and only if all of the conditions were fulfilled at that time, the occurrence will be broadcast to the spectator. Circumstances like equal to, greater than or less than, and so on are often used in programming. The rule will apply to a single event in this scenario whenever it is implemented and the summarized fault connected with the wearable device must be equivalent to the possibility of erratum rate for that specific data origin.

(2) The purpose of joins is to coordinate occurrences from various data sequences by utilizing fundamental logical behaviors like conjunction (and) along with disjunction (or) to accomplish this (or). As a result, the risk of a minor effect with each individual stream of data will be multiplied by the number of data streams combined, resulting in a risk of a large impact with each single stream of data. If there are occurrences, X1 and X2, together with a complicated occurrence are described as one in which X1 exceeds the threshold and X2 falls below the threshold, then the following sounds true:

(3) Third, Windows has a tool for extracting temporal patterns from incoming events, which may then be used to deduce the details of a complex event from the raw data. The following are the two most basic kinds of windows: casement and picture windows. We may select a time frame and then extract events that occur only within that time period using the Time Frame feature. When evaluating a complex event, it is critical to examine the connection between many events and the passage of time. If the temperature shift in a room is five degrees centigrade in an hour, it will indicate a separate denotation than the similar temperature shift in a single minute. The first survey may have occurred as a result of the heater being switched on, while the second observation may have occurred as a result of an actual fire. In order to specify the time frame, either a specific time window or a rolling time window may be utilized [25]. In addition, simple arithmetic operations, such as calculating the highest, lowest, or summation value, need the explanation of a time period. To the contrary of the time window, the tuple window determines how many times an event occurs depending on the number of occurrences that have been provided. Typical tuple window actions include the sum of every five samples, which is extremely frequent in real-world situations [26, 27]. The overall erratum would be equal to the total of the erratum rates of every single occurrence that occurs inside the window, regardless of the circumstance. As an example, consider the following definition of a rule: If occurrence X1 is more than threshold and event X2 is larger than threshold for n successive interpretations, then the rule is stated as follows: If event X1 is greater than threshold and if event X2 is greater than threshold for n consecutive

readings, then the rule is written as follows: It will be possible to determine how likely it is that the greatest error will occur in this scenario by using the formula: pdfF(sum) = m (pdfF(X1) pdfF(X2)), where m is the number of mistakes present in the sample. When all of these capabilities are combined, CEP rules may get more complex; nevertheless, the gross error may be computed by plainly restoring the capacity with various formulas. The probability of forecast erratum expressions for each data sequence, as a consequence, may be replaced in the formulae 3–5 to get an expression for the total likelihood of prediction error. This section will teach you how to calculate the formula for prediction error using the formula in the next section. Experiment-based evaluation is the third step [28]. The congestion statistics furnished by the Madrid city served as the basis for our assessment of the proposed strategy. There are a significant number of traffic sensors placed at permanent neighborhood around Madrid City to monitor a range of traffic parameters, especially average traffic frequency (quantity of conveyances per hour) and average conveyance velocity that are both directly related to the state of the traffic. The city of Madrid makes this information accessible via a RESTful service in xml format, which is provided by the city council. These data must be inspected spontaneously and in real time for detecting conveyance patterns along with generating complex occurrences like poor conveyance flow or congestion. Esper CEP is one of the most efficient clarifications in this layout since it has the ability of evaluating streaming information, making it the most cost-effective alternative. It is possible to set Esper rules, which can subsequently be used to construct complex events, using the EPL for pattern categorization. The technique 2 presents a pseudo code consisting of a single fundamental rule that may be used to infer a complex event from a simpler event (such as poor traffic or congestion). The data streams used in this example will include the speed limit and the intensity of traffic flow, among other things. The inclusion of data from other sources, such as weather predictions or social media, is feasible in a more complex algorithm. In situations when the usual traffic velocity along with median traffic movement are less than the criteria for every successive observations, the CEP generates a complex event, which is described as in this case, if the incoming data are expected data, as is the case with our technique, the complicated occurrence detected will occur in the long run as well, enabling traffic managers to carry out preventive operations to reduce traffic jam. This is a single instance of how CEP directives may be used in detecting more complicated occurrences by taking use of their inherent flexibility, which is only one of many possibilities [29].

In order to guarantee a fair examination of the results, four various sensing positions across the city of Madrid were selected at random, each with its own set of characteristics. To calculate the average window magnitude for learning the ML model in this research, we utilized the suggested Lomb Scargle technique, which was used in this work. On the basis of traffic speed readings, the period gram was created from a single data point. When we predicted traffic using different window widths on a single month of traffic data and calculated the analogous Mean Absolute Percentage Error (MAPE), we found that our method was accurate enough [30].

8.2 IoT Versus Cloud Computing

It is our intention to investigate the cloud service provided by GoDaddy and Amazon Web Services in this project (AWS). The Internet of Things (IoT) context is completed by integrating Internet of Things technologies. It is possible to save and retrieve data from the IoT, which is a major benefit of cloud services since it can be done from any place and at any time.

A major goal of the ML supported Statistical Analysis of IoT is to reduce costs. This is one of the primary goals of the project. There are significant cost savings to be had by analyzing information on the edge, that really is, on the SBC unit, and transmitting chosen data to internet and the cloud, rather than processing data in the data center (if applicable) [31].

Customer data centers and sites may be housed on GoDaddy Cloud Servers, which are virtual servers that operate on GoDaddy's distributed computing environment. Each designer, technology business enthusiast including IT professionals will be able to quickly create, test, and scale cloud arrangements with the help of GoDaddy Cloud Servers along with Cloud Applications, and they will be able to urge their clients to do the same. Domains, domain name services, and other GoDaddy products and APIs are all compatible with Cloud Servers.

By using the Name System, which is available through the internet, customers may manage and maintain newer and surviving regions and sub-domains with the help of the Name System. We now go on to the second Cloud-based Service discussed in this post, which is the Amazon Web Service (AWS) IoT, which offers a secure linking interface for the Raspberry Pi to communicate with the rest of the world. The Embedded-C application on the Raspberry Pi can send MQTT messages to the AWS IoT Cloud, which is accessible via the AWS IoT Gateway. To access the various sensor data, Python-based apps, on the other hand, might be developed. 90 services are accessible, including the capacity to send SMS and emails as well as the option to monitor weather conditions and subscribe to certain services, among other things. When using the MQTT publish subscribe method, the messages transmitted and received may be stored in NoSQL databases for later retrieval. This will be followed by a further phase, which will include integrating the current degree of system combination with a multi-cloud federated habitat, which will be the succeeding track in the project [32].

8.3 Assessment with Intelligent IoT

For comparing the presentation of AMWR and various other regression algorithms, many innovative regression algorithms from the Python ML package scikit-learn were used to assess the accomplishment of AMWR and various other regression algorithms. For the purposes of this example, it may be shown that AMWR surpasses several regression algorithms since it accurately monitors the incoming data sequences. Essentially, there may be two elements that contribute to the high level of accuracy provided by AMWR. AMWR takes into account the model complexity when new data are made available and retrains the model based on this new information. Because the length of the training window is so less, it is capable of retraining along with forecasting events in real time that are extremely near to the actual moment of the event. Whenever the prediction error starts to increase (which is a frequent occurrence), the length of the prediction window is decreased for maintaining the extent of confidence. Depending on how much MAPE builds up over time at a given location, data characteristics at the sensing site are important to understand. When there are more variations in the data and a high standard deviation, the accuracy of the predicted readings will be decreased as a result of the increased variability. In an effort to get the probability density curves for expected traffic speed and intensity, the prediction error was computed and presented as a histogram using one-month data in order to obtain the prediction error. In general, a histogram is a graph of data that can be utilized to evaluate the probability distribution of the data it contains [33].

The Gaussian distribution was applied to the erroneous data via the application of curve fitting mechanisms, and the parametric distribution for both the erroneous data and the control data was found. When it came to the bulk of the data in the error propagation histogram, the Gaussian distribution performed well, but when it came to the extremes of the error histogram, the Gaussian distribution performed horribly. As a consequence, an improved fit of the curve for inaccuracy modeling was still needed. As a result of its wide tail, the Student's t distribution can be utilized to better model outliers than the normal distribution. The Student's t distribution also includes a degree-of-freedom parameter that may be altered in order to adapt the distribution's shape to the nature of the erroneous producing data. As a result, the Student's t distribution may be utilized to further enhance the modeling of data, including erroneous generation, even further [34].

The creation and evaluation of machine learning models in our proposed architecture have been carried out using the scikit-learn Python package. Although it is capable of handling fairly larger datasets by mounting up, it is not financially efficient and has a definite limitation on the quantity of incoming data that it may operate at one time. It is also not particularly reliable. In the wake of the Internet of Things, there has been an enormous influx of big data, and we may be processing data from hundreds of millions of sensors at the city level, according to some estimates. The upshot of this was that we broadened our job and included machine learning constituents in Spark MLlib, an Apache Spark machine learning framework. This enabled us to address the issue and make our system really scalable as a result of our efforts (as opposed to scaling up) [35]. Apache Spark is a large data processing framework that has made significant contributions to the development of the field. It is capable of processing massive amounts of data from a variety of data sources. As a consequence of this capacity, it is quickly growing in favor among users. When used in iterative applications with a large number of machine learning algorithms, it performs especially well. Because of the Resilient Distributed Datasets (RDDs) idea, which Spark maintains, it is possible to retain RDDs in memory without demanding redundancy while still maintaining fault tolerance. Besides that, Spark may comprehend data from any repository device that implements the Hadoop File System API, like HDFS, Amazon S3, and OpenStack Swift, among other storage systems and technologies. In the accompanying paper, we provide detailed details on the bulk-scale execution of our suggested technique:

Our suggested framework facilitates a general predictive explanation that can be used for a wide range of Internet of Things applications, as shown in this paper. Different components involved may be quickly and easily customized to suit the requirements of a certain application with reasonable simplicity. The use of different sensors to monitor the health of patients is another instance. These devices generate a significant quantity of data, which must be surveyed and connected together as quickly as possible for ensuring the welfare of the patients who are utilizing the devices in the first place [36]. Whenever a victim's heart rate or blood pressure begins to climb, our system may determine the upward tendency and forecast it in advance, enabling it to be treated before it reaches a potentially dangerous level. When combined with various data origins, like a victim's physical structure or food behavior, CEP has the ability to identify a likely complex event by comparing the projected values with the actual values (health caveat for victims). A unique best training window must be assigned to each data stream, and this window will be different for each stream. In addition, although many Internet of Things data sequences include the various element of periodicity, which is not every time the case in all instances. In these types of circumstances, the baseline size for the training window may be determined. Large training windows require more training time than narrow training windows. According to the requirements of the scenario that is being utilized, the default length will be calculated. For example, in a health monitoring scenario, real time is defined as less than 10 s, while in an ITS scenario, a delay of up to 2 min would still be considered real time, and vice versa. We used open source components that are effortlessly obtainable and may be expanded to serve bulk-scale implementations with little effort [37].

According to the researchers, the scalability and authenticity of sensor data are the two most significant challenges facing IoT sensor networks. A variety of sensor data measurement and data methods are used to solve these problems. These strategies include data collection techniques as well as data cleansing matters, information administration, and information retrieval, along with data mining. When it comes to achieving the desired outcomes, machine learning along with deep learning techniques represent an important part in the process that includes information gathering and decision-making. According to the researchers, sensor data from the Internet of Things require an effective method for extracting useful statistics from the data. Using Internet of Things sensor data analysis, it is necessary for the machine learning algorithms to be performed inside the sensor implanted CPU. It necessitates the modification of algorithms as well as the development of a data structure that is effective in dealing with the forms of real IoT sensor information. To handle the different characteristics of sensor data, the authors suggested the Gaussian Mixture Model (GMM) as a clarification, which was accepted by the community. Additional work was done to develop real-time hardware and software collaborations, as well as continual machine learning algorithms, in order to train data and classify the resulting data for Internet of Things (IoT)-dependent implementation [38].

Deep learning algorithms: The deep learning mechanism was suggested by the researchers for feature extraction of IoT sensor records and used the deep learning methodology. The IoT sensor dataset contains ambiguous characteristics, which must be clarified via real-time deep learning-dependent categorization in order to be correct. In contrast, deep neural networks are computationally costly to run when used in conjunction with sensor boards that are limited in their resource availability. As a result, the authors suggested a spectral-domain preprocessing method, after which deep learning methods were implemented [39].

The use of a neural network for the processing and analysis of IoT sensor data: Artificial neural networks when trained using supervised learning methods are particularly well suited for issues involving comply and pattern recognition. One or more hidden layers are included in the architecture of ANN, as well as an activation function, an output layer, or one or more hidden units. Consisting of a network layer that performs convolution operations on two-dimensional about one sensor input, deep neural networks (CNN) are a kind of artificial neural network. The convolution operator is often utilized to extract patterns from dataset using a convolution neural network. The appropriate CNN variant is selected based on the data that is made accessible. The picture data utilized for image sensor statistical analysis are well suited for CNN, which is why it is so popular. The majority of Internet of Things devices, such as drone, smart vehicles, smart-phones, and other similar gadgets, are provided with camera. Many Internet of Things applications, such as flood or landslide prediction via drone pictures, forest fire forecast through satellite imagery, and traffic management, make use of vehicle cameras. CNN takes a 2D or 1D picture, voice, or signal and extracts the high-level characteristics from it by using a succession of hidden layers to create a 3D representation. The convolution layer is among the hidden layers, as is an entirely linked pooling layer present at the conclusion of the pipeline. The convolution layer contains a group of filters called as a learnable variable that is the heart of the CNN. It filters higher dimensional records to a low-dimensional data that aid in extracting the most suitable necessary features from the input picture by extracting the most ideal one who can handle from the incoming picture [40].

Known as recurrent neural networks (RNNs), these networks are capable of learning from sequence or time-series data. Prediction of certain jobs, like recognizing the chauffeur's role in intelligent cars, recognizing certain shifting patterns, or predicting the energy usage of a home setting, can be dependent on prior specimen. RNN will be the most appropriate option in these circumstances. It is capable of dealing with streams of varying extents. RNNs are particularly ably adapted for forecasting time sequences sensor records.

Both the current sample and the sample mentioned before are used as input to an RNN. With another way of putting it, the result of an RNN at process t1 in time has an impact on the output of the RNN at step t. Every neuron is furnished with a feedback loop, which replaces the output power as an incoming for the later phase in the computation. An RNN's internal memory may be described in the following way:

every neuron in an RNN has an internal storage capacity that retains the computation results from the past inputs. Long short-term memory is a type of RNN that has the ability to focus back in time for a longer span of time prior to making a forecast. The LSTM algorithm is capable of retrieving and identifying characteristics from sensor data in a timely manner for prediction.

Auto encoders (AE) are a kind of neural network, which has the identical amount of incoming and outgoing layers as it has output layers, and they are linked via a sequence of hidden layers. At the output layer, the auto encoders are capable of constructing an input. Because of this characteristic, auto encoders are widely employed in industrial IoT for a variety of applications, including defect revelation in hardware appliances, abnormality identification in the accomplishment of manufacturing lines, and so on. Generating adversarial networks (GANs) are composed of two types of neural networks, such as the conceptual and discriminative networks, and their primary goal is to generate enhanced-caliber data. They operate on the basis of the minimum–maximum game concept, in which a single network attempts to enhance the estimate function while the remaining network attempts to reduce it.

When using GAN in IoT practices, it is necessary to generate completely new datasets from the original dataset that was made accessible. Localization derivation and wayfinding in graph-based network are two examples of GAN's broad applications that have been proposed. In these implementations, the GAN generator network component estimates all of the potential viable routes, which last between two nodes using the GAN generator network framework. The classifier module of GAN is responsible for identifying the most efficient route between both the origin and the destination nodes. GANs are extensively utilized in assistive technology for people with disabilities. In addition, the authors address the use of GAN in the conversion of picture to auditory applications for visually handicapped people in their paper. Another option is to build specific statistics in text form from an original picture that has been provided. The authors used GAN for computer vision applications, with the goal of identifying the fabricated celebrity from a collection of various images of the genuine celebrity, which was created by the authors.

The Internet of Things sensor network-based applications are characterized by dynamic variables, different social categories, and real-time response processes. As a result, there is a need for a middleware layer between IoT-dependent programs and the actual IoT sensor records. Furthermore, the scalability handles the massive quantities of data, which are generated by the Internet of Things sensor network. Connectivity of IoT sensor networks with different developing mechanization like big data, fog computing, and edge-dependent data analytics are needed to address problems like scalability and real-time development in dynamic environments.

Cloud-dependent Data Analytics: The researchers suggested cloud-dependent data analysis for the IoT, which they described as follows: An ordered and dispersed paradigm in data transforming approaches is required in order to conduct effective data analysis. There are many virtual computers associated with a distant cloud data center that are used to duplicate this technique. The cloud-based analytics approach can, therefore, manage dynamic information retrieval and scalability problems without the need for any previous data knowledge on the part of the user.

Cluster-dependent functioning includes fragmenting more complicated analytical procedures into smaller, more manageable jobs and performing them in separate clusters, thus decreasing the amount of computing power required.

To further manage the enormous amount of data produced by the Internet of Things sensors, effective cloud-based solutions require the use of big data and parallel processing distributed system technologies, both of which are based on cloud computing. It is the researchers' concern that large amounts of higher velocity and complicated perceiving datasets produced by IoT sensor arrangements be stored in a secure manner. These articles discussed data fusion methods that combine IoT and massive sensor data stored on a distant cloud server, allowing the system to offer effective care for IoT applications as a result. The curtain of IoT data sources into the cloud has been shown to solve a variety of problems, including sensor network scalability, metadata management, data compression, storage systems, data analysis, and data visualization. The researchers addressed the problem of data collection for IoT devices that are resource limited and dispersed.

The potential of in situ data analysis, along with context-aware and real-time computing, in order to alleviate network congestion was also evaluated and the results of fog and edge computing, and was found to be promising. In this case, security camera sensors were taken into consideration in order to achieve end-to-end optimization. We looked into a variety of feature extraction approaches as well as different classification algorithms. We also looked into the suggested processing depth as well as the amplification of gain via efficient methods. When comparing the experimental results to other designs, it was discovered that the power consumption was reduced by 4.3 times.

8.4 Future Scope for Intelligent IoT

It is a difficult job to convert data into knowledge when dealing with maximum scale, higher-throughput data processing. This is particularly true when using the pipelining of present and future computer frameworks in data mining. The fact that these data may be interpreted in a variety of ways as showing a degree of uncertainty is also significant. Both the expression of application data access needs and the supply of programming language abstractions that take use of parallelism are essential. IoT will cover the topic of big data analytics on a large scale.

In recent years, academics have been more interested in machine learning ideas and techniques, believing that they may help them in generating more relevant findings. There are benefits and drawbacks to each tool, and the development of more effective methods to cope with the issues that emerge while working with huge quantities of data is required. The capacity of a tool to deal with a range of problems, such as noisy data, ambiguity, and instability, along with missing figures, among other things, determines its efficacy.

Listed below are the most significant lessons from the topic:

In recent years, the proliferation of smart gadgets and sensors has led to a rise in the amount of data produced. It is still early days for the interaction between big data and the IoT, which is a result of the massive quantities of data that must be processed, transformed, and analyzed on a regular basis.

There was much discussion on the link between business data analytics and the Internet of Things, as well as different research subjects, data analysis possibilities in the IoT paradigm, difficulties, and business data analytics tools, to name a few.

A distinct approach is taken by each Big Data platform, according to the findings; some are built for batch processing, while others thrive in real-time analytics and machine learning.

Several distinct methods were used in the course of the investigation. Statistical analysis, data mining, automated learning, intelligent analysis, cloud computing, and other techniques were among them, among others. Academics should pay more attention to these methods in the future since they are effective and efficient in addressing large data issues.

8.5 Conclusion

It is feasible to analyze anomalous occurrences in the environment using sensor data collected as a time series. This is made possible by the data collected by the sensors. It is possible to use the textual and numerical information gathered by the sensors in conjunction with statistical tools and methods to analyze the data obtained. The trigger points in the data series may be used to assess how well the other sensors were functioning at the time of the trigger point. Also remarkable is how well reverse engineering methods work when it comes to detecting someone's presence in their environment. Because the presence of someone provides logically supportive evidence, as shown by the Boolean values from the PIR movement sensor, the presence of someone may be utilized to prove that there is anything wrong with the system. It is possible to verify the presence of someone nearby when a PIR motion sensor detects movement. When attempting to track down a specific person, a probability distribution is used. While numerical and textual data are insufficient for sensor analysis, multimedia data may be used as a confirmatory test in conjunction with numerical and textual data. Being able to work with the digital pictures and video streams that will be captured as part of this effort will be a fascinating experience, and they will offer invaluable physical support for statistical analysis of the endeavor. The use of a pay-as-you-go approach for multimedia data repository along with transmission on the cloud environment is recommended. The answer in a cloud-based Internet of Things system is edge computation, which lowers the cost of storage by reducing the amount of data stored. As detailed in this article, a suggested and executed framework for anticipating complicated occurrences in proactive Internet of Things requisitions has been proposed and shown. The real-time and historical data rates are integrated in our proposed architecture, which takes use of CEP and machine learning to improve performance (ML). It was necessary to identify the most often encountered barriers to merging each technique, and then put our suggested clarification into action by overcoming those threats. Here, the authors have proposed a forecast technique named AMWR for near real-time data. The machine learning model is trained using a moving window rather than a fixed window, which enables it to work properly on dynamic IoT data instead of using a fixed window. Using real-world traffic data, it was shown that the prediction method was accurate to within 96% of the actual value of the parameter. A real-scenario use case from the field of transportation infrastructure technology was used to demonstrate the viability of the proposed architecture, in which upload speed information about the condition of traffic allows system administrators to control traffic in a more efficient manner than is currently available. Our studies using machine learning-based predictions in conjunction with CEP have shown that they have an additional benefit over current options in that they provide high-accuracy prior notice to traffic managers about traffic events that are occurring. More importantly, because of the generalization of the network framework, the identical sequence may also contribute to enhanced performance in other Internet of Things networks, like monitoring products in the supply chain or intelligent healing, to mention a few examples. Further down the road, we would want to assess our framework for usage in other Internet of Things implementations, such as those in which early predictions of complex occurrences may help to develop proactive problem-solving methods.

References

1. Biswal AK, Singh D, Pattanayak BK, Samanta D, Yang M (2021) IoT-Based smart alert system for drowsy driver detection. Wirel Commun Mob Comput 2021:13, Article ID 6627217. https://doi.org/10.1155/2021/6627217
2. Pramanik S, Samanta D, Dutta S, Ghosh R, Ghonge M, Pandey D (2020) Steganography using improved LSB Approach and asymmetric cryptography. In: 2020 IEEE international conference on advent trends in multidisciplinary research and innovation (ICATMRI), Buldhana, India, 2020, pp 1–5. https://doi.org/10.1109/ICATMRI51801.2020.9398408.
3. Maheswari M, Geetha S, kumar SS, Karuppiah M, Samanta D, Park Y (2021) PEVRM: probabilistic evolution based version recommendation model for mobile applications. IEEE Access. https://doi.org/10.1109/ACCESS.2021.3053583
4. Kumar R, Kumar R, Samanta D, Paul M, Kumar V (2017) A combining approach using DFT and FIR filter to enhance impulse response. In: 2017 International conference on computing methodologies and communication (ICCMC), Erode, India, 2017, pp 134–137. https://doi.org/10.1109/ICCMC.2017.8282660
5. Gomathy V, Padhy N, Samanta D et al (2020) Malicious node detection using heterogeneous cluster based secure routing protocol (HCBS) in wireless adhoc sensor networks. J Ambient Intell Human Comput 11:4995–5001. https://doi.org/10.1007/s12652-020-01797-3
6. Ghosh G, Samanta D, Paul M, Janghel NK (2017) Hiding based message communication techniques depends on divide and conquer approach. In: 2017 international conference on computing methodologies and communication (ICCMC), Erode, 2017, pp 123–128. https://doi.org/10.1109/ICCMC.2017.8282658
7. Sivakumar P, Nagaraju R, Samanta D et al (2020) A novel free space communication system using nonlinear InGaAsP microsystem resonators for enabling power-control toward smart cities. Wireless Netw 26:2317–2328. https://doi.org/10.1007/s11276-019-02075-7

8. Samanta D, Sanyal G (2012) A novel approach of SAR image classification using color space clustering and watersheds. In: 2012 4th international conference on computational intelligence and communication networks, Mathura, India, 2012, pp 237–240. https://doi.org/10.1109/CICN.2012.27.
9. Khamparia A, Singh PK, Rani P, Samanta D, Khanna A, Bhushan B (2020) An internet of health things-driven deep learning framework for detection and classification of skin cancer using transfer learning. Trans Emerg Telcommun Technol 2020:e3963. https://doi.org/10.1002/ett.3963
10. Hossain MA, Samanta D, Sanyal G (2012) Statistical approach for extraction of panic expression. In: 2012 4th international conference on computational intelligence and communication networks, Mathura, India, 2012, pp 420–424. https://doi.org/10.1109/CICN.2012.189
11. Althar RR, Samanta D (2021) The realist approach for evaluation of computational intelligence in software engineering. Innov Syst Softw Eng. https://doi.org/10.1007/s11334-020-00383-2
12. Singh RK, Begum T, Borah L, Samanta D (2017) Text encryption: character jumbling. In: 2017 International conference on inventive systems and control (ICISC), Coimbatore, India, 2017, pp 1–3. https://doi.org/10.1109/ICISC.2017.8068691
13. Guha A, Samanta D (2021) Hybrid approach to document anomaly detection: an application to facilitate RPA in title insurance. Int J Autom Comput 18:55–72. https://doi.org/10.1007/s11633-020-1247-y
14. Agarwal M, Sarkhel D, Samanta D (2018) Architecture of 'loop' without 'for' & 'while.' In: 2018 2nd international conference on inventive systems and control (ICISC), Coimbatore, India, 2018, pp 491–494. https://doi.org/10.1109/ICISC.2018.8399121
15. Samanta D, Sivaram M, Rashed A, Boopathi CS, Amiri IS, Yupapin P (2020) Distributed feedback laser (DFB) for signal power amplitude level improvement in long spectral band. J Opt Commun. https://doi.org/10.1515/joc-2019-0252
16. Chakrabarti S, Samanta D (2015) Notice of removal: a novel approach to digital image steganography of key-based encrypted text. In: 2015 International conference on electrical, electronics, signals, communication and optimization (EESCO), Visakhapatnam, India, 2015, pp 1–6. https://doi.org/10.1109/EESCO.2015.7254009
17. Pramanik S, Samanta D, Bandyopadhyay S, Ghosh R (2021) A new combinational technique in image steganography. Int J Inf Secur Priv (IJISP) 15(3). ISSN: 1930–1650|EISSN: 1930–1669
18. Rao KR, Samanta D, Somashekara MT, Gurunath R, Paul A (2019) Automatic segmentation based graphical interface for recognition of tomography image analysis of damage cell. In: 2019 3rd international conference on inventive systems and control (ICISC), Coimbatore, India, 2019, pp 52–55. https://doi.org/10.1109/ICISC44355.2019.9036343
19. Gurunath R, Agarwal M, Nandi A, Samanta D (2018) An overview: security issue in IoT network. In: 2018 2nd international conference on I-SMAC (IoT in Social, Mobile, Analytics and Cloud) (I-SMAC), Palladam, India, 2018, pp 104–107. https://doi.org/10.1109/I-SMAC.2018.8653728
20. Ghosh G, Samanta D, Paul M (2016) Approach of message communication based on twisty "Zig-Zag." In: 2016 International conference on emerging technological trends (ICETT), Kollam, 2016, pp 1–5. https://doi.org/10.1109/ICETT.2016.7873676
21. Dhanush V, Mahendra AR, Kumudavalli MV, Samanta D (2017) Application of deep learning technique for automatic data exchange with air-gapped systems and its security concerns. In: 2017 International conference on computing methodologies and communication (ICCMC), Erode, India, 2017, pp 324–328. https://doi.org/10.1109/ICCMC.2017.8282701
22. Hossain MA, Samanta D, Sanyal G (2012) Extraction of panic expression depending on lip detection. In: 2012 International conference on computing sciences, Phagwara, India, 2012, pp 137–141. https://doi.org/10.1109/ICCS.2012.35
23. Hossain MA, Samanta D, Sanyal G (2012) A novel approach for panic-face extraction based on mutation. In: 2012 IEEE International conference on advanced communication control and computing technologies (ICACCCT), Ramanathapuram, India, 2012, pp 473–477. https://doi.org/10.1109/ICACCCT.2012.6320825

24. Szilagyi I, Wira P (2016) Ontologies and semantic web for the internet of things—a survey, IECON 2016—42nd annual conference of the IEEE industrial electronics society. Florence 2016:6949–6954. https://doi.org/10.1109/IECON.2016.7793744
25. Raptis TP, Passarella A (2017) A distributed data management scheme for industrial IoT environments. In: IEEE 13th international conference on wireless and mobile computing, networking and communications (WiMob), pp 196–203. https://doi.org/10.1109/WiMOB.2017.8115846
26. Uy NQ, Nam VH (2019) A comparison of AMQP and MQTT protocols for Internet of Things. In: 6th NAFOSTED conference on information and computer science (NICS), Hanoi, Vietnam, pp 292–297. https://doi.org/10.1109/NICS48868.2019.9023812
27. Wang X, Ellul J, Azzopardi G (2020) Elderly fall detection systems: a literature survey. Front Robot AI. https://doi.org/10.3389/frobt.2020.00071
28. Wukkadada B, Wankhede K, Nambiar R, Nair A (2018) Comparison with HTTP and MQTT in Internet of Things (IoT). In: International conference on inventive research in computing applications (ICIRCA), Coimbatore, pp 249–253. https://doi.org/10.1109/ICIRCA.2018.8597401
29. Xiao S, Liu T, Wang X, Liu X, Zhou C (2020) Tailoring the absorption bandwidth of Graphene at critical coupling. Phys Rev B. https://doi.org/10.1103/PhysRevB.102.085410
30. Xingyuan W, Suo G (2020) Image encryption algorithm for synchronously updating boolean networks based on matrix semi-tensor product theory. Inf Sci 507:16–36. https://doi.org/10.1016/j.ins.2019.08.041
31. Xu X, Zhong M, Wan J et al (2016) Health monitoring and management for manufacturing workers in adverse working conditions. J Med Syst 40(222). https://doi.org/10.1007/s10916-016-0584-4
32. Yacchirema DC, Sarabia-Ja´come D, Palau CE, Esteve M (2018) A smart system for sleep monitoring by integrating IoT with big data analytics. IEEE Access 6:35988–36001
33. Yahaya AS, Javaid N, Fahad A, Rehman A, Ullah I, Shahid A, Shafiq M (2020) Blockchain based sustainable local energy trading considering home energy management and demurrage mechanism. Sustainability 12:3385. https://doi.org/10.3390/su12083385
34. Yang C (2020) The inequity of conscientious objection: refusal of emergency contraception. Nurs Ethics 27(6). https://doi.org/10.1177/0969733020918926
35. Yuan X, Wang Y, Liu J, Xu X, Yuan X (2018) Experimental and numerical study of airflow distribution optimization in high-density data center with flexible baffles. Build Environ 140:128–139. https://doi.org/10.1016/j.buildenv.2018.05.043
36. Zhang C, Liu Z (2019) Application of big data technology in agricultural internet of things. Int J Distrib Sens Netw 15:10. https://doi.org/10.1177/1550147719881610
37. Zhang P, Yin ZY, Jin FY, Chan THT (2020) A novel hybrid surrogate intelligent model for creep index prediction based on particle swarm optimization and random forest. Eng Geol 265. https://doi.org/10.1016/j.enggeo.2019.105328
38. Jalasri M, Lakshmanan L (2018) A survey: integration of IoT and fog computing. In: 2018 2nd international conference on green computing and internet of things (ICGCIoT), Bangalore, India, pp 235–239. https://doi.org/10.1109/ICGCIoT.2018.8753010
39. Jerald F, Anand M, Deepika N (2019) Design of an industrial IoT architecture based on MQTT protocol for end device to cloud communication. Int J Recent Technol Eng 7(6S2):552–554
40. Karthigha M, Latha L, Sripriyan K (2020) A comprehensive survey of routing attacks in wireless mobile ad hoc networks. In: 2020 International conference on inventive computation technologies (ICICT), Coimbatore, India, pp 396–402. https://doi.org/10.1109/ICICT48043.2020.9112588

Index

D. Samanta and A. Banerjee, *Computationally Intensive Statistics for Intelligent IoT*, Studies in Autonomic, Data-driven and Industrial Computing,
https://doi.org/10.1007/978-981-16-5936-2